Omics Technologies for Clinical Diagnosis and Gene Therapy

Medical Applications in Human Genetics

Edited by

Syeda Marriam Bakhtiar

Department of Bioinformatics and Biosciences
Faculty of Health and Life Sciences
Capital University of Science and Technology
Islamabad
Pakistan

&

Erum Dilshad

Department of Bioinformatics and Biosciences
Faculty of Health and Life Sciences
Capital University of Science and Technology
Islamabad
Pakistan

Omics Technologies for Clinical Diagnosis and Gene Therapy

Editors: Syeda Marriam Bakhtiar and Erum Dilshad

ISBN (Online): 978-981-5079-51-7

ISBN (Print): 978-981-5079-52-4

ISBN (Paperback): 978-981-5079-53-1

need for a court order if at any point you breach any terms of this License Agreement. In no event will any delay or failure by Bentham Science Publishers in enforcing your compliance with this License Agreement constitute a waiver of any of its rights.

3. You acknowledge that you have read this License Agreement, and agree to be bound by its terms and conditions. To the extent that any other terms and conditions presented on any website of Bentham Science Publishers conflict with, or are inconsistent with, the terms and conditions set out in this License Agreement, you acknowledge that the terms and conditions set out in this License Agreement shall prevail.

Bentham Science Publishers Pte. Ltd.
80 Robinson Road #02-00
Singapore 068898
Singapore
Email: subscriptions@benthamscience.net

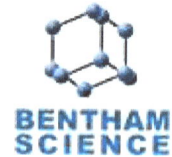

CONTENTS

FOREWORD

Human diseases especially genetic disabilities have always been a focus of research. Research on genetics and molecular genetics has contributed extensively to improving the overall quality of life and management of patients suffering from genetic diseases. With the onset of Omics and Next generation technologies (NGS), the dream of personalized medicine has almost come to reality. Technological advances in the domains of genomics, transcriptomics, proteomics and metabolomics have enabled scientists to explore the genetic and molecular causes in extraordinary detail. These technologies have contributed immensely to advancements related to early and efficient diagnosis, which have revolutionized clinical practices. Despite the contribution of these technologies, it is always felt that none of these technologies alone have the potential to cope with the biological complexity of human diseases. The integration of multiple technologies and a combination of diverse data types is the new approach that has the potential to provide a more comprehensive understanding of biological systems controlling the onset, progression and impact of diseases.

Initially, the focus of research has been on the early diagnosis and methods by which the symptoms of the disease could be eased off. Gene Therapy, personalized medicine, and precision medicine are very promising concepts but there have always been concerns about the access of the general public to these approaches as well as the application for diverse genetic diseases including rare and common diseases, multifactorial diseases including cancers. Omics Technologies have not only provided the scientists with better opportunities for correct diagnosis but also expanded the options for treatment including gene therapy, pharmacogenomics, single-cell omics, regenerative medicine, stem cell technologies and many more. Integrative approaches utilizing engineering and informatics have also widened the knowledge base required for appropriate treatment and management approaches.

This book compiled and edited by scientists working in various domains of genomics and human genetics will not only provide the researchers with new approaches in conventional methods of genetics-based diagnosis and counselling but will also open new avenues for further exploration of genetic causes and treatment options. This book is a great effort to document state-of-the-art techniques and technologies for disease prediction and early diagnosis to disease treatment and prognosis using integrative Omics.

Shahid Mahmood Baig
Department of Biological and Biomedical Sciences,
Agha Khan University, Karachi
Pakistan
Chairman, Pakistan Science Foundation

PREFACE

Human inherited disorders have been the focus of attention for a long time. Various books have been written with a focus on classical genetic approaches, clinical diagnostic strategies, and counselling, management strategies. With the emergence of Next-generation techniques, a new era was started and lots of developments have occurred in Human Genetics. The perspective has also been widened with emerging OMICS technologies. An integrated approach is being used not only for diagnosis but also for management and therapeutic purposes. This book is an effort to highlight and compile various emerging areas of OMICS technology and its application in the diagnosis and management of human genetic disorders.

The book is planned with three areas of research and implementation i.e., Diagnosis covering conventional strategies to next-generation platforms. This section focuses on the role of Insilco analysis, databases and multi-omics of single-cell which will help in designing better management strategies. Section II covers management and therapeutic interventions starting with genetic counselling and then including more specific techniques such as pharmacogenomics and personalized medicine, gene editing techniques and their applications in gene therapies and regenerative medicine. Section III focuses on case studies and discusses the applications and success of all the above-mentioned strategies on selected human disorders.

Syeda Marriam Bakhtiar
Department of Bioinformatics and Biosciences
Faculty of Health and Life Sciences
Capital University of Science and Technology
Islamabad
Pakistan

&

Erum Dilshad
Department of Bioinformatics and Biosciences
Faculty of Health and Life Sciences
Capital University of Science and Technology
Islamabad
Pakistan

List of Contributors

Adnan Haider	Department of Biological Sciences, National University of Medical Sciences, Rawalpindi, Pakistan
Alvina Gul	Atta-ur-Rahman School of Applied Biosciences (ASAB), National University of Sciences and Technology (NUST), Islamabad, Pakistan
Amina Basheer	Department of Industrial Biotechnology,Atta-ur-Rahman School of Applied Biosciences (ASAB), National University of Sciences and Technology (NUST), Islamabad, Pakistan
Amjad Ali	Department of Industrial Biotechnology,Atta-ur-Rahman School of Applied Biosciences (ASAB), National University of Sciences and Technology (NUST), Islamabad, Pakistan
Ammara Siddique	Atta-ur-Rahman School of Applied Biosciences (ASAB), National University of Sciences and Technology (NUST), Islamabad, Pakistan
Amna Naheed Khan	Department of Bioinformatics and Biosciences, Faculty of Health and Life Sciences, Capital University of Science and Technology (CUST), Islamabad, Pakistan
Anam Naz	Institute of Molecular Biology and Biotechnology (IMBB), The University of Lahore (UOL), Lahore, Pakistan
Aqsa Ikram	Institute of Molecular Biology and Biotechnology (IMBB), The University of Lahore (UOL), Lahore, Pakistan
Ambrin Fatima	Department of Biological and Biomedical Sciences, The Aga Khan University, Karachi, Pakistan
Areena Suhail Khan	Department of Biosciences, COMSATS University Islamabad, Park Road, Islamabad, Pakistan
Atif Ali Khan Khalil	Department of Biological Sciences, National University of Medical Sciences, Rawalpindi, Pakistan
Attiya Kanwal	International Islamic University Islamabad (IIUI), Islamabad, Pakistan
Ayaz Khan	National Institute for Biotechnology and Genetic Engineering College, Pakistan Institute of Engineering and Applied Sciences (NIBGE-C, PIEAS), Faisalabad, Pakistan
Aysha Saeed	Department of Biotechnology, Kinnaird College for Women, Lahore, Pakistan
Bibi Nazia Murtaza	Department of Zoology, Abbottabad University of Science and Technology, Abbottabad, Pakistan
Bisma Rauff	Department of Biomedical Engineering, University of Engineering and Technology (UET), Narowal Campus, Lahore, Pakistan
Bushra Bano	Institute of Basic Medical Sciences, Khyber Medical University, Peshawar, Pakistan
Erum Dilshad	Department of Bioinformatics and Biosciences, Faculty of Health and Life Sciences, Capital University of Science and Technology (CUST), Islamabad, Pakistan

Faiza Naseer Shifa College of Pharmaceutical Sciences, Shifa Tameer-e-Millat University, Islamabad, Pakistan

Fakhra Nazir Department of Bioinformatics and Biosciences, Capital University of Science and Technology, Islamabad (CUST, Islamabad), Pakistan
Department of Biosciences, COMSATS University Islamabad, Sahiwal, Pakistan

Fatima Shahid Department of Industrial Biotechnology, Atta-ur-Rahman School of Applied Biosciences (ASAB), National University of Sciences and Technology (NUST), Islamabad, Pakistan

Fazli Subhan Department of Biological Sciences, National University of Medical Sciences, Rawalpindi, Pakistan

Hafiza Noor Ul Ayan National Institute for Biotechnology and Genetic Engineering College, Pakistan Institute of Engineering and Applied Sciences (NIBGE-C, PIEAS), Faisalabad, Pakistan
Institute for Cardiogenetic, University of Lubeck, Lubeck, Germany

Hajra Qayyum Department of Biosciences and Bioinformatics, Capital University of Science and Technology, Islamabad, Pakistan

Hayeqa Shahwar Awan Department of Industrial Biotechnology,Atta-ur-Rahman School of Applied Biosciences (ASAB), National University of Sciences and Technology (NUST), Islamabad, Pakistan

Hira Kazmi Centre for Human Genetics, Hazara University Mansehra, Pakistan

Humna Masood Institute of Biochemistry and Biotechnology, University of Veterinary and Animal Sciences-UVAS, Lahore, Pakistan

Huma Tariq Department of Zoology, Hazara University, Manshera, Pakistan

Ilyas Ahmad Institute for Cardiogenetic, University of Lubeck, Lubeck, Germany

Iram Anjum Department of Biotechnology, Kinnaird College for Women, Lahore, Pakistan

Iqra Bashir Department of Bioinformatics and Biosciences, Faculty of Health and Life Sciences, Capital University of Science and Technology (CUST), Islamabad, Pakistan

Komal Aslam Department of Biotechnology, Kinnaird College for Women, Lahore, Pakistan
Department of Biotechnology, Lahore College for Women University, Lahore, Pakistan

Mahnoor Ejaz Atta-ur-Rahman School of Applied Biosciences (ASAB), National University of Sciences and Technology (NUST), Islamabad, Pakistan

Mahnoor Asif National Institute for Biotechnology and Genetic Engineering College, Pakistan Institute of Engineering and Applied Sciences (NIBGE-C, PIEAS), Faisalabad, Pakistan

Maria Iqbal National Institute for Biotechnology and Genetic Engineering College, Pakistan Institute of Engineering and Applied Sciences (NIBGE-C, PIEAS), Faisalabad, Pakistan
Centogene GmbH, Rostock, Germany

Maria Shabbir Healthcare Biotechnology, Attaur Rehman School of Applied Biosciences, National University of Science and Technology, Islamabad, Pakistan

Marriam Bakhtiar	Department of Bioinformatics and Biosciences, Faculty of Health and Life Sciences, Capital University of Science and Technology (CUST), Islamabad, Pakistan
Muhammad Faheem	Department of Biological Sciences, National University of Medical Sciences, Rawalpindi, Pakistan
Muhammad Ilyas	Centre for Omic Sciences, Islamia College University Peshawar, Pakistan Department of Bioengineering, University of Engineering and Applied Sciences, Swat, Pakistan
Muhammad Jawad Hassan	Department of Biological Sciences, National University of Medical Sciences, Rawalpindi, Pakistan
Muhammad Tariq	National Institute for Biotechnology and Genetic Engineering College, Pakistan Institute of Engineering and Applied Sciences (NIBGE-C, PIEAS), Faisalabad, Pakistan
Muhammad Maaz	Department of Bioinformatics and Biosciences, Faculty of Health and Life Sciences, Capital University of Science and Technology (CUST), Islamabad, Pakistan
Muhammad Saad Khan	Centre for Bioresource Research, Islamabad, Pakistan
Muneeba Ishtiaq	Department of Bioinformatics and Biosciences, Capital University of Science and Technology, Islamabad (CUST, Islamabad), Pakistan
Muhammad Naeem	Department of Biological Sciences, National University of Medical Sciences, Rawalpindi, Pakistan
Narjis Khatoon	Department of Bioinformatics and Biosciences, Capital University of Science and Technology, Islamabad (CUST, Islamabad), Pakistan
Naveed Altaf Malik	National Institute for Biotechnology and Genetic Engineering College, Pakistan Institute of Engineering and Applied Sciences (NIBGE-C, PIEAS), Faisalabad, Pakistan
Naveed Altaf Malik	National Institute for Biotechnology and Genetic Engineering College, Pakistan Institute of Engineering and Applied Sciences (NIBGE-C, PIEAS), Faisalabad, Pakistan
Rabbiah Manzoor Malik	Department of Bioinformatics and Biosciences, Capital University of Science and Technology, Islamabad (CUST, Islamabad), Pakistan Wah Medical College, WahCantt, Pakistan
Raees Khan	Institute of Basic Medical Sciences, Khyber Medical University, Peshawar, Pakistan
Syeda Seema Waseem	National Institute for Biotechnology and Genetic Engineering College, Pakistan Institute of Engineering and Applied Sciences (NIBGE-C, PIEAS), Faisalabad, Pakistan
Shahid Mahmood Baig	National Institute for Biotechnology and Genetic Engineering College, Pakistan Institute of Engineering and Applied Sciences (NIBGE-C, PIEAS), Faisalabad, Pakistan
Sadia Nawaz	Institute of Biochemistry and Biotechnology, University of Veterinary and Animal Sciences-UVAS, Lahore, Pakistan

Shumaila Zulfiqar National Institute for Biotechnology and Genetic Engineering College, Pakistan Institute of Engineering and Applied Sciences (NIBGE-C, PIEAS), Faisalabad, Pakistan
Department of Biotechnology, Kinnaird College for Women, Lahore, Pakistan

Shafaq Ramzan National Institute for Biotechnology and Genetic Engineering College, Pakistan Institute of Engineering and Applied Sciences (NIBGE-C, PIEAS), Faisalabad, Pakistan

Shahid Mahmood Baig National Institute for Biotechnology and Genetic Engineering College, Pakistan Institute of Engineering and Applied Sciences (NIBGE-C, PIEAS), Faisalabad, Pakistan

Syeda Marriam Bakhtiar Department of Biosciences and Bioinformatics, Capital University of Science and Technology, Islamabad, Pakistan

Sabba Mehmood Department of Biological Sciences, National University of Medical Sciences, Rawalpindi, Pakistan

Shifa Tariq Ashraf Department of Industrial Biotechnology, Atta-ur-Rahman School of Applied Biosciences (ASAB), National University of Sciences and Technology (NUST), Islamabad, Pakistan

Sajjad Ahmed Department of Zoology, Hazara University, Manshera, Pakistan

Shumaila Azam Department of Bioinformatics and Biosciences, Capital University of Science and Technology, Islamabad, Pakistan

Sahar Fazal Department of Bioinformatics and Biosciences, Capital University of Science and Technology, Islamabad, Pakistan

Sana Elahi Department of Bioinformatics and Biosciences, Capital University of Science and Technology (CUST), Islamabad, Pakistan

Sarmad Mehmood Department of Pathology, CMH Institute of Medical Sciences, Bahawalpur, Pakistan

Sajjad Haider Department of Chemical Engineering, King Saud University, Riyadh, Saudi Arabia

Syed Babar Jamal Department of Biological Sciences, National University of Medical Sciences, Rawalpindi, Pakistan

Uzma Abdullah University Institute of Biochemistry and Biotechnology, PMAS-Arid Agriculture University, Rawalpindi, Pakistan

Zafar Ali Centre for Biotechnology and Microbiology, University of Swat, Swat, Pakistan

CHAPTER 1

Next-Generation Technologies for Rare Inherited Disorders

Hira Kazmi[1] and **Muhammad Ilyas**[2,3,*]

[1] *Centre for Human Genetics, Hazara University Mansehra, Pakistan*

[2] *Centre for Omic Sciences, Islamia College University Peshawar, Pakistan*

[3] *Department of Bioengineering, University of Engineering and Applied Sciences, Swat, Pakistan*

Abstract: Rare inherited disorders have become a major public health concern in recent years. Owing to a lack of resources, poorly planned primary and basic health care, and inadequate political structures, treatment, and management policies are daunting challenges in many countries. As a result, these diseases need particular attention, especially in less developed areas, where these disorders remain unnoticed. Similarly, the effect of such severe disorders on underprivileged populations is expected to be devastating. Identifying certain genetic markers can provide a valuable explanation for disease etiology, molecular characterization, and pathogenesis. In this chapter, we highlight the importance of next-generation sequencing to explore and recognize the role of novel causative genes in developing successful treatments for the most prevalent rare genetic disorders. DNA methylation and transcriptome markers have been shown to aid in the prediction of common diseases; however, this has not been tested on rare genetic disorders. Since the rate of rare inherited disorders is higher in developing countries, we believe that these populations can provide us with much stronger clues for the genetic and environmental association. These markers, along with other parameters, can be used to systematically build machine learning models to improve risk prediction; this approach has the potential to reshape how we predict disease risk and save many lives around the world.

Keywords: Clinical genomics, Genetic counseling, Next-generation sequencing, Prenatal diagnosis, Rare inherited diseases.

1. INTRODUCTION

Rare disorders affect more than 300 million people worldwide, with a diagnosis of less than 0.2 million people [1]. Around 80% of these disorders are genetic in

* **Corresponding author Muhammad Ilyas**: Centre for Omic Sciences, Islamia College University Peshawar, Pakistan and Department of Bioengineering, University of Engineering and Applied Sciences, Swat, Pakistan; E-mail: milyas@icp.edu.pk

Syeda Marriam Bakhtiar and Erum Dilshad (Eds.)

origin and have no treatment at all. Identification of such disease variants in patients can now be done with greater accuracy and lower cost by using whole genome/exome sequencing [2]. Despite this, researchers and policymakers are still grappling with the problems involving the use and interpretation of genotype data. Genetic variations have been used in molecular diagnostic research in the past, but with a few loci [3]. With lower cost, faster, and more precise sequencing technologies, it is easier to perform diagnostic tests at the single nucleotide level. Researchers around the world have created more sophisticated methods to study the role of variants and their associated environment in complex diseases using human genome data generated by the 1000 genome project and other genome research groups [4]. Clinical researchers are now using genome-wide studies to advance diagnostics and provide improved decision-making tools for patients. This is how genomics' impact on health care ushered in a new era of genetic medicine, also known as personalized medicine. It takes a reasonable amount of time and money to get results from a lab to a professional clinic. According to genetic specialists, it takes more than ten years for the pharmaceutical industry to conduct medical research based on FDA policies [5]. The genome-wide study contributes to the possibility of developing diseases that are widespread in the world's population. These common diseases include diabetes, hypertension, cancer, and cardiovascular diseases [6]. Comprehensive knowledge of the genetic structure of such disorders will help detect the vital mechanism of cells and, in the long run, improve our understanding of how various factors affect an individual's health.

Genetic studies have revolutionized many fields of research, with the total economic value of the human genome project estimated to be 796 billion USD [7]. Until recently, it was time-consuming and costly to carry out tests to detect pathogenic mutations. The recent boom in Next-Generation Sequencing (NGS) technologies has been a key to low-cost, fast, and reliable performance for molecular diagnostics. After the publication of the human genome, the main challenge for researchers working in the field of medical genetics has been to translate and use this mass of data in a clinical setting. However, genetic characterizations, which include transcriptomic and epigenomic studies of populations with unusual genetic disorders, are not yet properly investigated in the demographic and epidemiological studies of rare inherited diseases. Genes and variants that may be used as markers for the pre-diagnostic testing of such disorders should be identified. This will potentially benefit patients and families with such neglected and devastating disorders through pre-screening, genetic counseling, and carrier screening, and will provide a step toward fully personalized medicine and therapy [8].

1.1. Whole Genome/Exome Sequencing

Next-generation sequencing (NGS) technology has become the most groundbreaking research achievement in the science world. It refers to a series of modern DNA sequencing procedures which are making significant progress in the sequencing of millions of genomic fragments by employing particularly parallel reactions [9, 10]. The cost of sequencing a genome with NGS technology is cheaper as compared to the Sanger sequencing method [11]. The costs have plunged in the last few years, quickly exceeding Moore's Law, the standard benchmark for the declining cost of technology [12] (Fig. **1.1**). Numerous technologies, including cutting-edge chemistries, amplification methodologies, and efficient and high-resolution microscopy, have been redesigned to make this possible. In recent years, genome-wide studies using microarray technology have made significant progress [13]. Microarray chip approaches were initially used for gene expression analysis, but they later found widespread use in the analysis of copy number alterations, microRNA studies, mapping of binding sites for protein-protein and DNA-protein interactions, and genotyping of single nucleotide variants [14]. However, NGS technology has made significant advances and is expected to replace the majority of microchip platforms in the long term [15].

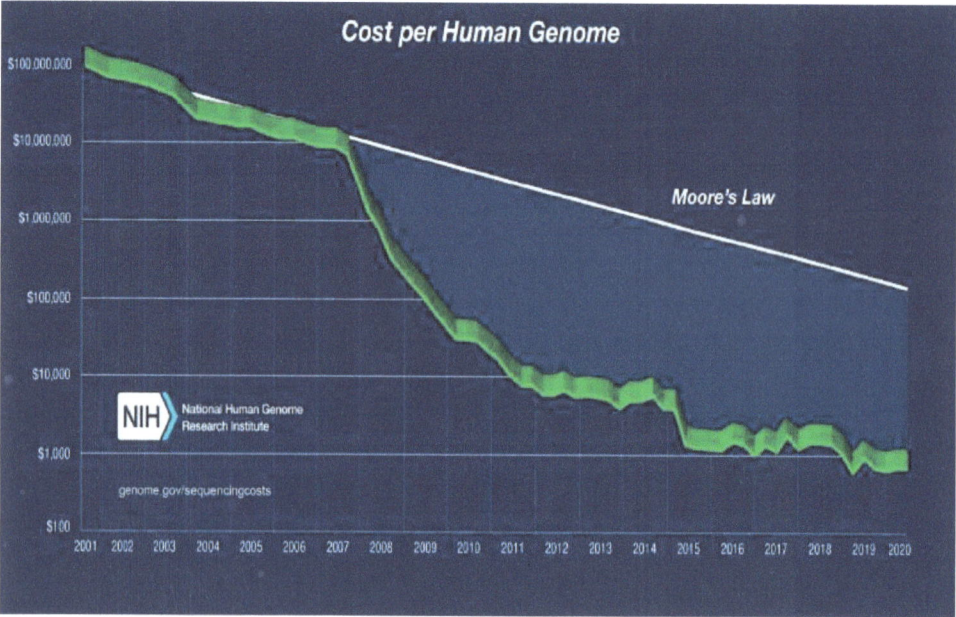

Fig. (1.1). Cost per genome data - August 2020. Data obtained from National Human Genome Research Institute (https://www.genome.gov).

NGS offers ultra-high throughput and speed for sequencing using massively parallel sequencing, and meets the requirements of depth information regarding genomes. Various platforms are available for NGS including Illumina, ion torrent, solid, and many more. All these platforms work on the workflow comprising, library preparation, sequencing, and data analysis. Library preparation is different for each platform and is the most crucial step as the efficiency of the sequencing depends on this step. The library is usually generated by fragmenting the sequences and attaching adaptor sequencing keeping the multiplexing in consideration. For sequencing, most of the NGS platforms use sequencing by synthesis approach or a modified version such as paired-end sequencing. After the sequencing step, the instrument performs base calling by identifying nucleotides, the data generated is then analyzed, normalized, and annotation is performed by bioinformatics.

Emerging genomics techniques, such as next-generation sequencing (NGS), have been widely used in research settings, and they also offer significant benefits in clinical settings. Despite NGS-based genetic testing's remarkable success in improving the diagnosis of genetic variants in rare diseases, there is still a translational gap between clinical implementation and NGS-based genetic testing. Many factors contribute to the suboptimal implementation of NGS technologies in the detection of rare diseases.

In order to make NGS-based genetic testing to be valid and implemented, the patient value can be clearly explained by providing the physician with the tools for better decision making. In this case, there is often minimal real-world proof that supports NGS based genetic testing. The unavailability of sequencing equipment and high cost for many researchers at this time are still unaffordable; however, due to competing market forces, a significant decline is expected in the coming years.

Before NGS can achieve its potential for patients, clinics and society, there are several obstacles to overcome. The main argument is whether genetics based on NGS will produce reliable and reproducible results to aid in the detection of rare diseases [16]. To deal with this, the goal of genetic testing in the detection of rare diseases must be clarified. Secondly, the relationship between genetic testing service providers, clinicians, and patients must be seamless and coordinated.

Since the introduction of NGS technology, several applications have emerged that have proven to be effective in diagnosing a variety of rare diseases in both research and clinical realm. Various genetic testing programs have been developed globally and the market value is estimated to be 22 billion USD in 2024 [17]. There are more than 10,000 diagnostic tests available from about 500 institutions located in Europe that are largely focused on the detection of the defined causative gene [18]. These screening methods served a variety of clinical purposes. About 86% of the genetic screening tests are for postnatal analysis. Somatic genetics for pediatric cancer and antenatal diagnosis accounted for 5.24% and 5.05% of all diagnostic measurements, respectively. It was not shocking that due to its technical immaturity, pre-implant diagnosis comprised less than 1% of the diagnostic tests available.

Besides, Sanger sequencing is still commonly adopted by the community (55%) as a critical orthogonal verification technique [18, 19]. This panel-based sequencing progressed gradually to the dominant sector (14%) [20]. Almost 90% of all the genetic studies available are diagnostic tests for the detection of genetic mutations, such as SNV, duplication and deletion in the coding area. Such screening tests can be utilized for the diagnosis of thousands of genes linked with rare diseases. These rare diseases include neurological conditions, developmental disorders, inborn metabolic disorders, eye disorders, and bone diseases (Table **1.1**).

Table 1.1. Details of rare inherited diseases databases and their web addresses.

Sr. No.	Title	Description	Database
1	Orphanet	Orphanet is a resource for information on rare diseases and orphan drugs, with over 6,000 diseases covered.	www.orpha.net
2	Online Mendelian Inheritance in Man (OMIM)	OMIM is a database of human genes and genetic disorders, with a focus on their relationship.	http://www.ncbi.nlm.nih.gov/omim
3	Gene Reviews	It focuses on the application of molecular genetic testing in the diagnosis, management, and genetic counseling of patients.	http://www.ncbi.nlm.nih.gov/sites/GeneTests/review?db=GeneTests

(Table 1) cont.....

Sr. No.	Title	Description	Database
4	Genetics Home Reference	It provides details about genetic disorders and the genes or chromosomes that are linked to them.	http://ghr.nlm.nih.gov/
5	National Organization for Rare Disorders (NORD)	The rare disease database contains over 1200 reports.	www.rarediseases.org
6	Genetic Alliance	It includes over 1,000 disease-specific advocacy groups.	www.geneticalliance.org
7	Genetic Mutation Database of Rare Diseases	It gives physicians access to a virtual encyclopedia of genetic information at their fingertips, allowing for more accurate and efficient diagnosis of rare diseases.	https://www.centogene.com
8	GDRD	This database is intended for educational or research purposes only, and should not be used for direct diagnostic purposes or medical decision-making without the review of a genetics professional.	https://db.cngb.org/gdrd/

1.2. Transcriptomics (RNA-Seq) of Rare Diseases

The accessibility of the entire euchromatic sequence (GRCh37/hg19) allowed researchers to quickly identify disease-causing mutations in over 2850 genes responsible for a wide range of Mendelian disorders as well as statistically important associations between over 1000 loci and over 150 complex diseases and traits [21]. However, the study of human genetic diseases is a challenging task – particularly for multi-factorial diseases –due to the limited contribution of several genes in the phenotype, and frequently due to unknown gene-gene and gene-environment interactions [22].

Approximately 88% (Single Nucleotide Polymorphisms (SNPs)) of genetic variants that contribute to complex diseases and genome wide association (GWAS) traits are located in intronic or intergenic regions [23]. This study strongly suggests that these nucleotide changes are more likely to have unintended consequences by changing gene expression rather than protein activity. Loci with such ability are referred to as expression quantitative trait loci (eQTL). Several studies have conclusively shown that inherited polymorphisms cause gene expression variation and that global gene expression analyses – which do not involve a priori hypothesis – offer a comprehensive approach to the analysis of complex traits and disease pathogenesis [24].

Even though many human genetic disorders have a deep genetic understanding, most research has yet to provide important insights as to the actual contribution or functional significance of certain DNA polymorphisms in the disease's genesis. In this instance, comprehensive transcriptome analysis is quickly becoming a key player, as it is an important discovery method for putting existing genetic knowledge about numerous diseases into context [25].

For transcriptomic analysis, RNA seq is becoming a state-of-the-art technique by detecting transcript isoforms, gene fusions, SNP variants and provides researchers with information regarding changes in response to therapeutics and environmental changes. The techniques involve modifications in NGS technologies to make it more focused regarding targeted RNA sequencing, Single-Cell RNA seq, ultra low input RNA seq, RNA exome capture sequencing and in some cases total RNA sequencing. Ribosome profiling is also done using RNA sequencing. RNA seq helps scientists to determine variants expressed in specific disease state and also helps in identifying gene expression signatures, as well as small RNAs regulating gene expressions.

1.3. DNA Methylation (Methyl-Seq) in Rare Diseases

DNA methylation is one of the first epigenetic changes observed in humans [26]. DNA methyltransferases (DNMT) transfer a methyl group from S-adenyl methionine to the fifth carbon of cytosine residues, forming 5-methylcytosine, a common post-replication modification found in cytosines of the CpG dinucleotide sequence (5mC) [27]. Demethylation is a complex process that can be either active or passive. TET enzymes oxidize 5mCs, allowing DNA methylation at particular loci to be eliminated [28].

The 5mC is converted into 5-hydroxymethylcytosine (5hmC) and 5-formylcytosine (5fC) via step-by-step oxidation in the presence of water, oxygen, and -ketoglutarate, yielding carbon dioxide and succinate. Both 5fC and 5caC can then be substituted with unmodified cytosine using thymine DNA glycosylase's base-excision repair [29].

Although all cells in a multicellular organism have the same genome, the diversity of cell types suggests that genome information is used in the different tools for establishing precise expression programs that determine cell identity [30]. A variety of processes, including epigenetic mechanisms, influence the dynamic regulation of gene expression. Epigenetics has a variety of definitions that stem from the need to fill the gap between genetics and development. It's often compared to several layers of instructions that control the genome's functions and coordinate cell fate decisions.

Complex disorders are characterized by altered epigenetic landscapes, but determining whether they are a cause or a result of disease can be difficult [31]. The finding of inherited epigenetic machinery was a major innovation in medical genetics [32]. These findings help to address gaps in our understanding of epigenetic mechanisms, their activities, and roles in body growth and development, as well as to learn more about the etiology of a variety of human diseases.

Because of the growing body of evidence revealing the importance of DNA methylation in common diseases, scientists have begun to use it as a biomarker to detect epigenetic changes linked to disease [33]. This population-based epidemiology method is said to be capable of investigating the role of epigenetics in common diseases and discovering novel risk factors that may be missed by traditional epigenetic epidemiological methods like the Genome-Wide Association Study (GWAS). This epigenetic epidemiologic process is also known as epigenome-wide association study (EWAS) [34]. Despite the fact that epigenetic epidemiology studies are promising and conceptually straightforward, there are some particular obstacles to this approach.

DNA methylation sequencing depends on bisulphate conversion for the detection of unmethylated cytosines. OCR is used for the identification of converted bases and later NGS modifications exploits amplicon methyl-seq and target enrichment. This method not only provides methylation patterns of CpG, CHH and CHG regions but also covers the emerging regions of interests in human genome important for Epigenomics RoadMap Consortium.

1.4. Long-Reads Sequencing for Rare Inherited Disorders

Long-read sequencing, also known as third generation sequencing, has several benefits over short-read sequencing [9]. Though a short-read sequencer can produce readings of up to 600 bases, long-read sequencing technology can produce readings of more than 10 kb on a regular basis [35]. Short-read sequencing is a low-cost, high-precision approach that supports a wide range of analysis tools and pipelines. However, natural nucleic acid polymers, on the other hand, are eight orders long, and sequencing these short-amplified fragments makes rebuilding and numbering the original molecules more difficult. Thus, the long reads enhanced de-novo assembly, mapping certainty, isoform analysis of transcripts, and structural variations detection. In addition, DNA and RNA sequencing of native molecules removes amplification errors and maintains basic modifications. These capabilities, in combination with ongoing improvements in precision, cost, and throughput have begun to open up a wide array of applications for genomic model and non-model organisms. Long read sequencing is a highly accurate approach and a modification of NGS to sequence the genomes with highly repetitive elements, which otherwise are very challenging.

Long-read sequencing is dominated by two techniques: Oxford Nanopore Technologies (ONT) nanopore sequencing and Pacific Biosciences (PacBio) single-molecular real-time (SMRT) sequencing [36]. The SMRT and nanopore sequencing technologies were first released in 2011 and 2014, respectively, and since then have proven to be useful in a variety of applications. These platforms generate data that is qualitatively different from that generated by the second generation, requiring the use of advanced analysis tools. Over the last decade, the study of pathogenic mutations in rare genetic diseases has focused on massively parallel short-read sequencers that sequence coding regions or the entire genome [37]. Nevertheless, using these methods, the current diagnosis rate is around 50%, and there are still several rare genetic disorders with unidentified causes. There could be several reasons for this, but one possibility is that the responsible mutations are located in regions of the genome that are difficult to sequence using traditional methods (*e.g.* , tandem repeat expansion or complex chromosomal structural aberrations). Despite the inconveniences of the cost and the shortage of conventional approaches, various studies have examined pathogenic genome changes using long read sequencing techniques. The results of such studies give us hope that using long-read sequencers to identify causative mutations in unsolved genetic disorders will help us better understand human genomes and diseases [38]. Such methods will also be applied to individuals with inherited disorders in prospective molecular diagnostics and therapeutic strategies in the future.

1.5. The International Rare Diseases Research Consortium

The International Rare Disease Consortium (IRDiRC) was established in 2010 to promote international research cooperation and funding in the field of rare disorders, with the goal of discovering 200 new treatments and methods to diagnose the majority of rare disorders by 2020 [39]. The IRDiRC is aimed to speeding up the advancement of research on rare diseases through international cooperation and collaboration to allow people with all rare diseases to be diagnosed and to contribute to developing new treatments for rare disorders. The IRDiRC has grown to include over 50 funding agencies and patient advocacy groups from 20 countries with the objective of improving diagnosis and treatment for individuals with rare disorders (https://irdirc.org).

CONCLUSION AND RECOMMENDATIONS

Next-generation Sequencing approaches have greatly advanced the identification of rare inherited diseases and therefore have become a genetic testing tool for several disease groups. They have made significant progress towards understanding many of the genetic factors that underpin inherited disorders in humans, such as the discovery of disease-causing mutations. Though, the road ahead is still long, particularly in the case of complex diseases, and 'the more we investigate, the more complicated it becomes.' Nonetheless, multiple experiments have conclusively shown that SNPs discovered by GWAS, and located beyond genes' coding regions can trigger gene expression fluctuation, highlighting the importance of transcriptome and epigenetic studies in several rare diseases.

A public training program, including improving research capacity, training, and collaboration should be developed for public health and genomic research.

- There must be new multidisciplinary scientific collaborations and data and approaches that must be shared with researchers worldwide. This will establish datasets, knowledge and fundamental understanding of the genetic basis of rare, inherited diseases.
- There is an urgent need for holistic treatment covering the scope of the health, social and everyday needs of individuals dealing with a rare disease and their families.
- Prenatal screening testing and genetic counselling services should be available in hospitals, especially in places where consanguineous marriages are very common.
- Policymakers, health care professionals, and the general public need to be aware of common and rare genetic diseases.

- Clinicians are either actual or potential opinion leaders, so they must be well aware of the emerging technologies related to clinical genetics.
- Problems related to rare genetic disorders should be discussed openly at seminars, conferences, and workshops.
- Advanced or introductory classes in medical/human genetics should be included in educational institutions' curricula, including medical colleges.
- The government should support research communities in every way possible so that scientists can get a better understanding of all rare diseases.

CONSENT FOR PUBLICATION

Not applicable.

CONFLICT OF INTEREST

The author declares no conflict of interest, financial or otherwise.

ACKNOWLEDGEMENTS

Declared none.

REFERENCES

[1]   Šimić G. Rare diseases and omics-driven personalized medicine. Croat Med J 2019; 60(6): 485-7.
[http://dx.doi.org/10.3325/cmj.2019.60.485] [PMID: 31894912]

[2]   Bamshad MJ, Ng SB, Bigham AW, *et al.* Exome sequencing as a tool for Mendelian disease gene discovery. Nat Rev Genet 2011; 12(11): 745-55.
[http://dx.doi.org/10.1038/nrg3031] [PMID: 21946919]

[3]   Posey JE, Rosenfeld JA, James RA, *et al.* Molecular diagnostic experience of whole-exome sequencing in adult patients. Genet Med 2016; 18(7): 678-85.
[http://dx.doi.org/10.1038/gim.2015.142] [PMID: 26633545]

[4]   Cardon LR, Bell JI. Association study designs for complex diseases. Nat Rev Genet 2001; 2(2): 91-9.
[http://dx.doi.org/10.1038/35052543] [PMID: 11253062]

[5]   van Dijk EL, Auger H, Jaszczyszyn Y, Thermes C. Ten years of next-generation sequencing technology. Trends Genet 2014; 30(9): 418-26.
[http://dx.doi.org/10.1016/j.tig.2014.07.001] [PMID: 25108476]

[6]   Koene RJ, Prizment AE, Blaes A, Konety SH. Shared Risk Factors in Cardiovascular Disease and Cancer. Circulation 2016; 133(11): 1104-14.
[http://dx.doi.org/10.1161/CIRCULATIONAHA.115.020406] [PMID: 26976915]

[7]   Bennett ST, Barnes C, Cox A, Davies L, Brown C. Toward the $1000 human genome. Pharmacogenomics 2005; 6(4): 373-82.
[http://dx.doi.org/10.1517/14622416.6.4.373] [PMID: 16004555]

[8]   Castellani C, Macek M Jr, Cassiman JJ, *et al.* Benchmarks for Cystic Fibrosis carrier screening: A European consensus document. J Cyst Fibros 2010; 9(3): 165-78.
[http://dx.doi.org/10.1016/j.jcf.2010.02.005] [PMID: 20363197]

[9]   Kumar KR, Cowley MJ, Davis RL. Next-Generation Sequencing and Emerging Technologies. Semin Thromb Hemost 2019; 45(7): 661-73.

[http://dx.doi.org/10.1055/s-0039-1688446] [PMID: 31096307]

[10] Ari Ş, Arikan M. Next-generation sequencing: Advantages, disadvantages, and future. Plant Omics: Trends and Applications. Cham: Springer International Publishing 2016; pp. 109-35.
[http://dx.doi.org/10.1007/978-3-319-31703-8_5]

[11] Zhang Z, Liu G, Chen Y, *et al.* Comparison of different sequencing strategies for assembling chromosome-level genomes of extremophiles with variable GC content. iScience 2021; 24(3): 102219.
[http://dx.doi.org/10.1016/j.isci.2021.102219] [PMID: 33748707]

[12] Park ST, Kim J. Trends in Next-Generation Sequencing and a New Era for Whole Genome Sequencing. Int Neurourol J 2016; 20(2) (Suppl. 2): S76-83.
[http://dx.doi.org/10.5213/inj.1632742.371] [PMID: 27915479]

[13] Grant SFA, Hakonarson H. Microarray technology and applications in the arena of genome-wide association. Clin Chem 2008; 54(7): 1116-24.
[http://dx.doi.org/10.1373/clinchem.2008.105395] [PMID: 18499899]

[14] Mullany LE, Wolff RK, Herrick JS, Buas MF, Slattery ML. SNP Regulation of microRNA Expression and Subsequent Colon Cancer Risk. PLoS One 2015; 10(12): e0143894.
[http://dx.doi.org/10.1371/journal.pone.0143894] [PMID: 26630397]

[15] Jia B, Xu S, Xiao G, Lamba V, Liang F. Learning gene regulatory networks from next generation sequencing data. Biometrics 2017; 73(4): 1221-30.
[http://dx.doi.org/10.1111/biom.12682] [PMID: 28294287]

[16] Liu Z, Zhu L, Roberts R, Tong W. Toward clinical implementation of next-generation sequencing-based genetic testing in rare diseases: Where are we? Trends Genet 2019; 35(11): 852-67.
[http://dx.doi.org/10.1016/j.tig.2019.08.006] [PMID: 31623871]

[17] Perakslis E, Coravos A. Is health-care data the new blood? Lancet Digit Health 2019; 1(1): e8-9.
[http://dx.doi.org/10.1016/S2589-7500(19)30001-9] [PMID: 33323242]

[18] Javaher P, Nyoungui E, Kääriäinen H, *et al.* Genetic screening in Europe. Public Health Genomics 2010; 13(7-8): 524-37.
[http://dx.doi.org/10.1159/000294998] [PMID: 20203479]

[19] Crossley BM, Bai J, Glaser A, *et al.* Guidelines for Sanger sequencing and molecular assay monitoring. J Vet Diagn Invest 2020; 32(6): 767-75.
[http://dx.doi.org/10.1177/1040638720905833] [PMID: 32070230]

[20] Lee HCH, Lau WL, Ko CH, *et al.* Flexi-Myo panel strategy: Genomic diagnoses of myopathies and muscular dystrophies by next-generation sequencing. Genet Test Mol Biomarkers 2020; 24(2): 99-104.
[http://dx.doi.org/10.1089/gtmb.2018.0185] [PMID: 30907627]

[21] Ward LD, Kellis M. Interpreting noncoding genetic variation in complex traits and human disease. Nat Biotechnol 2012; 30(11): 1095-106.
[http://dx.doi.org/10.1038/nbt.2422] [PMID: 23138309]

[22] Hahn LW, Ritchie MD, Moore JH. Multifactor dimensionality reduction software for detecting gene-gene and gene-environment interactions. Bioinformatics 2003; 19(3): 376-82.
[http://dx.doi.org/10.1093/bioinformatics/btf869] [PMID: 12584123]

[23] Costa V, Aprile M, Esposito R, Ciccodicola A. RNA-Seq and human complex diseases: recent accomplishments and future perspectives. Eur J Hum Genet 2013; 21(2): 134-42.
[http://dx.doi.org/10.1038/ejhg.2012.129] [PMID: 22739340]

[24] Stranger BE, Stahl EA, Raj T. Progress and promise of genome-wide association studies for human complex trait genetics. Genetics 2011; 187(2): 367-83.
[http://dx.doi.org/10.1534/genetics.110.120907] [PMID: 21115973]

[25] Parkhomchuk D, Borodina T, Amstislavskiy V, *et al.* Transcriptome analysis by strand-specific

sequencing of complementary DNA. Nucleic Acids Res 2009; 37(18): e123.
[http://dx.doi.org/10.1093/nar/gkp596] [PMID: 19620212]

[26] Jin Z, Liu Y. DNA methylation in human diseases. Genes Dis 2018; 5(1): 1-8.
[http://dx.doi.org/10.1016/j.gendis.2018.01.002] [PMID: 30258928]

[27] Bellizzi D, D'Aquila P, Scafone T, *et al.* The control region of mitochondrial DNA shows an unusual CpG and non-CpG methylation pattern. DNA Res 2013; 20(6): 537-47.
[http://dx.doi.org/10.1093/dnares/dst029] [PMID: 23804556]

[28] Xu GL, Wong J. Oxidative DNA demethylation mediated by Tet enzymes. Natl Sci Rev 2015; 2(3): 318-28.
[http://dx.doi.org/10.1093/nsr/nwv029]

[29] Bochtler M, Kolano A, Xu GL. DNA demethylation pathways: Additional players and regulators. BioEssays 2017; 39(1): e201600178.
[http://dx.doi.org/10.1002/bies.201600178] [PMID: 27859411]

[30] Whyte WA, Orlando DA, Hnisz D, *et al.* Master transcription factors and mediator establish super-enhancers at key cell identity genes. Cell 2013; 153(2): 307-19.
[http://dx.doi.org/10.1016/j.cell.2013.03.035] [PMID: 23582322]

[31] Eichler EE, Flint J, Gibson G, *et al.* Missing heritability and strategies for finding the underlying causes of complex disease. Nat Rev Genet 2010; 11(6): 446-50.
[http://dx.doi.org/10.1038/nrg2809] [PMID: 20479774]

[32] Portela A, Esteller M. Epigenetic modifications and human disease. Nat Biotechnol 2010; 28(10): 1057-68.
[http://dx.doi.org/10.1038/nbt.1685] [PMID: 20944598]

[33] Muka T, Koromani F, Portilla E, *et al.* The role of epigenetic modifications in cardiovascular disease: A systematic review. Int J Cardiol 2016; 212: 174-83.
[http://dx.doi.org/10.1016/j.ijcard.2016.03.062] [PMID: 27038728]

[34] Birney E, Smith G D, Greally J M. Epigenome-wide association studies and the interpretation of disease-omics. PLoS genetics 2016; 12(6): e1006105.
[http://dx.doi.org/10.1371/journal.pgen.1006105]

[35] Rhoads A, Au KF. PacBio sequencing and its applications. Genomics Proteomics Bioinformatics 2015; 13(5): 278-89.
[http://dx.doi.org/10.1016/j.gpb.2015.08.002] [PMID: 26542840]

[36] Karl MM. Insights into old and new acetogens: transformation barriers and genomics (Doctoral dissertation, Universität Ulm).

[37] Mitsuhashi S, Matsumoto N. Long-read sequencing for rare human genetic diseases. J Hum Genet 2020; 65(1): 11-9.
[http://dx.doi.org/10.1038/s10038-019-0671-8] [PMID: 31558760]

[38] Majewski J, Schwartzentruber J, Lalonde E, Montpetit A, Jabado N. What can exome sequencing do for you? J Med Genet 2011; 48(9): 580-9.
[http://dx.doi.org/10.1136/jmedgenet-2011-100223] [PMID: 21730106]

[39] Lochmüller H, Torrent i Farnell J, Le Cam Y, *et al.* IRDiRC Consortium Assembly. The International Rare Diseases Research Consortium: Policies and Guidelines to maximize impact. Eur J Hum Genet 2017; 25(12): 1293-302.
[http://dx.doi.org/10.1038/s41431-017-0008-z] [PMID: 29158551]

CHAPTER 2

Genetic Testing for Rare Genetic Disorders

Muhammad Tariq[1,*], Naveed Altaf Malik[1], Ilyas Ahmad[2], Syeda Seema Waseem and **Shahid Mahmood Baig[1]**

[1] *National Institute for Biotechnology and Genetic Engineering College, Pakistan Institute of Engineering and Applied Sciences (NIBGE-C, PIEAS), Faisalabad, Pakistan*

[2] *Institute for Cardiogenetic, University of Lubeck, Lubeck, Germany*

[3] *Cologne Center for Genomics (CCG), University of Cologne, Germany*

Abstract: Rare genetic disorders affect a significant proportion of the global population. A large number of these patients are either misdiagnosed or remain undiagnosed which can have potentially adverse effects, including failure to provide anticipatory prognosis and identify potential treatment. With the completion of HGP, genetic testing has fast grown into a diagnostic discipline introducing new and cost-effective diagnostic tests with reasonable accuracy and specificity. NGS technologies, in particular, changed the field of genetic diagnosis by sequencing the entire genome or subset thereof in a single test and accomplishing diagnosis of virtually all diseases, either congenital or late-onset. These technologies have opened up new opportunities and unique challenges. This chapter discusses the importance of genetic testing, its scope, various technologies and approaches and, finally, the opportunities and challenges accompanying the new age genetic tests.

Keywords: aCGH, ARMS-PCR, Genetic disorders, Genetic testing, Massive Parallel Sequencing, NGS, Targeted Gene Panels, WES.

1. INTRODUCTION

Mendelian disorders are more commonly known as rare inherited disorders, especially among researchers working on these disorders. Around 7000 of these disorders are currently known of which a substantial number of disorders are life-threatening or chronically debilitating [1]. Ironically, however, 40 to 82 of every 1000 live births have one or another genetic disorder [2]. If a total load of genetic disorders constituted by all the inherited disorders together is considered, as much as 8% of the world population presents with a genetic disorder before adolescence [3].

---
[*] **Corresponding author Muhammad Tariq:** National Institute for Biotechnology and Genetic Engineering College, Pakistan Institute of Engineering and Applied Sciences (NIBGE-C, PIEAS), Faisalabad, Pakistan; E-mail: tariqpalai@gmail.com

Syeda Marriam Bakhtiar and Erum Dilshad (Eds.)

Thus, taken together, the so-called rare genetic disorders are not very rare! Moreover, these disorders are amongst the most difficult to diagnose in clinical practice owing to their genetic heterogeneity [4]. For instance, mutations in more than 150 genes have been implicated in inherited hearing loss only [5]. Thus, a large number of patients are either misdiagnosed or remain undiagnosed. This lack of diagnosis can fail to identify any potential therapeutic intervention and assess the risk of recurrence of the disorder in future pregnancies. Therefore, the completion of the Human Genome Project (HGP) in 2003 was heralded as the dawn of an era of genomic medicine [6] wherein individual genetic information will be used for making clinical decisions and delivery of personalized medicine [7]. Promises of rapid detection of mutations and improved diagnosis and prognosis made by proponents of this project fueled patients' desire for a rapid and accurate molecular diagnosis of their disease [8].

But until appropriate genetic tests are available for individual patients, access to the complete human genome alone cannot materialize the dream of personalized genomic medicine.

1.1. Genetic Testing and Its Scope

Ever since the first DNA test in the late 70s [9], genetic testing has fast grown to become an established diagnostic discipline today. Within the last few decades, genetic testing of disease-causing variants has been extensively used in clinical diagnosis and carrier screening of a large number of inherited disorders. In addition, it has also been used for prenatal diagnosis of the fetus in families with a history of a severe disease. Genetic testing is the procedure that detects variations in DNA to determine a patient's predisposition to develop diseases and disabilities. Although genetic tests were in use before, their applications increased by an order of several magnitudes after the completion of HGP, changing our medical practice for good (reproductive medicine and oncology, for instance) [10]. Today, these applications span a variety of medical disciplines, such as newborn screening for highly penetrant disorders; diagnostic and carrier testing for inherited disorders; screening for adult onset and complex multifactorial disorders; and evaluation of drug dosage, selection and response in pharmacogenetic testing [11].

In this chapter, we discuss the genetic test and its types, and its importance in the diagnosis of rare genetic disorders. The utility of a particular genetic test, in the clinic, depends on the degree of genetic heterogeneity of the disease being investigated and prospects for therapeutic intervention. The selection of genetic tests and platforms is also guided by the nature of the disease, patient's age, family history and available specimen. Some of the tests can rapidly detect gene variants previously implicated in similar, or the same, diseases (allele-specific tests) while others are tailor-made for examining the entire coding sequence of one or more genes in search of as yet undiscovered causative variants; each strategy has its strengths and weaknesses [12]. Prenatal whole genome sequencing (WGS), for instance, is useful for detecting carrier status in a large number of heterogeneous rare disorders [13], whereas in single-gene disorders, such as beta-thalassemia, molecular diagnosis can be accomplished in routine by simple and low-cost PCR amplification [14].

1.2. Screening and Diagnostic Testing

A genetic test is different from other clinical tests in that the routine clinical test is purely diagnostic and is meant to select appropriate interventions for a patient. However, a genetic test can serve both as a screening test and as a diagnostic test. As a screening test, it can be used to screen asymptomatic individuals to identify those predisposed to disease or screen for a mutation with potential risk to an unborn child (fetus). As a diagnostic test, it is used to testify the presence of an active disease process. Predictive testing can assess a healthy individual's risk of developing a disease, way before its onset, although it cannot predict its onset and severity [15]. The primary objective of a screening test is to identify individuals who can benefit from further diagnostic testing. Diagnostic tests have higher sensitivity and specificity and specifically, look for a particular clinical condition [16].

1.3. Why Genetic Testing?

For a family with a history of a genetic disorder, genetic testing enables the parents to make decisions during pregnancy based on the information provided by the test, coupled with genetic counselling. An expecting family can, for instance, decide to terminate or continue their pregnancy based on the result of a prenatal genetic test [17]. Postnatal genetic tests are not only useful for inaccurate diagnosis but may also advise on the prognosis of the disease. It has an important influence on a patient's management and therapy decisions. Moreover, a genetic diagnosis can spare further diagnostics and lessen emotional and financial burdens on patients and their families [18].

2. TESTING TECHNOLOGIES

As a natural corollary of the explosion of molecular discoveries during the past few decades, clinicians need to keep up-to-date on research in molecular biology, genetics and genomics so that they understand and interpret the pathophysiology of diseases and how to incorporate genetic testing into their practice in a practical and effective way [12]. When deciding on which test to employ, clinicians, and of course researchers, need to Fig out if they should take a targeted approach or sequence the entire genome or a subset thereof. A clinician expects a laboratory professional to find one or more genetic variants that underlie a particular disease condition, using an appropriate platform which is rapid and economic but also reliable. In the following section, we have listed some of the most popular testing technologies that have been, and are being, widely used for genetic testing of rare inherited disorders.

2.1. Detection of Targeted Allele Specific Mutation

The detection of PCR amplified DNA fragments by restriction digestion, hybridization or visualization through gel documentation has been one of the most economical and, hence, widely used approaches for diagnosing in clinical settings. Detection of PCR products is simple, rapid and reliable for the detection of disease-causing variants [11]. It is, therefore, amenable to the throughput of multiple samples, as is usually desired in clinical molecular diagnostics. Allele-specific ARMS (amplification refractory mutation detection system)-PCR (Fig. **2.1**), for instance, involves a single PCR followed by gel electrophoresis. It is designed for detecting single base changes or small deletions using allele-specific primers which allow the amplification of test DNA only if the target allele is present in the test sample. The presence or absence of a product, following ARMS-PCR, indicates the presence or absence of the corresponding allele and is, thus, diagnostic [19].

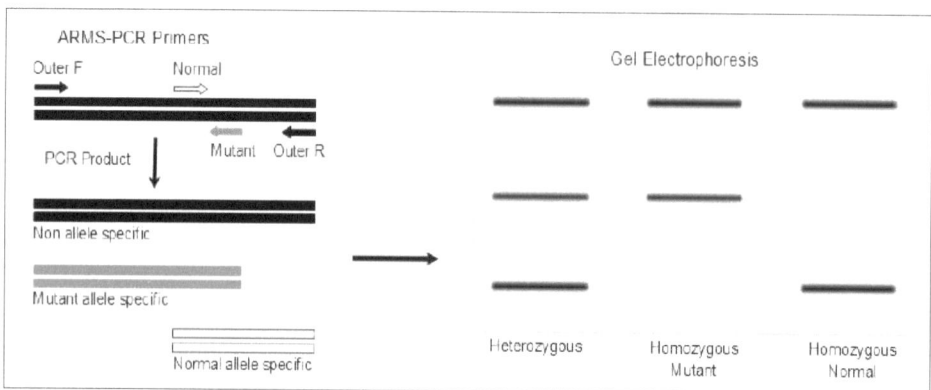

Fig. (2.1). Conceptual diagram of allele specific ARMS-PCR assay. Amplification of the product using allele/genotype specific primers (Normal and Mutant) corresponds to the presence or absence of the disease-causing variant. The Outer primers (Outer F and Outer R), not only enriches the target fragment for the two allele specific primers, it also works as a control to check if the PCR reaction was successful.

We have used ARMS PCR for prenatal diagnosis in a pilot project aimed at the identification of *HBB* gene variants causing beta-thalassemia in Pakistani patients. In order to increase the throughput, ARMS-PCR was multiplexed to detect more than one variant in a single PCR reaction [14]. Employing the same technique, we also conducted prenatal diagnosis of hereditary brain tumor by genotyping disease causing *PMS2* gene variants in first trimester chorionic villus samples (CVS) among families with a history of the disease [17]. This was the first ever prenatal diagnosis of inherited brain tumor by genetic testing. Diseases caused by pathogenic repeats, for instance Fragile X syndrome, are routinely diagnosed using PCR amplification of the fragment containing repeat expansions [20].

In the first ever DNA test in 1978, Kan and Dozy exploited polymorphism in the digestion pattern a DNA fragment that contains the beta globin structural gene resulting from a variation in the recognition site of *Hpa I* restriction endonuclease, ~5 kb from the 3' end of the gene. Restriction digestion of the fragments with normal sequence produces a fragment of 7.6 kb whereas those with the altered recognition site produce either 7 or 13 kb long fragment. This difference in the digestion fragments is, therefore, diagnostic [9]. Similarly, *Eae I* restriction digestion was found to be even more efficient at diagnosing Hb Q-India compared to ARMS-PCR [21].

Since these approaches target only a predefined set of variants, these are unable to detect any other variant(s) in the gene which are of clinical relevance in connection with the disease under investigation. Notwithstanding this limitation, targeted mutation detection, by restriction analysis or PCR, is cost-effective and will continue to play a pivotal role in clinical diagnosis in resource deficient laboratories and in low-income countries where the mass application of cutting-edge modern technologies is beyond affordability.

2.2. Gene-specific Sanger Sequencing

Owing to its low error rate, dideoxy chain termination sequencing, more known as Sanger sequencing, is regarded as a gold standard for identifying point mutations or small deletions [22]. Sequencing of the entire human genome as a reference was, in fact, inspired and accomplished up to ~3 billion nucleotides, using this technology [23]. In Sanger sequencing, the amplified DNA fragment is purified and extended by DNA polymerase from a primer adjacent to the target sequence using a mix of normal deoxy- and labeled dideoxy nucleotides. Every time the polymerase incorporates a fluorescently labelled complementary dideoxynucleotide, the growing chain terminates. The resulting mixture of fluorescently labelled DNA strands of varying lengths is resolved by capillary electrophoresis to determine nucleotide sequence [24]. After PCR with designed primers for amplification of specific fragments, Sanger sequencing exploits chain termination by ddNTPs, which are radiolabeled. The sequencer detects the radiolabeling of ddNTP and chromogram is generated.

Sanger sequencing has the advantage to detect all the variants in a DNA fragment being investigated and is, therefore, able to detect rare and novel variants not included in, for example, ARMS-PCR panels for a single gene disorder such as beta-thalassemia [25]. Similarly, direct sequencing of a single *FGFR2* gene is a cost-effective genetic test to confirm or rule out Apert's Syndrome [11]. In addition, it could be an effective first-line approach for diagnosing genetically heterogeneous disorders wherein one or a few gene variants are more prevalent than others and where exome sequencing (see Genetic Testing in the NGS Era) is not an option because of its high cost or unavailability. For instance, there are >25 genes reported to cause microcephaly [26], however, direct sequencing of only three of these (*ASPM, WDR62* and *MCPH1*) can detect causative variants in 9 out of 10 microcephaly patients [27]. Sanger sequencing is highly sensitive and specific with the lowest error rate among all the sequencing technologies but has its own limitations. The method is time-consuming; sequencing of the human genome reference sequence, for instance, took 13 years [28]. Its utility is limited to sequencing targeted DNA regions and it is unable to detect sequences beyond the focused region. It fails to detect most structural variations and, hence, for the diagnosis of a number of disorders where structure alterations are likely to be involved, direct sequencing alone is not sufficient. However, until next generation technologies improve their error rates and cost, Sanger sequencing will continue to be the most reliable sequencing technology in genetic testing.

2.3. Testing for Structural Variations

DNA rearrangements (deletions, duplications, inversions, insertions, and translocations) involving 50 nucleotides, or more, are known as structural variations [29]. Deletions and duplications exceeding 1 kb in size are also called copy-number variations (CNVs) [30]. Structural variations are important drivers of human genome evolution and are, therefore, implicated in several inherited disorders [31, 32]. Gene-sized or larger genetic aberrations are routinely tested for by fluorescence *in situ* hybridization (FISH) [33]. For FISH, labelled probes are designed for sequence complementary to the target region. The basic protocol includes slide preparation and pretreatment, denaturation of probe and target, hybridization, washing and analysis. FISH is a robust cytogenetic technique used for the visualization of nucleic acid sequences in their native (*in situ*) context in a single cell. It can be performed on RNA within cells, DNA in metaphase mitotic cells or in interphase nuclei from cells in the non-mitotic phases of the cell cycle.

In the clinical laboratory, FISH probes are used to target repetitive or unique DNA sequences, entire chromosome arms, or whole chromosomes [34].

However, FISH can only target a few loci at a time and that too with a limited resolution; small deletions, typically in a few kb, can hardly be detected. Therefore, the technique has been phased out in genetic testing, replaced slowly and gradually by array comparative genomic hybridization (aCGH). aCGH is a high throughput method and its strength lies in its ability to detect hundreds or thousands of discrete genomic imbalances (CNVs) to a resolution of even as low as 1 kb, in a single assay [35, 36]. Sampled and reference genomes, uniquely labelled with fluorescent dyes, are co-hybridized to an array matrix containing cloned DNA. The array may consist of whole genome or a subset thereof, arrayed on a glass slide. Deletion or duplications (CNVs) are quantified by analyzing the ratios of fluorescent signals [37]. aCGH has undoubtedly enhanced the resolution and sensitivity of genomic rearrangement detection, however, it is unable to detect balanced translocations and genomic inversions.

2.4. Genetic Testing in the NGS Era

For a genetic test to be used in a routine, it must first be democratized by reducing its cost and increasing its throughput so that everyone can afford and access it. The completion of HGP in 13 years costing $ ~3 billion meant that despite automation Sanger sequencing was not amenable to achieve the desired throughput to sequence the whole genome at a low cost affordable for genetic testing [38]. However, the availability of a reference genome inspired further inventions and improvements in sequencing technologies which resulted in high throughput sequencing machines, popularly known as next generation sequencing (NGS) platforms. Genomic DNA is randomly sheared into small fragments of varying lengths. Since the sample has multiple copies of genomic DNA, the same segment of DNA is fragmented in several different ways. These fragments are then amplified to produce NGS library with hundreds of copies of each fragment [39]. Typically, NGS library is massively parallel sequenced on any of the several platforms. During this sequencing *en masse*, the sequencing platform uses library fragments to determine the sequence, which is captured base-by-base by the instrument in a process termed sequencing by synthesis.

Rapid sequencing of the whole genome through these platforms is reshaping medical genomics by removing the necessity to prioritize candidate genes for sequencing. Genome sequencing is devised to cover both coding and noncoding genomic regions, therefore, there is no enrichment of any subset of the genome and, hence, no pre-sequencing sample preparation. This means that instead of the traditional approach wherein positional mapping was followed by Sanger sequencing, the disease identification process has been reduced to a single step (whole genome sequencing) and, therefore, allows application of this technology at mass scale [40]. Additionally, by virtue of its increased quantitative accuracy, data can also be analyzed for structural variants (including CNVs) in both hetero- and euchromatin regions [41]. In 2010, the mutational status of a fetus was determined from the maternal plasma DNA, proving both the sensitivity and efficiency of this technique for clinical genetic testing [42]. However, whole genome sequencing is the costliest of the NGS technologies and offers minimum average depth of coverage. Limitations in the interpretation of noncoding variants and variants of unknown significance also question the utility of this application. Majority of the published genome sequencing studies have, therefore, focused on the coding subset of the genome because approximately 85% of the known causative variants for rare disorders are protein coding [43].

Two different enrichment strategies have been in use to target the protein coding part of genome; disease-targeted gene panel sequencing and whole exome sequencing (WES). Gene panel sequencing aims to detect causative variants in a select set of genes which have known or suspected associations with the disease under investigation. Customized panels are designed by a thorough review of the literature and cross referencing publicly available databases such as The Human Genome Mutation Database (http://www.hgmd.org) and Online Mendelian Inheritance in Man (http://www.ncbi.nlm.nih.gov/omim/). NGS library is enriched for genomic regions containing target genes using oligonucleotide probes that hybridize to specified targets. The captured fragments are amplified to maximize the number of enriched fragments before sequencing *en masse*. A customized gene panel of 146 known hearing loss genes was used to successfully detect all known nuclear gene variants, which is a testimony of the accuracy and reliability of the targeted gene panel sequencing [44].

Selecting a limited set of genes results in a higher depth of coverage thereby increasing sensitivity and specificity of gene testing, especially in the case of dominantly inherited disorders where the causative variants are expected to be heterozygous. Since the role of targeted genes is already established, interpretation of the identified variants is easier. Targeting fewer genes means laboratories can use desktop sequencers and diagnose more patients per instrument. However, it also means that they will be outdated rather quickly as new studies implicate new disease genes during the time the gene panel is conceived, developed and validated for clinical utilization [45]. Another limitation of gene panels is that a clear diagnosis of the phenotype for which to develop a panel, is a prerequisite, *e.g.* , hearing loss and retinal diseases could be easily diagnosed. For heterogeneous disorders, for instance, neurodevelopmental disorders and other overlapping neurological presentations, the development of panels is limited by the selection of target genes. For these, and similar, disorders a smart alternative is sequencing the <2% coding subset of the genome, referred to as the whole exome.

For WES, only fragments encompassing the specified target exons are enriched from the NGS library using any of the commercially available oligonucleotide probes. These fragments are then amplified and sequenced on an NGS platform of choice [46]. Thus, unlike gene panels, exome sequencing is not limited to the detection of known pathogenic genes only and in case a new causative gene is discovered, a retrospective analysis of the exome data will find it. *In silico* analysis of WES and gene panel sequencing shows that the former covers more than 98% of the variants detected on the latter [45]. In our own experience, WES can find some of the very rare gene variants for genetic deafness which are rather unlikely to be included in common hearing loss gene panels and are, thus, prone to missed [47]. Similarly, compared to whole-genome sequencing, WES decreases both cost and turnaround time by focusing only on less than 2% of the genome and is still capable of finding more than 8 out of 10 disease-causing variants [43]. For patients who remain without a diagnosis, clinical application of WES has successfully diagnosed the disease by detecting causative variants in over 25% of the cases referred by clinicians [48, 49]. In neurogenetic anomalies, patients and their families are exposed to so called "diagnostic odysseys" because of a long time and cost that diagnosis costs. The use of WES in a series of 40 consecutive patients resulted in a diagnostic yield of 40% costing 60% less than the diagnostic workup prior to WES [50].

However, WES does have its inherent limitations. These include its inability to detect CNVs, translocations and trinucleotide repeats (repeat expansions, tandem repeat size), to name a few. Then there are regions in the genome with poor depth/coverage, particularly GC rich areas which WES fails to sequence adequately [51]. While some of the limitations are inherent to this technology, others are likely to be resolved with prospective improvements in technology; for instance, longer read length will improve sequencing quality in the repeat-dense regions. The detection rate of whole genome sequencing is only 7% higher and reanalyzing of WES is always recommended till the cost of former approximates that of the latter [52].

3. INCIDENTAL FINDINGS

Clinical NGS has the potential for identifying genetic variants beyond the scope of the initial purpose of testing but clinically relevant, nonetheless. Such results are referred to as incidental or secondary findings (ISFs). Whether or not to report these findings to the ordering clinicians or patients has been a matter of vigorous debate ever since the extension of NGS from research to clinical laboratories. Traditionally clinicians have sought genetic testing for patients with indication of disease or a positive family history. However, with clinical NGS, patients seeking a genetic test for a particular condition undergo a genetic test for all other disease-causing gene variants, this, in principle, compromises patient's preferences and the right to choose whether to test for conditions other than initially intended. Opponents argue that unless there is strong evidence of benefit to the patients or family, incidental finding need not be reported in clinical sequencing. But since these genes' variants are not intended for, there is a possibility that these variants are false positive in the initial analysis requiring additional validation, such as Sanger sequencing. Proponents believe that any of the disease-causing variants can be of clinical value and, therefore, in order to prevent harm, it is a fiduciary duty of clinicians and laboratory personnel to inform patients and their families about certain incidental findings; this principle supersedes concerns about autonomy.

The American College of Medical Genetics and Genomics (ACMG) recommends that after a clinical NGS, a minimum list of conditions and gene variants be evaluated in every clinical sequencing and results shared with the clinician who referred the patients for genetic testing. The concerned clinician can then assess these findings since s/he has access to patient's clinical data, medical and family history and any prior diagnostic workup [53].

4. FUTURE PROSPECTS AND CHALLENGES

The application of clinical NGS is rapidly transforming genomic medicine. With declining costs and continuous technological improvements, these technologies will soon serve as the first step in genetic testing in rare disease diagnosis. Modern sequencing technologies have the potential to screen the entire genome or its subset in a single genetic test. Thus, the overall cost and turnaround time of disease diagnosis has been reduced by several orders of magnitude during the last decade. Similarly, the existing capability of performing NGS on cell free DNA [13, 54] is expected to be routinely used for prenatal diagnosis, in the near future. The application of single cell technology, using several cells simultaneously, offers more accuracy than cell free DNA and can, at the same time, evaluate for sequencing errors or placental mosaicism [55].

However, in addition to technical limitations and challenges mentioned in previous sections, NGS has brought a new scenario with itself. Previously, a patient looking for diagnosis of a particular disease was ready, to some extent at least, for undesirable findings. But with NGS based genetic tests, healthy individuals, diagnosed for variants that might predispose them to a late-onse-

-disease, for instance, find it emotionally challenging to adapt to such incidental findings. This new scenario brings unprecedented challenges of medical and genetic counselling. This situation, therefore, demands behavioral and counseling research to devise effective clinical approaches to meet this challenge [56]. In addition, with the NGS technology shifting from laboratories to clinics, clinicians will be required to equip themselves with knowledge in genetics and genomics to be able to interpret findings in the context of patient's clinical data and family history.

CONCLUDING REMARKS

Emerging technologies have modernized diagnosis and cost-effective genetic tests with reasonable sensitivity, specificity and turnaround time are now available for a variety of rare genetic disorders. However, currently available tests have their limitations and challenges. Therefore, further research is still needed to determine best practices for clinical implementation of emerging technologies in connection to interpretation, turnaround time and appropriate counseling of patients and their families. Unlike other diagnostic tests, a sequenced genome is a resource, and not just a test, which will be interpreted and used over the life time of the patient. It is, therefore, imperative to deposit findings of genetic tests in a publicly available centralized database so as to help improve interpretation of as yet uncharacterized genetic variants.

CONSENT FOR PUBLICATION

Not Applicable.

CONFLICT OF INTEREST

The author declares no conflict of interest, financial or otherwise.

ACKNOWLEDGEMENTS

Declared none.

REFERENCES

[1]   Amberger JS, Bocchini CA, Schiettecatte F, Scott AF, Hamosh A. OMIM.org: Online Mendelian Inheritance in Man (OMIM®), an online catalog of human genes and genetic disorders. Nucleic Acids Res 2015; 43(D1): D789-98.
      [http://dx.doi.org/10.1093/nar/gku1205] [PMID: 25428349]

[2]   Christianson A L, *et al.* Global report on birth defects: the hidden toll of dying and disabled children. March of Dimes Birth Defects Foundation 2006.

[3]   Baird PA, Anderson TW, Newcombe HB, Lowry RB. Genetic disorders in children and young adults: a population study. Am J Hum Genet 1988; 42(5): 677-93.

[PMID: 3358420]

[4]   Tucker T, Marra M, Friedman JM. Massively parallel sequencing: the next big thing in genetic medicine. Am J Hum Genet 2009; 85(2): 142-54.
[http://dx.doi.org/10.1016/j.ajhg.2009.06.022] [PMID: 19679224]

[5]   Azaiez H, Booth KT, Ephraim SS, *et al.* Genomic Landscape and Mutational Signatures of Deafness-Associated Genes. Am J Hum Genet 2018; 103(4): 484-97.
[http://dx.doi.org/10.1016/j.ajhg.2018.08.006] [PMID: 30245029]

[6]   Guttmacher AE, Collins FS. Welcome to the genomic era. N Engl J Med 2003; 349(10): 996-8.
[http://dx.doi.org/10.1056/NEJMe038132] [PMID: 12954750]

[7]   Ginsburg GS, Willard HF. Genomic and personalized medicine: foundations and applications. Transl Res 2009; 154(6): 277-87.
[http://dx.doi.org/10.1016/j.trsl.2009.09.005] [PMID: 19931193]

[8]   Burke W. Genetic Testing. N Engl J Med 2002; 347(23): 1867-75.
[http://dx.doi.org/10.1056/NEJMoa012113] [PMID: 12466512]

[9]   Kan YW, Dozy AM. Polymorphism of DNA sequence adjacent to human beta-globin structural gene: relationship to sickle mutation. Proc Natl Acad Sci USA 1978; 75(11): 5631-5.
[http://dx.doi.org/10.1073/pnas.75.11.5631] [PMID: 281713]

[10]   Sequeiros J, Paneque M, Guimarães B, *et al.* The wide variation of definitions of genetic testing in international recommendations, guidelines and reports. J Community Genet 2012; 3(2): 113-24.
[http://dx.doi.org/10.1007/s12687-012-0084-2] [PMID: 22368105]

[11]   Katsanis SH, Katsanis N. Molecular genetic testing and the future of clinical genomics. Nat Rev Genet 2013; 14(6): 415-26.
[http://dx.doi.org/10.1038/nrg3493] [PMID: 23681062]

[12]   Drack AV, Lambert SR, Stone EM. From the laboratory to the clinic: molecular genetic testing in pediatric ophthalmology. Am J Ophthalmol 2010; 149(1): 10-17.e2.
[http://dx.doi.org/10.1016/j.ajo.2009.08.038] [PMID: 20103038]

[13]   Kitzman JO, Snyder MW, Ventura M, *et al.* Noninvasive whole-genome sequencing of a human fetus. Sci Transl Med 2012; 4(137): 137ra76.
[http://dx.doi.org/10.1126/scitranslmed.3004323] [PMID: 22674554]

[14]   Mahmood Baig S, Sabih D, Rahim MK, *et al.* β-Thalassemia in Pakistan. J Pediatr Hematol Oncol 2012; 34(2): 90-2.
[http://dx.doi.org/10.1097/MPH.0b013e31823752f3] [PMID: 22258353]

[15]   Constantin CM, Faucett A, Lubin IM. A primer on genetic testing. J Midwifery Womens Health 2005; 50(3): 197-204.
[http://dx.doi.org/10.1016/j.jmwh.2005.01.001] [PMID: 15894997]

[16]   Stoler JM. Prenatal and Postnatal Genetic Testing: Why, How, and When? Pediatr Ann 2017; 46(11): e423-7.
[http://dx.doi.org/10.3928/19382359-20171023-01] [PMID: 29131922]

[17]   Baig SM, Fatima A, Tariq M, *et al.* Hereditary brain tumor with a homozygous germline mutation in PMS2: pedigree analysis and prenatal screening in a family with constitutional mismatch repair deficiency (CMMRD) syndrome. Fam Cancer 2019; 18(2): 261-5.
[http://dx.doi.org/10.1007/s10689-018-0112-4] [PMID: 30478739]

[18]   Weber YG, Biskup S, Helbig KL, Von Spiczak S, Lerche H. The role of genetic testing in epilepsy diagnosis and management. Expert Rev Mol Diagn 2017; 17(8): 739-50.
[http://dx.doi.org/10.1080/14737159.2017.1335598] [PMID: 28548558]

[19]   Little S. Amplification-refractory mutation system (ARMS) analysis of point mutations. Curr Protoc Hum Genet 2001; 9(9.8).

[20]   Wallace AJ. Detection of unstable trinucleotide repeats. Methods Mol Med 1996; 5: 37-62.
[PMID: 21374511]

[21]   Khalil MSM, Henderson S, Schuh A, Hussein MRA, Old J. The first use of EaeI restriction enzyme in
DNA diagnosis of Hb Q-India. Int J Lab Hematol 2011; 33: 492-7.
[http://dx.doi.org/10.1111/j.1751-553X.2011.01316.x] [PMID: 21435192]

[22]   Bakker E. Is the DNA sequence the gold standard in genetic testing? Quality of molecular genetic tests
assessed. Clin Chem 2006; 52(4): 557-8.
[http://dx.doi.org/10.1373/clinchem.2005.066068] [PMID: 16595822]

[23]   Lander ES, Linton LM, Birren B, *et al.* International Human Genome Sequencing Consortium. Initial
sequencing and analysis of the human genome. Nature 2001; 409(6822): 860-921.
[http://dx.doi.org/10.1038/35057062] [PMID: 11237011]

[24]   Anderson MW, Schrijver I. Next generation DNA sequencing and the future of genomic medicine.
Genes (Basel) 2010; 1(1): 38-69.
[http://dx.doi.org/10.3390/genes1010038] [PMID: 24710010]

[25]   Old J, Henderson S. Molecular diagnostics for haemoglobinopathies. Expert Opin Med Diagn 2010;
4(3): 225-40.
[http://dx.doi.org/10.1517/17530051003709729] [PMID: 23488532]

[26]   Shaheen R, Maddirevula S, Ewida N, *et al.* Genomic and phenotypic delineation of congenital
microcephaly. Genet Med 2019; 21(3): 545-52.
[http://dx.doi.org/10.1038/s41436-018-0140-3] [PMID: 30214071]

[27]   Morris-Rosendahl D, Kaindl A, Zaqout S. Autosomal Recessive Primary Microcephaly (MCPH): An
Update. Neuropediatrics 2017; 48(3): 135-42.
[http://dx.doi.org/10.1055/s-0037-1601448] [PMID: 28399591]

[28]   Pareek CS, Smoczynski R, Tretyn A. Sequencing technologies and genome sequencing. J Appl Genet
2011; 52(4): 413-35.
[http://dx.doi.org/10.1007/s13353-011-0057-x] [PMID: 21698376]

[29]   Sudmant PH, Rausch T, Gardner EJ, *et al.* 1000 Genomes Project Consortium. An integrated map of
structural variation in 2,504 human genomes. Nature 2015; 526(7571): 75-81.
[http://dx.doi.org/10.1038/nature15394] [PMID: 26432246]

[30]   Freeman JL, Perry GH, Feuk L, *et al.* Copy number variation: New insights in genome diversity.
Genome Res 2006; 16(8): 949-61.
[http://dx.doi.org/10.1101/gr.3677206] [PMID: 16809666]

[31]   Perry GH, Yang F, Marques-Bonet T, *et al.* Copy number variation and evolution in humans and
chimpanzees. Genome Res 2008; 18(11): 1698-710.
[http://dx.doi.org/10.1101/gr.082016.108] [PMID: 18775914]

[32]   Weischenfeldt J, Symmons O, Spitz F, Korbel JO. Phenotypic impact of genomic structural variation:
insights from and for human disease. Nat Rev Genet 2013; 14(2): 125-38.
[http://dx.doi.org/10.1038/nrg3373] [PMID: 23329113]

[33]   Gu J, Smith JL, Dowling PK. Fluorescence In Situ Hybridization Probe Validation for Clinical Use.
Methods Mol Biol 2017; 1541: 101-18.
[http://dx.doi.org/10.1007/978-1-4939-6703-2_10] [PMID: 27910018]

[34]   Tsuchiya KD. Fluorescence *in situ* hybridization. Clin Lab Med 2011; 31: 525-42.

[35]   Coppinger J, Alliman S, Lamb AN, Torchia BS, Bejjani BA, Shaffer LG. Whole-genome microarray
analysis in prenatal specimens identifies clinically significant chromosome alterations without increase
in results of unclear significance compared to targeted microarray. Prenat Diagn 2009; 29(12): 1156-
66.
[http://dx.doi.org/10.1002/pd.2371] [PMID: 19795450]

[36]   Park JH, Woo JH, Shim SH, *et al.* Application of a target array Comparative Genomic Hybridization to prenatal diagnosis. BMC Med Genet 2010; 11(1): 102.
[http://dx.doi.org/10.1186/1471-2350-11-102] [PMID: 20576126]

[37]   Park SJ, Jung EH, Ryu RS, *et al.* Clinical implementation of whole-genome array CGH as a first-tier test in 5080 pre and postnatal cases. Mol Cytogenet 2011; 4(1): 12.
[http://dx.doi.org/10.1186/1755-8166-4-12] [PMID: 21549014]

[38]   Scott AR. Technology: Read the instructions. Nature 2016; 537(7619): S54-6.
[http://dx.doi.org/10.1038/537S54a] [PMID: 27602740]

[39]   O'Daniel JM, Lee K. Whole-genome and whole-exome sequencing in hereditary cancer: impact on genetic testing and counseling. Cancer J 2012; 18(4): 287-92.
[http://dx.doi.org/10.1097/PPO.0b013e318262467e] [PMID: 22846728]

[40]   Gilissen C, Hoischen A, Brunner HG, Veltman JA. Disease gene identification strategies for exome sequencing. Eur J Hum Genet 2012; 20(5): 490-7.
[http://dx.doi.org/10.1038/ejhg.2011.258] [PMID: 22258526]

[41]   Rehm HL, Bale SJ, Bayrak-Toydemir P, *et al.* Working Group of the American College of Medical Genetics and Genomics Laboratory Quality Assurance Commitee. ACMG clinical laboratory standards for next-generation sequencing. Genet Med 2013; 15(9): 733-47.
[http://dx.doi.org/10.1038/gim.2013.92] [PMID: 23887774]

[42]   Lo YMD, Chan KCA, Sun H, *et al.* Maternal plasma DNA sequencing reveals the genome-wide genetic and mutational profile of the fetus. Sci Transl Med 2010; 2(61): 61ra91.
[http://dx.doi.org/10.1126/scitranslmed.3001720] [PMID: 21148127]

[43]   Botstein D, Risch N. Discovering genotypes underlying human phenotypes: past successes for mendelian disease, future approaches for complex disease. Nat Genet 2003; 33(S3) (Suppl.): 228-37.
[http://dx.doi.org/10.1038/ng1090] [PMID: 12610532]

[44]   Tekin D, Yan D, Bademci G, *et al.* A next-generation sequencing gene panel (MiamiOtoGenes) for comprehensive analysis of deafness genes. Hear Res 2016; 333: 179-84.
[http://dx.doi.org/10.1016/j.heares.2016.01.018] [PMID: 26850479]

[45]   LaDuca H, Farwell KD, Vuong H, *et al.* Exome sequencing covers >98% of mutations identified on targeted next generation sequencing panels. PLoS One 2017; 12(2): e0170843.
[http://dx.doi.org/10.1371/journal.pone.0170843] [PMID: 28152038]

[46]   Bamshad MJ, Ng SB, Bigham AW, *et al.* Exome sequencing as a tool for Mendelian disease gene discovery. Nat Rev Genet 2011; 12(11): 745-55.
[http://dx.doi.org/10.1038/nrg3031] [PMID: 21946919]

[47]   Zhou Y, Tariq M, He S, Abdullah U, Zhang J, Baig SM. Whole exome sequencing identified mutations causing hearing loss in five consanguineous Pakistani families. BMC Med Genet 2020; 21(1): 151.
[http://dx.doi.org/10.1186/s12881-020-01087-x] [PMID: 32682410]

[48]   Yang Y, Muzny DM, Reid JG, *et al.* Clinical whole-exome sequencing for the diagnosis of mendelian disorders. N Engl J Med 2013; 369(16): 1502-11.
[http://dx.doi.org/10.1056/NEJMoa1306555] [PMID: 24088041]

[49]   Yang Y, Muzny DM, Xia F, *et al.* Molecular findings among patients referred for clinical whole-exome sequencing. JAMA 2014; 312(18): 1870-9.
[http://dx.doi.org/10.1001/jama.2014.14601] [PMID: 25326635]

[50]   Córdoba M, Rodriguez-Quiroga SA, Vega PA, *et al.* Whole exome sequencing in neurogenetic odysseys: An effective, cost- and time-saving diagnostic approach. PLoS One 2018; 13(2): e0191228.
[http://dx.doi.org/10.1371/journal.pone.0191228] [PMID: 29389947]

[51]   Benjamini Y, Speed TP. Summarizing and correcting the GC content bias in high-throughput

sequencing. Nucleic Acids Res 2012; 40(10): e72.
[http://dx.doi.org/10.1093/nar/gks001] [PMID: 22323520]

[52]   Alfares A, Aloraini T, subaie LA, *et al.* Whole-genome sequencing offers additional but limited clinical utility compared with reanalysis of whole-exome sequencing. Genet Med 2018; 20(11): 1328-33.
[http://dx.doi.org/10.1038/gim.2018.41] [PMID: 29565419]

[53]   Green RC, Berg JS, Grody WW, *et al.* American College of Medical Genetics and Genomics. ACMG recommendations for reporting of incidental findings in clinical exome and genome sequencing. Genet Med 2013; 15(7): 565-74.
[http://dx.doi.org/10.1038/gim.2013.73] [PMID: 23788249]

[54]   Fan HC, Gu W, Wang J, Blumenfeld YJ, El-Sayed YY, Quake SR. Non-invasive prenatal measurement of the fetal genome. Nature 2012; 487(7407): 320-4.
[http://dx.doi.org/10.1038/nature11251] [PMID: 22763444]

[55]   Jelin AC, Vora N. Whole Exome Sequencing. Obstet Gynecol Clin North Am 2018; 45(1): 69-81.
[http://dx.doi.org/10.1016/j.ogc.2017.10.003] [PMID: 29428287]

[56]   Biesecker LG. Opportunities and challenges for the integration of massively parallel genomic sequencing into clinical practice: lessons from the ClinSeq project. Genet Med 2012; 14(4): 393-8.
[http://dx.doi.org/10.1038/gim.2011.78] [PMID: 22344227]

CHAPTER 3

Preimplantation, Prenatal, and Postnatal Diagnosis

Sadia Nawaz[1,*] and **Humna Masood**[1]

[1] *Institute of Biochemistry and Biotechnology,University of Veterinary and Animal Sciences-UVAS, Lahore-54000, Pakistan*

Abstract: Pre-implantation genetic diagnosis (PGD) is a practical alternate evolving approach to prenatal diagnosis and termination of pregnancies in families with a high risk of Mendelian monogenetic and polygenetic disorders. Pre-implantation genetic diagnosis testing is continuing to extend immensely, along with a novel genetic analysis and *in vitro* fertilization approaches are in practice in the medical field throughout the world. However, PGD is regarded as ethically sensitive because repetitive termination of pregnancy causes huge psychological effects on the couples, and also because the low rate of pregnancy and birth makes it unreliable compared to prenatal testing. But it is also helpful in achieving additional goals *e.g.*, improved embryo and gender selection, overcoming the chances of birth of a child with an unknown genetic defect, better understanding of epigenomic regulations and reduction in the monetary burden of society. This chapter focuses on PGD, its procedure, utility and advantages, goals and objectives and the various issues surrounding it. We also discuss the future of this technology at the end of the chapter.

Keywords: Mendelian monogenetic and Polygenetic disorder, Prenatal diagnosis, Preimplantation genetic diagnosis.

1. INTRODUCTION

With the advent of new technologies in genomics, there is an opportunity to resolve or overcome the challenges of genetics and reproductive sciences. It helps to analyze recessive, dominant or X-linked disorders which are the cause of incurable early or late-onset phenotypes or morbidities. For this purpose, different diagnostic methods such as pre-implantation, prenatal and postnatal are offered to prevent the transmission of these genetic anomalies from parents to offspring. These diagnoses are done before or just after birth for the identification of the genetic basis of the disease, which opens up new possibilities to overcome and treat a disease completely or to some extent.

* **Corresponding author Sadia Nawaz**: Institute of Biochemistry and Biotechnology, University of Veterinary and Animal Sciences-UVAS, Lahore-54000, Pakistan; E-mails: sadia.nawaz@uvas.edu.pk and shamiryar@hotmail.com

Syeda Marriam Bakhtiar and Erum Dilshad (Eds.)
All rights reserved-© 2022 Bentham Science Publishers

In this chapter, we briefly overview pre-implantation genetic diagnosis (PGD), prenatal diagnosis (PND), postnatal diagnosis, chromosomal abnormalities, and monogenic and polygenic diseases. We also discuss the diagnostic methods which could be employed before or after birth for the identification of genetic disorders in infants or adults.

1.1. Preimplantation Genetic Diagnosis (PGD)

Medical advances have allowed scientists to achieve preimplantation genetic diagnosis (PGD) clinically, which helps in the selection of genetically unaffected embryos before implantation in the uterus [1]. PGD was first ideated by Robert Edward in the mid-1960s. In 1968, Gardner and Edward conducted experiments for the production of animals of desired sex [2]. By using the sex-specific chromatin patterns, they were able to identify rabbit sex chromatin in the blastocyst stage and then transfer it to the uterus [3]. Later on, it became the first successful PGD test in humans. In the mid-90s, the first preimplantation genetic consultant Alan H. Handyside and his colleagues applied PGD for an X-linked disorder, cystic fibrosis (CF), in Hammersmith Hospital, Landon [4]. Preimplantation genetic diagnosis has advantages over prenatal diagnosis because some families with a high risk of genetically defected progeny in the future choose not to terminate a pregnancy after prenatal genetic testing. Therefore, the basic aim of preimplantation genetic diagnosis is to have healthy offspring and to avoid the invasive termination of pregnancy if the embryo is affected. PGD has applications in three groups of genetic anomalies. The first group comprises patients who are at high risk of transmission of monogenic disorder to their progeny *e.g.* Duchenne muscular dystrophy (DMD) and CF *etc.* The second group consists of families with imbalanced chromosomal abnormalities *e.g.*, translocation, where the number of affected offspring's birth and abortions could be reduced by using PGD. The third group includes patients having aneuploidy in children due to advanced maternal age [5].

Furthermore, there are three professional and highly qualitative laboratories involved in PGD [5] and their details are as follows:

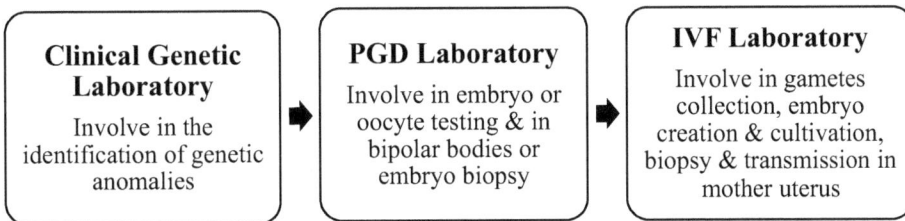

Fig (3.1). Conceptual diagram of professional laboratories involved in pre-implantation diagnosis.

1.1.1. PGD and In vitro Diagnostic Procedures

For the preimplantation genetic diagnostic procedure, family counselling and evaluation are concisely done by IVF members. Afterwards, a variety of procedures can be used for obtaining zygote or oocytes *e.g.*, ovarian hyper-stimulation, *in vitro* fertilization (IVF) techniques *e.g.*, intra-cytoplasmic sperm injection.

1.1.2. Phases of PGD

Embryo biopsy and genetic diagnosis are two phases of PGD; their details are given below.

1.1.3. Embryo Biopsy

PGD biopsy is carried out in two steps: the first step is puncturing the zona-pellucida (a membrane that is present in the surrounding of embryo or oocyte) and the second is the removal of cells from the embryo. The membrane can be breached or punctured by using chemical, mechanical or laser techniques. Different biopsy methods have been reported which are given below [6]:

PB (Polar Body) Biopsy is the first stage of biopsy in which the two polar bodies are removed sequentially or simultaneously. On the 0th day, the first PB is removed from the oocyte in the sequential biopsy method. Then on the 1st day, the second PB is removed after fertilization [7, 8].

Blastomere (Cleavage Stage) Biopsy: The mitotic division of the human zygote occurs after every 24 hours. So, two cells (blastomeres) can be biopsied on the 3rd day without disturbing embryo development and metabolism. Blastomere aspiration and zona-pellucida puncturing are done by using a micro-manipulator [9].

Trophectoderm (Blastocyst) Biopsy: Without harming inner cell mass, 10 to 30 cells in the blastocyst stage can be biopsied on 5th or 6th day. The breaching of zona pellucida is done on the 3rd day and then on the 5th day, cells are removed for preimplantation genetic diagnosis [10].

1.1.4. Genetic Diagnostic Analysis

Different diagnostic techniques such as PCR, FISH, micro-array and next generation sequencing *etc.* are used in PGD. Details are given in the second part of this chapter.

1.2. Prenatal Diagnosis (PND)

Prenatal diagnosis deals with the determination of either maternal or fetal condition [11]. In 1950, the first prenatal diagnosis was performed with the help of ultrasound to identify abnormalities in the fetus Later, in 1970, real time gray scale imaging was used for improving prenatal diagnosis. Nowadays, the age of gestation, number of the fetus, fetus condition testing and malformation evaluation can be done by ultrasonography with invasive and therapeutic diagnostic procedures [12].

1.2.1. In Vivo Procedure of PND

The prenatal diagnostic procedure is sub-divided into two parts:

1.2.2. Sampling of Fetus Cells

For prenatal diagnostic testing, fetus cells can be obtained from three different stages of pregnancy. These are;

Choriocentesis: in which, fetus cells are usually removed within 10-18 weeks of gestation from the transvaginal route with the help of forceps or by inserting a needle from the trans-abdominalroute.

Amniocentesis: In this process, fetus cells can be removed within 14-16 weeks of gestation from amniotic fluid.

Cordocentesis: Before 21 weeks of gestation, percutaneous-fetus blood can be taken from the umbilical vein.

Now non-invasive PND methods are used for diagnostic purposes. These methods are preferred for having a low risk of damaging fetus cells. They are;

The analysis of fetus cells from mother blood is done within 6-8 weeks of gestation. Although it is difficult for finding appropriate fetus cells in mother's blood.

Free RNA or DNA analysis from mother blood allows for finding X-linked diseases (especially in males) and also helps in determining Rh-group-typing in case of any fetus damage.

1.2.3. Genetic Diagnostic Analysis

This diagnostic analysis is divided into two groups and their details are given below:

DNA analysis is for finding mutations within the genes commonly transmitted from parents to their offsprings.

Chromosomal analysis includes aneuploidy and chromosomal morphological modification testing for finding chromosomal aberrations [13]. Further details of prenatal diagnostic techniques will be discussed in the second part of this chapter.

1.3. Postnatal Diagnosis

Postnatal diagnosis is associated with the examination and determination of a disease after birth. After birth, the first postnatal examination is performed within 1 to 2 hours for the confirmation of the condition of the newborn. Again, another examination is done before discharging mother and baby from the hospital. If the baby's birth takes place at home, then the first postnatal diagnosis should be done as soon as possible (within 24-48 hours after birth). Postnatal diagnosis is necessary for early diagnosis of genetic disorders particularly if it is prevalent in their families. At least 4 postnatal examinations are required within the first six weeks. It is reported that renal abnormalities in infants can be detected and identified using postnatal evaluation. Various types of renal abnormalities in infants are reported to be detected through antenatal sonogram. The most common abnormality found is hydronephrosis (also termed as renal pelvic dilation). Its prevalence is estimated to be 0.5% to 1%. Two grading systems are reported to be used for hydronephrosis *i.e.*, anterior posterior diameter (APD), and society for fetal urology (SFU). Furthermore, the post evaluation of infants with any abnormality must be started with physical examination [14].

1.3.1. Chromosomal Abnormalities

Traditionally, hereditary disorders are divided into three groups: monogenic disorders (Mendelian diseases), polygenic or multifactorial disorders and diseases that occur due to chromosomal abnormalities or aberrations. In chromosomal abnormalities, a part of chromosome or whole chromosome is duplicated, altered or deleted. Approximately 11 out of 150 live births have these problems [15]. Various factors such as advanced maternal age, environmental factors, multiple abortions, inherited genetic disorder history and consanguineous marriages are reported to be responsible for influencing genetic errors and various diseases or conditions *i.e.*, congenital abnormalities, intellectual and developmental disabilities arise due to such abnormalities. They are classified into two types *i.e.*, numerical or structural.

Numerical chromosomal abnormalities occur when either the whole chromosome is missing or there are an extra number of chromosomes *i.e.*, 45, or

47 chromosomes *e.g.*, Down syndrome (21 trisomy), Turner syndrome (X monosomy), Klinefelter syndrome (XXY), and XXX. It may occur in sex chromosomes or autosomes.

Structural (morphological) chromosomal abnormalities are those abnormalities that occur because of a missing, translocated, duplicated or inverted specific portion or section of the individual chromosome. It may appear due to chromosomal breakage and incorrect rejoining *e.g.*, ring chromosome which is formed due to the joining of the broken ends of chromosome in a circular way. It occurs in sex chromosomes, autosomal chromosomes or in both [16].

1.3.2. Monogenic (Mendelian) Diseases

Monogenic disorders arise due to a single mutation that causes severe or life-threatening diseases which may be inherited from their parents to their children [17]. They are relatively infrequent but disturb a considerable population especially those in rural areas of developing countries. The World Health Organization (WHO) evaluated that approximately every 1-10 in 1000 births are globally affected by monogenic diseases. The main reason for the prevalence of these disorders is consanguineous marriages. The inherited pattern in large families can be traced by pedigree analyses. About 7000 types of monogenic disorders are reported *e.g.*, DMD, α-1-antitrypsin deficiency, Friedreich ataxia, cystic fibrosis, familial amyloid polyneuropathy, atypical hemolytic uremic syndrome-1, Fragile X Syndrome, osteogenesis imperfecta, retinoblastoma, *etc* [18]. On the basis of their inheritance, pattern monogenic disorders are classified into the following three subgroups.

Dominant autosomal diseases occur because of the mutation or impairment within a single autosomal gene (total 22 autosomal chromosomes in humans) and as a result, a visible phenotypic disorder appears.

Recessive autosomal diseases occur due to the impairment of homozygous individual genes (both alleles of the gene) *e.g.*, phenylketonuria and sickle cell anemia.

Sex-linked chromosomal diseases appear due to mutation of the sex (X & Y) chromosomes. The inheritance pattern of the sex chromosomal gene is the same as the inheritance pattern of the autosomal chromosomal gene. But the difference is only found in the inheritance pattern of X and Y chromosomes genes because X chromosome genes have the same pattern of inheritance as autosomal genes while Y chromosomes have very nearly no gene [19].

1.3.3. Polygenic Diseases

Polygenic disorders are associated with the joint contribution of more than one gene which may either act independently or interact with other genes in causing a particular disease. They occur more frequently in humans as compared to monogenic disorders and possess socio-economic impact. The genes responsible for the development of polygenic diseases are reported to be Figd out by using two strategies *i.e.*, by determining the role of specific gene(s) followed by the role of their respective protein involved in the pathogenesis of diseases using linkage analysis and association studies; and whole genome sequencing using different markers which are distributed over the entire genome [20]. Some of the polygenic diseases reported include Alzheimer's disease, Parkinson's disease, Schizophrenia, and several cardiovascular diseases [21].

2. PREIMPLANTATION, PRENATAL, AND POSTNATAL DIAGNOSTIC TECHNIQUES

Different techniques are used for the identification of unbalanced chromosomal, monogenic and polygenic disorders. Their details are given below.

2.1. Array Comparative Genomic Hybridization (aCGH)

Array comparative genomic hybridization (aCGH) is the most reliable molecular technique for preimplantation genetic diagnosis, as well as for prenatal and postnatal diagnosis. Using aCGH, comprehensive chromosomal screening can be carried out [1, 22] which allows the detection of quantitative deviation of chromosomal copy numbers such as trisomy and monosomy. It also detects the quantitative deviation of unbalanced chromosomes *i.e.*, translocations. In aCGH, the labelled DNA of test and control samples is hybridized to DNA microarray, which is followed by array scanning, imaging, and evaluation of the intensities of both the test and control hybridization signals with respect to each probe. Then, a plot of acquired data is generated through a computer program. This whole technique is performed under a microscope. The limitation of this technique is that it cannot detect the quantitative deviations of translocation and inversion in a balance-chromosomal re-arrangement [2, 23]. This is a microarray-based cytogenetic technology used to evaluate loss and gains resulting in chromosomal copy number change in chromosomal sequences. It requires whole genomic DNA from patients and controls, which is then fluorescently labelled and co-hybridized with nucleic acid targets.

2.2. Fluorescence *In Situ* Hybridization (FISH)

FISH is used in various cytogenetic testings. It is basically a technique in which fluorescent probe (DNA fragment) is hybridized with the specific region of chromosome at interphase or metaphase stage producing signals. These signals are then visualized through fluorescent microscopy [24, 25].

There are different types of fluorescent probes used for the identification of chromosomal abnormalities *e.g.*, centromere probes used for the identification of trisomy, monosomy and marker chromosome origin, various sets of probes implied for chromosomal sub-telomeric region identification and others used for the identification of a particular genomic region. Currently DNA probes for chromosome 21, 18, 16, 15, 14, 13, X and Y are simultaneously used for PGD analysis. FISH also enables analysis of the chromosomal abnormalities related to frequent miscarriages. The detection rate is approximately 70% for aneuploidies [26]. Furthermore, FISH technique supports high resolution analysis of specified location [3, 27].

2.3. Next Generation Sequencing (NGS)

Next generation sequencing is a cost-effective emerging technique providing high throughput and high-resolution base pair information for genetic studies within 12 hours [4, 27]. There are two main methods of NGS for aneuploidy screening. In the first method, whole DNA of cells biopsied from embryos is released, amplified, broken into short fragments, and then subjected to NGS. The chromosomal origin of fragments is then identified which further allows the determination of chromosomal aneuploidy. In another method, the whole genomic DNA is not amplified, but there is an amplification of some fragments of specific loci using PCR. Then the obtained amplified DNA fragments are subjected to NGS and evaluated for the detection of chromosomal aneuploidy [28]. NGS is also used for prenatal and postnatal diagnosis. In PGD, NGS is used to identify unbalanced chromosome derivatives, and partial chromosomal aneuploidies in an embryo [5, 29]. Previously NGS was used for the cytogenetic analysis of cells with great precision and accuracy [4]. But now preimplantation genetic testing with the use of NGS increases the chances of pregnancy as well as NGS technique has an ability to identify mosaic embryos and facilitating the exclusion of abnormal/ mosaic embryos [30].

2.4. Whole Genome Amplification (WGA)

WGA is used for the analysis of the whole genome of a cell. It depends on MDA (multiple displacement amplification). MDA gives result within a few hours by using minimum quantity of DNA. It opens up new ways for other technologies *e.g.*, DNA microarray and preimplantation genetic haplotyping (PGH) [31]. It is the most robust method for amplification of an entire genome and requires very amount of DNA as a template. Various modified versions include MDA *i.e.*, Multiple Displacement Amplification, DOP-PCR *i.e.*, Degenerate Oligonucleotide PCR and PEP *i.e.*, Primer Extension Preamplification.

3. PRENATAL AND POSTNATAL DIAGNOSTIC TECHNIQUES FOR CHROMOSOMAL ABNORMALITIES, MONOGENIC, AND POLYGENIC DISEASES

3.1. Methylation PCR

Methylation PCR is a simple, fast, cost-effective, and non-invasive procedure to identify the methylation status of DNA in order to diagnose diseases linked with unusual DNA methylation [6, 32]. Methylation PCR is used to detect allele methylation even at minute level *i.e.*, less than 1%, and could be employed in several specimens including paraffin-embedded specimens and body fluids. In methylation PCR, the DNA to be used is treated with sodium bisulfite, and primers are required for amplification. In addition to this, methylation PCR can provide both qualitative and quantitative results in order to identify DNA methylation changes to diagnose diseases such as cancer [33].

3.2. Amniocentesis

Amniocentesis method is a prenatal genetic diagnosis that is used for monitoring the fetus position in mother's uterus. It is performed during the gestation period of 15 to 20 weeks at which approximately 200ml of amniotic fluid is available. In this, a needle having 22-gauge is allowed to pass into the amniotic fluid using the trans-abdominal approach with the help of ultrasound, and amniotic fluid of the desired quantity is aspired which is further used in the genetic diagnosis of various diseases. Furthermore, amniocentesis is performed efficiently and precisely on twin gestation by the injection of needle into the first sac followed by the injection of needle into the second sac for fluid aspiration with an assistance of ultrasonography [7, 34].

3.3. Karyotyping

Karyotyping particularly spectral karyotyping is used for the detection of chromosomal copy number and gross translocations in chromosomes. In this, a microscopic slide with metaphase chromosomes spread is subjected to hybridization of a chromosome-specific probe set having up to 5 fluorescent dyes, which results in chromosome specific as well as unique combinations. Then the detection is carried out using an interferometer. In addition to this, fragments of chromosomes in spectral karyotyping are identified as individual fragments, which is a limitation of some other diagnostic methods or tools [35].

3.4. Multiplex Ligation Dependent Probe Amplification (MLPA)

Multiplex ligation dependent probe amplification (MLPA) being a reliable and effective diagnostic tool identifies region-specific genetic abnormalities of various disorders. MLPA uses a simple PCR based assay and detects a change in DNA copy number of approximately 45 loci at a time [36]. Probes used in MLPA have two oligonucleotides which hybridize with the sequence of interest, then further amplified in PCR using a specific set of forward and reverse primers and quantified using capillary gel electrophoresis. For prenatal identification of chromosomal aneuploidies in chromosome X, Y, 13, 18, and 21, MLPA with P095 is used. Aneuploidy probe mix is a rapid detection method for the samples obtained from chorionic villi and uncultured amniotic fluid. However, female tri-ploidies, inversions, translocations, and low-grade mosaicism cannot be detected through MLPA [8, 37].

3.5. Restriction Fragment Length Polymorphism (RFLP)

Restriction fragment length polymorphism (RFLP) is also used for the detection of genetic disorders such as monogenic and polygenic disorders by allowing the analysis of different fragments length of DNA to identify the polymorphism which is responsible for various genetic abnormalities such as Down syndrome, *etc.* Due to polymorphism which appears because of the phenomena of deletion or insertion of DNA sequences between 2 cut sites, DNA fragments of various sizes are generated using restriction enzymes. This is why it is known as restriction fragment length polymorphism. RFLP can be used for detection purpose with the help of southern blotting [9, 38].

3.6. Quantitative Fluorescence Polymerase Chain Reaction (QF-PCR)

Quantitative fluorescent PCR (QF-PCR) is used in the prenatal diagnosis of genetic disorders such as chromosomal aneuploidies. The analysis using QF-PCR is cost-effective, less time consuming, and appropriate for automation; and can identify the abnormalities mostly detected by conventional karyotyping. QF-PCR also reduces laboratories' workload by dealing with a large number of test samples at the same time, thus providing results of multiple samples in a very short time. In order to detect aneuploidies in chromosome 13, 18, 21, X, and Y, a study was conducted in which STR markers were used to perform QF-PCR. The primers were labelled with fluorochromes which produced fluorescence and PCR products and results were examined using a software program. The ratios reported between 0.8 to 1.4 were suggested normal and the values below or above this ratio indicated trisomy. On the other hand, it is reported that QF-PCR is unable to detect and identify mosaicism at small level *i.e.* if aneuploidy exists in less than 20% of cells [10, 39].

3.7. Cell Free Fetal DNA Analysis

Cell free fetal DNA (cffDNA) analysis also known as noninvasive prenatal testing, is targeted for pregnancies of women (at high risk). Using this analysis, aneuploidies and chromosomal micro-deletions are detected in embryos. In cffDNA testing, the fragments of cell free fetal DNA are isolated from maternal blood. Thereafter, the proportion of fragments (of DNA) from both the target chromosomes *i.e.*, 13, 18, and 21, and reference chromosomes is compared. The limitation of cffDNA analysis is that the detection rate is associated with the cell free fetal DNA proportion which is further affected by maternal, placental, as well as fetal factors. Moreover, the false positive results in cffDNA analysis are due to maternal aneuploidy, maternal copy number variations, maternal obesity, or maternal malignancies. Furthermore, cffDNA techniques are of various types *i.e.*, massive parallel sequencing in which the cell free DNA is sequenced randomly; chromosome selective sequencing in which preselected fragments of cffDNA are sequenced; and single nucleotide polymorphism-based sequencing in which SNPs are targeted and genotype-based analytic method is used [40, 41].

3.8. Chromosomal Microarray Analysis

Chromosomal microarray analysis (CMA) is a technique used to detect aneuploidies and copy number variants across the whole genomic DNA extracted from prenatal samples. Compared to karyotyping, CMA has high resolution in detecting and identifying deletions or repetitions of sequences down to 100kb. This high-resolution property of CMA increases the chances of detecting variants with variable phenotypes, and late-onset disorders, thereby, allowing parents to decide whether or not to terminate pregnancy [42].

3.9. Chorionic Villus Sampling

This technique is performed during the gestation period of 10 to 13 weeks in order to determine and diagnose chromosomal and genetic disorders of fetus. Due to chorionic villus sampling, the patients are able to decide either to terminate pregnancy or not if results appear abnormal or normal, respectively. Prior to this sampling procedure, ultrasound examination was carried out to identify cervical-uterine angle, gestational age, fetus number, and location of placenta. In this, tissue sample is taken from either cervix, abdomen, transvaginal, or transcervical. In transcervical chorionic sampling, a few chorionic villi are extracted using a catheter which enters the uterus and directed to the placenta from the cervix with the help of ultrasound. Then the obtained villi are determined and detected due to the characteristic branching morphology. Then, further, chromosomal and DNA analysis of cells is performed using other techniques *i.e.*, FISH (fluorescent *in situ* hybridization) [43].

4. FUTURE CHALLENGES IN PREIMPLANTATION, PRENATAL AND POSTNATAL DIAGNOSIS

The future challenge in preimplantation, prenatal and postnatal diagnosis is to overcome the chances of birth of infants with genetic defects by knowing the genetic makeup and altering them accordingly where the particular defect is present. But various ethical issues arise regarding embryo or fetal protection. Some countries *e.g.*, Ireland, Switzerland and Germany do not allow preimplantation genetic diagnosis. In these countries, prenatal diagnosis is allowed but not regulated because it is carried out at the embryonic level and has the potential to cause embryo or fetal disruption, ultimately leading to the termination of pregnancy in mothers. Misdiagnosed cases are also reported due to the technical limitations of these technologies. Furthermore, various treatments like gene therapy, RNA interference, *etc.*, which are preferred or prescribed in the UK and European countries to remove a particular genetic defect after diagnosing a particular disease have very less chances of acceptance by human body [44].

5. FUTURE PROSPECTS

The future of PGD, PND, and postnatal diagnosis lies in creating and introducing new advanced clinical approaches, procedures, and technologies that are appropriate for genetic analysis during and after the development of an embryo. The following goals would also be accomplished using preimplantation, prenatal, and postnatal diagnosis:

- Prevention of abnormalities which are associated with chromosomes.
- Successful treatment of Mendelian mitochondrial associated, and multifactorial diseases.
- Epigenome and epigenomic regulations in the genome of an embryo or infant would be understood quite well [45].

CONCLUDING REMARKS

Every year, a number of genetic cases are reported that are diagnosed by preimplantation, prenatal and postnatal genetic diagnostic techniques. PGD is an effective genetic tool from the patient's perspectives as compared to PND. Biopsies in PGD can be performed at early embryonic stages *i.e.*, cleavage stage, morula stage, or blastocyst stage for the identification of monogenic diseases, polygenic diseases, balanced and imbalanced chromosomal rearrangement. Several techniques such as next generation sequencing, aCGH, FISH, RFLP, cell free fetal DNA, amniocentesis, methylation PCR, QF-PCR, multiplex ligation dependent probe amplification, karyotyping, CMA, and chorionic villus sampling are used for PGD, prenatal, and postnatal evaluation. However, high cost of PGD as well as low rate of pregnancy and birth make it unreliable as compared to prenatal testing. On the other hand, various ethical issues arise regarding embryo or infant protection during the conduction of these procedures, but various goals can also be accomplished such as prevention of genetic abnormalities, possible treatments for diseases, and better understanding of epigenomic regulations in infants. To conclude, PGD, prenatal, and postnatal diagnoses serve as a promising method to identify and detect a genetic defect before or after birth in humans.

CONSENT FOR PUBLICATION

Not Applicable.

CONFLICT OF INTEREST

The author declares no conflict of interest, financial or otherwise.

ACKNOWLEDGEMENTS

Declared none.

REFERENCES

[1]   Griffin DK, Handyside AH, Penketh RJA, Winston RML, Delhanty JDA. Fluorescent in-situ hybridization to interphase nuclei of human preimplantation embryos with X and Y chromosome specific probes. Hum Reprod 1991; 6(1): 101-5.
        [http://dx.doi.org/10.1093/oxfordjournals.humrep.a137241] [PMID: 1874942]

[2]   Johnson LA. Gender preselection in mammals: an overview. Dtsch Tierarztl Wochenschr 1996; 103(8-9): 288-91.
        [PMID: 8840588]

[3]   Nichols J, Gardner RL. Effect of damage to the zona pellucida on development of preimplantation embryos in the mouse. Hum Reprod 1989; 4(2): 180-7.
        [http://dx.doi.org/10.1093/oxfordjournals.humrep.a136868] [PMID: 2918072]

[4]   Handyside AH, Kontogianni EH, Hardy K, Winston RML. Pregnancies from biopsied human preimplantation embryos sexed by Y-specific DNA amplification. Nature 1990; 344(6268): 768-70.

[http://dx.doi.org/10.1038/344768a0] [PMID: 2330030]

[5] Stadler ZK, Gallagher DJ, Thom P, Offit K. Genome-wide association studies of cancer: principles and potential utility. Oncology (Williston Park) 2010; 24(7): 629-37.
[PMID: 20669800]

[6] Verlinsky Y, Cieslak J, Ivakhnenko V, Lifchez A, Strom C, Kuliev A. Preimplantation Genetics Group. Birth of healthy children after preimplantation diagnosis of common aneuploidies by polar body fluorescent *in situ* hybridization analysis. Fertil Steril 1996; 66(1): 126-9.
[http://dx.doi.org/10.1016/S0015-0282(16)58399-X] [PMID: 8752623]

[7] Strom CM, Ginsberg N, Rechitsky S, *et al.* Three births after preimplantation genetic diagnosis for cystic fibrosis with sequential first and second polar body analysis. Am J Obstet Gynecol 1998; 178(6): 1298-306.
[http://dx.doi.org/10.1016/S0002-9378(98)70336-9] [PMID: 9662315]

[8] Harper JC. Preimplantation genetic screening. J Med Screen 2018; 25(1): 1-5.
[http://dx.doi.org/10.1177/0969141317691797] [PMID: 28614992]

[9] Hardy K, Martin KL, Leese HJ, Winston RML, Handyside AH. Human preimplantation development *in vitro* is not adversely affected by biopsy at the 8-cell stage. Hum Reprod 1990; 5(6): 708-14.
[http://dx.doi.org/10.1093/oxfordjournals.humrep.a137173] [PMID: 2254404]

[10] Kokkali G, Traeger-Synodinos J, Vrettou C, Stavrou D, Jones GM, Cram DS. D. S and K. Pantos, Blastocyst biopsy *versus* cleavage stage biopsy and blastocyst transfer for preimplantation genetic diagnosis of β-thalassaemia. Hum Reprod 2007; 22(5): 1443-9.
[http://dx.doi.org/10.1093/humrep/del506] [PMID: 17261575]

[11] Johnson LA, Welch GR, Keyvanfar K, Dorfmann A, Fugger EF, Schulman JD. Preimplantation diagnosis: Gender preselection in humans? Flow cytometric separation of X and Y spermatozoa for the prevention of X-linked diseases. Hum Reprod 1993; 8(10): 1733-9.
[http://dx.doi.org/10.1093/oxfordjournals.humrep.a137925] [PMID: 8300839]

[12] Carlson LM, Vora NL. Prenatal Diagnosis. Obstet Gynecol Clin North Am 2017; 44(2): 245-56.
[http://dx.doi.org/10.1016/j.ogc.2017.02.004] [PMID: 28499534]

[13] Nussbaum RL, McInnes RR, Thompson JS, Willard HF, Thompson MW, Boerkoel CF. Thompson & Thompson genetics in medicine e-book. > Elsevier Health Sciences 2015.

[14] Becker AM. Postnatal evaluation of infants with an abnormal antenatal renal sonogram. Curr Opin Pediatr 2009; 21(2): 207-13.
[http://dx.doi.org/10.1097/MOP.0b013e32832772a8] [PMID: 19663038]

[15] Nussbaum RL, McInnes RR, Thompson JS, Willard HF, Thompson MW, Boerkoel CF. Thompson & Thompson genetics in medicine e-book. Elsevier Health Sciences 2015.

[16] Alliance G. New York-Mid-Atlantic Consortium for Genetic and Newborn Screening Services. Understanding genetics: a New York, mid-Atlantic guide for patients and health professionals 2009.

[17] Consortium IHGS. International Human Genome Sequencing Consortium. Finishing the euchromatic sequence of the human genome. Nature 2004; 431(7011): 931-45.
[http://dx.doi.org/10.1038/nature03001] [PMID: 15496913]

[18] Fagiuoli S, Daina E, D'Antiga L, Colledan M, Remuzzi G. Monogenic diseases that can be cured by liver transplantation. J Hepatol 2013; 59(3): 595-612.
[http://dx.doi.org/10.1016/j.jhep.2013.04.004] [PMID: 23578885]

[19] Kakourou G, Dhanjal S, Daphnis D, *et al.* Preimplantation genetic diagnosis for myotonic dystrophy type 1: detection of crossover between the gene and the linked marker APOC2. Prenat Diagn 2007; 27(2): 111-6.
[http://dx.doi.org/10.1002/pd.1611] [PMID: 17192963]

[20] Lvovs D, Favorova OO, Favorov AV. A polygenic approach to the study of polygenic diseases. Acta

Nat (Engl Ed) 2012; 4(3): 59-71.
[http://dx.doi.org/10.32607/20758251-2012-4-3-59-71] [PMID: 23150804]

[21]   McCarroll SA, Hyman SE. Progress in the genetics of polygenic brain disorders: significant new challenges for neurobiology. Neuron 2013; 80(3): 578-87.
[http://dx.doi.org/10.1016/j.neuron.2013.10.046] [PMID: 24183011]

[22]   Christodoulou C, Dheedene A, Heindryckx B, *et al.* Preimplantation genetic diagnosis for chromosomal rearrangements with the use of array comparative genomic hybridization at the blastocyst stage. > Fertil Steril 2017; 107(1): 212-9.
[http://dx.doi.org/10.1016/j.fertnstert.2016.09.045]

[24]   Dahdouh EM, Balayla J, Audibert F, *et al.* Genetics Committee. RETIRED: Technical Update: Preimplantation Genetic Diagnosis and Screening. J Obstet Gynaecol Can 2015; 37(5): 451-63.
[http://dx.doi.org/10.1016/S1701-2163(15)30261-9] [PMID: 26168107]

[24]   Pinkel D, Gray JW, Trask B, van den Engh G, Fuscoe J, van Dekken H. Cytogenetic analysis by *in situ* hybridization with fluorescently labeled nucleic acid probes. Cold Spring Harb Symp Quant Biol 1986; 51(0): 151-7.
[http://dx.doi.org/10.1101/SQB.1986.051.01.018] [PMID: 3472711]

[25]   Shaffer LG, Bejjani BA. Development of new postnatal diagnostic methods for chromosome disorders. Semin Fetal Neonatal Med 2011; 16(2): 114-8.
[http://dx.doi.org/10.1016/j.siny.2010.11.001] [PMID: 21112262]

[26]   Bahçe M, Escudero T, Sandalinas M, Morrison L, Legator M, Munné S. Improvements of preimplantation diagnosis of aneuploidy by using microwave hybridization, cell recycling and monocolour labelling of probes. Mol Hum Reprod 2000; 6(9): 849-54.
[http://dx.doi.org/10.1093/molehr/6.9.849] [PMID: 10956558]

[27]   Treff NR, Fedick A, Tao X, Devkota B, Scott R T. Evaluation of targeted next-generation sequencing–based preimplantation genetic diagnosis of monogenic disease. Fertility and sterility. 2013; 99: pp. 1377-84. 2013; 99: pp.

[28]   Wells D. Next-generation sequencing: the dawn of a new era for preimplantation genetic diagnostics. Fertil Steril 2014; 101(5): 1250-1.
[http://dx.doi.org/10.1016/j.fertnstert.2014.03.006] [PMID: 24786744]

[29]   Zhang W, Liu Y, Wang L, *et al.* Clinical application of next-generation sequencing in preimplantation genetic diagnosis cycles for Robertsonian and reciprocal translocations. J Assist Reprod Genet 2016; 33(7): 899-906.
[http://dx.doi.org/10.1007/s10815-016-0724-2] [PMID: 27167073]

[30]   Friedenthal J, Maxwell SM, Munné S, *et al.* Next generation sequencing for preimplantation genetic screening improves pregnancy outcomes compared with array comparative genomic hybridization in single thawed euploid embryo transfer cycles. Fertil Steril 2018; 109(4): 627-32.
[http://dx.doi.org/10.1016/j.fertnstert.2017.12.017] [PMID: 29605407]

[31]   Muys J, Blaumeiser B, Janssens K, Loobuyck P, Jacquemyn Y. Chromosomal microarray analysis in prenatal diagnosis: ethical considerations of the Belgian approach. J Med Ethics 2020; 46(2): 104-9.
[http://dx.doi.org/10.1136/medethics-2018-105186] [PMID: 31527144]

[32]   Derks S, Lentjes MH, Hellebrekers DM, de Bruïne AP, Herman JG, van Engeland M. Methylation-specific PCR unraveled. Cell Oncol 2004; 26(5-6): 291-9.
[PMID: 15623939]

[33]   Zhan YX, Luo GH. DNA methylation detection methods used in colorectal cancer. World J Clin Cases 2019; 7(19): 2916-29.
[http://dx.doi.org/10.12998/wjcc.v7.i19.2916] [PMID: 31624740]

[34]   Galst JP, Verp MS. Prenatal and preimplantation diagnosis: the burden of choice. Springer. 2015.
[http://dx.doi.org/10.1007/978-3-319-18911-6]

[35]   Bakker B, van den Bos H, Lansdorp PM, Foijer F. How to count chromosomes in a cell: An overview of current and novel technologies. BioEssays 2015; 37(5): 570-7.
[http://dx.doi.org/10.1002/bies.201400218] [PMID: 25739518]

[36]   Jeuken J, Cornelissen S, Boots-Sprenger S, Gijsen S, Wesseling P. Multiplex ligation-dependent probe amplification: a diagnostic tool for simultaneous identification of different genetic markers in glial tumors. J Mol Diagn 2006; 8(4): 433-43.
[http://dx.doi.org/10.2353/jmoldx.2006.060012] [PMID: 16931583]

[37]   Schouten J, van Vught P, Galjaard RJ. Multiplex Ligation-Dependent Probe Amplification (MLPA) for Prenatal Diagnosis of Common Aneuploidies. Methods Mol Biol 2019; 1885: 161-70.
[http://dx.doi.org/10.1007/978-1-4939-8889-1_11] [PMID: 30506197]

[38]   Hames BD. Instant Notes in Biochemistry. Bios Scientific Pub.

[39]   Badenas C, Rodríguez-Revenga L, Morales C, *et al.* Assessment of QF-PCR as the first approach in prenatal diagnosis. J Mol Diagn 2010; 12(6): 828-34.
[http://dx.doi.org/10.2353/jmoldx.2010.090224] [PMID: 20889556]

[40]   Chen EZ, Chiu RWK, Sun H, *et al.* Noninvasive prenatal diagnosis of fetal trisomy 18 and trisomy 13 by maternal plasma DNA sequencing. PLoS One 2011; 6(7): e21791.
[http://dx.doi.org/10.1371/journal.pone.0021791] [PMID: 21755002]

[41]   Laberge A-M, Karalis A, Chakraborty P, Samuels ME. New Technologies in Pre-and Postnatal Diagnosis > In Maternal-Fetal and Neonatal Endocrinology. Springer 2020; pp. 941-69.
[http://dx.doi.org/10.1016/B978-0-12-814823-5.00053-2]

[42]   Muys J, Blaumeiser B, Janssens K, Loobuyck P, Jacquemyn Y. Chromosomal microarray analysis in prenatal diagnosis: ethical considerations of the Belgian approach. J Med Ethics 2020; 46(2): 104-9.
[http://dx.doi.org/10.1136/medethics-2018-105186] [PMID: 31527144]

[43]   Galst JP, Verp MS. . Prenatal and preimplantation diagnosis: the burden of choice. Springer 2015.
[http://dx.doi.org/10.1007/978-3-319-18911-6]

[44]   Corveleyn A, Zika E, Morris M, *et al.* Preimplantation Genetic Diagnosis in Europe. European Communities 2007; 114: 57-75.
[PMID: 18091772]

[45]   Pergament D, Ilijic K. The legal past, present and future of prenatal genetic testing: professional liability and other legal challenges affecting patient access to services. J Clin Med 2014; 3(4): 1437-65.
[http://dx.doi.org/10.3390/jcm3041437] [PMID: 26237611]

CHAPTER 4

Genetic Counseling in Inherited Disorders

Shumaila Zulfiqar[1,2]**, Muhammad Tariq**[1,*]**, Naveed Altaf Malik**[1]**, Ayaz Khan**[1]**, Shafaq Ramzan**[1]**, Maria Iqbal**[1,3]**, Iram Anjum**[2] **and Shahid Mahmood Baig**[1]

[1] *National Institute for Biotechnology and Genetic Engineering College, Pakistan Institute of Engineering and Applied Sciences (NIBGE-C, PIEAS), Faisalabad, Pakistan*

[2] *Department of Biotechnology, Kinnaird College for Women, Lahore*

[3] *Centogene GmbH, Rostock, Germany*

Abstract: In this chapter, we have focused on the journey of sorting genes and the connotation of genetic counseling started. In a literal sense, we will understand how genetic counseling could contribute to identifying pathogenicity and penetrance of genetic mutation/s in high-risk individual/s or populations. Great strides have been achieved in terms of diagnosis, management, and treatment of various genetic disorders due to rapid advancements in genetic research. The national Thalassemia Prevention Program of Cyprus has been one of the earliest and most celebrated successes in lowering the disease burden and improving life quality and survival rate in patients. The knowledge regarding gene/s and variant/s is quite instrumental for making important reproductive decisions and therapeutic interventions for both rare and common disorders. We also touch upon the associated ethical issues and challenges.

Keywords: Carrier screening, Eugenics, Genetic counseling, Genetic disorders, Genetic testing, Population screening.

1. INTRODUCTION

In 1902, Archibald E Garrod published a study in the journal *The Lancet,* suggesting an autosomal recessive mode of inheritance in a genetic disorder called alkaptonuria. This study enabled researchers to develop an association between genetic disorders and the laws of inheritance published by Gregor Mendel in 1865. From that point forward, our insight into genetic disorders has increased exponentially. Nonetheless, it does not mean that the history of genetic disorders began with the rediscovery of Mendel's laws toward

* **Corresponding author Muhammad Tariq**: National Institute for Biotechnology and Genetic Engineering (NIBGE-C), Faisalabad, Pakistan Institute of Engineering and Applied Sciences (PIEAS), Islamabad, Pakistan; E-mail: tariqpalai@gmail.com

Syeda Marriam Bakhtiar and Erum Dilshad (Eds.)

the start of the twentieth century. Earlier paintings, drawings and sculptures show evidence of patients with different conditions like achondroplasia, Robert's condition, hermaphroditism and neurofibromatosis. The famous X-linked blood disorder in Queen Victoria 's family had been known for a long time in the Middle Ages, referred to as "passio transition sanguinis" in the Talmud. Later in the nineteenth century, J L Schónlein named it "haemorrhophilia"; a term later transformed into the current "hemophilia". In 1866, British doctor, J Langdon Down, characterized mental retardation on the basis of different racial types; Caucasian, Ethiopian, Malaysian and Mongolian. The first three classes were not much persuading, therefore, their use was stopped gradually. However, Down's mongoloid idiot-ism, these days known as Down's syndrome, ended up being a well-characterized disorder. After 93 years of Down's paper publication, Lejeune found the reason for Down's condition: a little additional chromosome (chromosome 21) [1 - 5]. The scenario before the advent of modern medical science was completely different from today when complex cytogenetic analyses, proper diagnosis and management methods were unavailable. The only available option was to depict and analyze disease occurrence or reoccurrence verbally and communicate them to patients. Later, this method was referred to as genetic counseling.

The practice of advising people regarding genetic conditions started around the twentieth century, soon after William Bateson proposed that the new clinical and medical investigations of heredity be designated as "genetics". Heredity got interlaced with social changes and structured as a field of 'eugenics. Although eugenics was conceived with the intention to prevent inherited disorders, later development had deplorable results. Numerous states in the USA had laws ordering sterilization of the affected individuals, others were not permitted to move. By the 1930s, these policies were acknowledged by various different nations including Germany where the killing of the "genetically defective" persons was sanctioned in 1939 [6]. In 1992, a law was approved in Australia suggesting that parents of an affected child cannot have sterilization or hysterectomy by themselves to avoid defective child birth. Permission would be required from the court to do so. However, even after 10 years of this legislation, illegal sterilization of minors was noticed [7]. Edwin Black has termed the eugenic policies as "eugenics wars" and suggested a negative impact on people's life due to isolation, discrimination, genocide and violation of basic human rights. However, supporters of eugenics like Comfort proposed that it drives towards elimination of disease and a healthier society [8].

The term "genetic counseling" was formally coined in the post eugenic era by Sheldon Reed in his popular book *Counseling in Medical Genetics* published in 1955 [9, 10]. According to the World Health Organization, the first-ever genetic counseling service began at Heredity Clinic in the University of Michigan, USA in 1940. It is rather impossible to exactly speculate how the participating individuals would have acted regarding outcome of counseling (eugenic or dysgenic). Later, multiple genetic counseling centers were opened across the globe. (https://www.who.int/genomics/professionals/counselling). In 1963, phenylketonuria became the first ever genetic disorder for which a newborn screening was performed [11]. From then onwards, the idea prevailed that genetic counseling was used far earlier as genetic testing. The American Society of Human Genetics (ASHG) defines genetic counseling as a process of facilitating individuals to combat medical, psychological and familial implications of genetic disorders [12]. General objectives of genetic counseling, agreed upon by all professionals, are; 1. prevention of birth defects and genetic disorders, 2. promoting adaptation to a genetic condition without compromising on psychological well-being of counselees 3. counselees should make their own reproductive choices, however, decisions that reduce the impact of certain genetic condition/s should be encouraged [13].

With the collaboration between clinicians and geneticists, there has been an increase observed in genetic counseling . Human Genome Project opened new horizons to identify individuals carrying mutant allele/s responsible for inherited disorders before disease appearance. These advancements have broadened the prospects to delineate inherited disorders by analyzing human chromosomal abnormalities, providing facilities to analyze certain disorders in the first trimester of pregnancy (prenatal) and the initiation of screening programs for certain diseases in high-risk populations [14]. Various diagnostic centers provide services like karyotyping, dermatoglyphic analysis, syndrome recognition and biochemical tests related to the inborn errors of metabolism. Carrier screening and genetic counseling are offered to individuals with a positive family history of a certain genetic condition. Couples at risk of having affected children with genetic disorder(s) can be provided with reproductive options to avoid affected births. In this way, genetic counseling makes significant contributions to disease prevention as well as management.

As the initial step, the regular counseling process comprised a single interview where pedigree is prepared and a prediction/estimation of recurrence risk is provided to counselees. Later, as the psychological difficulties associated with counseling emerged, the research circle was expended to various other aspects including procedures, reasoning, psychodynamics and morals of advising. In some countries, the meeting and counseling are done by the same individual; in others, the counseling approach is a multiple tier process requiring interviews and multidisciplinary process. Mostly, the counselor lacks formal training in the methods/techniques of counseling, even if such trainings would be a benefit, but lack of training can lead to further complications [15]. Having the same counselor to take family history and do the counseling has the advantage that the first meeting offers the counselor some chance to become more acquainted with the counselees and set up some level of compatibility before entering the advanced stage of counseling. Complete components of the process have been summarized in Fig. (**4.1**) (adapted from Moharem-Elgamal *et al.* 2020) [16]. Genetic counselors only provide counseling and it is implied in the definition that counseling does not contain the diagnosis or clinical management of the patient's clinical condition [17]. For instance, amniocentesis is an obstetrical method, the biochemical or cytogenetic tests performed on the subsequent sample are diagnostic, the advice given to the parents is genetic counseling, and the termination of the pregnancy (if occurs) is management.

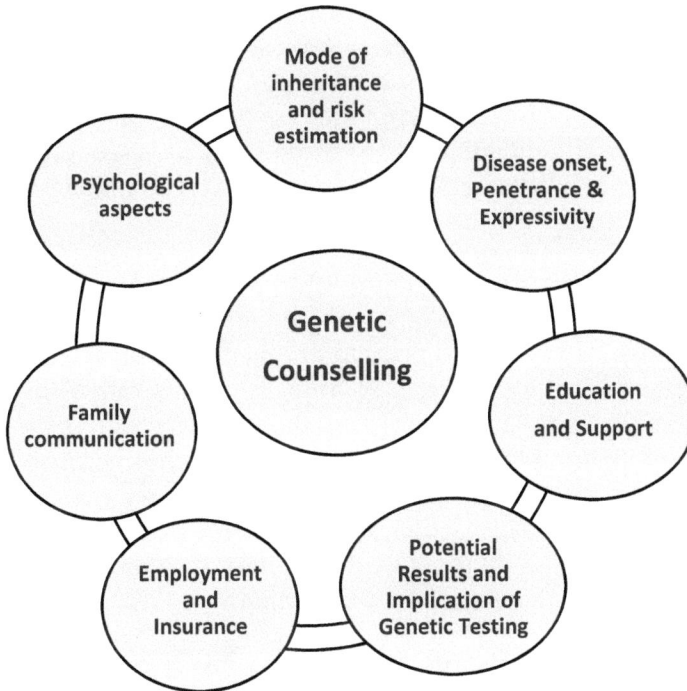

Fig. (4.1). Main components of Genetic Counseling.

2. POPULATION CARRIER SCREENING MECHANISM

The most common form of genetic disorders is recessively inherited disorders; a person is called a carrier if s/he carries a mutant copy of a gene. Carriers are asymptomatic and until they are genetically screened for a particular condition, or they have an affected child, they remain unaware of the fact that they possess a mutant gene. For disease manifestation in such, two copies of mutant alleles are required. But, when two carriers marry each other, the chances of having an affected child increase which enhances the requirements of carrier screening for such diseases to prevent further affected births and lowers disease burden in a family and, for that matter, in a population.

The first step in carrier screening is to take informed written consent. Professionals should brief the participants about the potential outcome (risks and benefits) of screening. The participants should be asked for their consent to participate in the screening program, and the results may be documented without revealing their identity. For diseased individuals, written informed consent should be obtained from legal guardian or from the participant (if mentally fit) [18]. The next step is to proceed for identification of mutation in the affected individual(s). Once a mutation is identified, other relatives will be screened for the same mutation. The main objective of carrier screening is to Fig out individuals who do not have any particular disease phenotype but possibly have one variant allele within a gene linked with the disorder [9]. If both partners are found heterozygous carriers of a genetic condition, counseling should be recommended depending on disease condition.

Every pregnant woman needs to be provided with complete information about procedure and possible outcomes of carrier screening. Ideally, carrier screening and counseling must be performed prior to pregnancy because this allows couples to make their reproductive decisions in time. It is imperative to get the family history of the patient, similarly, pedigrees should be prepared by taking family history indicating detailed information of ethnic background of relatives, rate of consanguinity, and the number of miscarriages and stillbirths (if any). Information, such as names, married females in the family should be noted in pedigree. Pedigree helps to infer a specific pattern of inheritance and makes risk estimate possible even if the diagnosis is uncertain.

The National Institute for Health and Clinical Excellence (NICE) guidelines suggest that high prevalence populaces could be screened for the most prevalent disorders. Screening refers to a process of detecting asymptomatic individuals from a population with the higher risk of disease or before the appearance of disease symptoms. This procedure is called population screening. The main types of population screening for genetic disorders are newborn screening and carrier screening. Studies suggest that the overall cost of prevention of a single genetic disorder, through screening, is far less than its treatment expenses [19]. Interestingly, there is no data available indicating how many genetic disorders have been prevented and how much money has been saved. But it could be estimated that the therapeutic cost of severely ill patients is quite high which could be reduced through genetic screening followed by genetic counseling [20].

2.1. Thalassemia a Case Study

In Cyprus, thalassemia was once a major health issue; one in every 230 children under 10 years old was having thalassemia. With 15% of the population carrying beta-thalassemia mutations and 10% alpha-thalassemia mutations, Cyprus had the highest frequencies of thalassemia disease alleles in the world [21]. To combat this disease, premarital screening was made compulsory and prenatal diagnosis was started in 1980s. In 1991, a10 years national Thalassemia Prevention Program was launched for population screening and counseling. The result was a rapid decrease in the number of affected births, from 18-20 to 6-7 per year. Between 1991 and 2001, only five children were born with thalassemia and in the next five years, no affected birth was reported. This was a huge success. In addition, with early screening and diagnosis, patients started effective iron chelation which resulted in improved life quality and survival rate [22]. Our own group at the National Institute for Biotechnology and Genetic Engineering (NIBGE) Faisalabad, Pakistan launched a pilot program on prenatal diagnosis of beta thalassemia in the southern parts of the Punjab province in Pakistan which has been successful in lowering the birth rate of affected children in at-risk families. However, for a country with approximately 9 million carriers, this is high time to launch a nationwide program for screening and prenatal diagnosis of beta thalassemia and other prevalent disorders [23].

It should be noted, however, that genetic screening and genetic testing are two different terms; with different aims and objectives. Affected individuals go through genetic testing to seek professional advice (also referred to as diagnostic testing). However, asymptomatic individuals may opt genetic screening to identify any mutations and potential disease risk. In certain cases, the individuals are already familiar with a specific diagnosis due to multiple affected individuals in their families. This type of testing, in such individuals, is called pre-symptomatic or predictive testing. Genetic counseling may bring about complete conclusions, improve understanding for the family and permit at-risk family members to have the alternatives like predictive testing. The key steps in predictive and symptomatic testing have been given in Fig. (**4.2**).

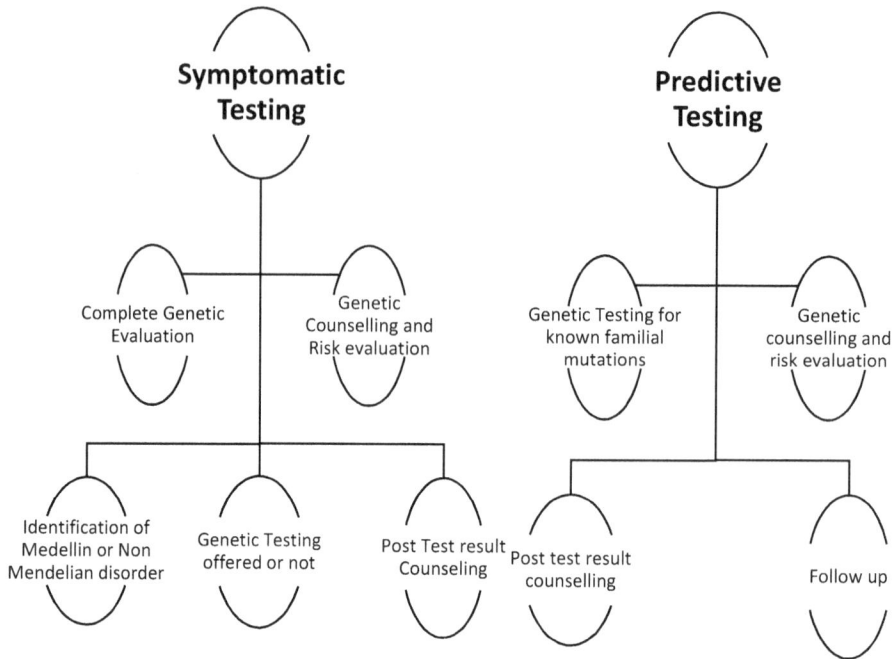

Fig. (4.2). Flow chart showing steps in Predictive and Symptomatic testing.

Detailed information regarding further tests and treatment is provided by screening providers to minimize associated risks or complications related to a disorder. The main objective of population screening is to correctly identify individuals from a group who have higher chances of disease manifestation. Once individuals at high risk for a disease are identified (screened), confirmatory (diagnostic) tests are then performed to detect disease with greater certainty. Yet, for population screening to be fruitful, a disease is required to meet various conditions. For instance:

a. In a population, a disease occurrence is higher and significant number of individuals carry the disease.
b. If the individuals carrying diseased genes are not identified, it could negatively affect individual's health.
c. The disorder must be treated or prevented though not necessarily cured.
d. Testing should be least invasive, effortlessly carried out and cost effective; and the testing technique must have been studied and scientifically verified to be correct, reliable and confirmed by follow-up testing.

3. RISK ESTIMATION

For estimation of disease risk, already published data regarding the concerned disease can be utilized. If the counselor has detailed information about a disease which is well characterized, many other questions irrespective of recurrence may arise. If the disease is well known to the counselor, s/he must have relevant data in hand. Counselees may ask questions like, *how long will a child with Down syndrome live?* And *what percentage of children with neurofibromatosis are mentally retarded?* Answering such questions require extensive research on clinical risks linked to such conditions. But if the counselor lacks information about the disease, which is quite rare, s/he may classify the disease in question as Mendelian or Non-Mendelian, by applying appropriate Mendelian laws to the particular family condition, can estimate the probability of recurrence. Risk estimation can be made by applying Bayesian algebra on data collected, for instance, the number of affected and unaffected individuals, age of disease onset in family members, *etc.* Empirical risk estimation from the literature should be considered in case of chromosomal and multifactorial disorders of unknown etiology [24, 25].

Although screening can decrease the risk of developing a genetic condition but it cannot offer a guarantee of protection. Screening tests will have both false positives and false negatives results These outcomes are mentioned in certain statistical predictive values. Positive and negative predictive values (PPV and NPV, respectively) show the extent of positive and negative results. Screening test results are followed by diagnostic test to determine whether an individual has the disorder and thus identify false positives (if present) [26]. Commonly, there is an irreducible minimum of false positive results (wrongly reported as having the condition) and false negative results (wrongly reported as not having the condition) [27].

Now let's imagine if the test result of a patient is positive what is the probability that the patient will develop a disease, or if test result comes out negative what are the chances that a patient does not have it. The ratio of sensitivity and specificity of results depict how well the proposed screening test performs against a decided 'Gold Standard' test. A gold standard level test is a diagnostic test or benchmark observed as conclusive. The gold test might be excessively upsetting for the patient, excessively illogical or too costly to be in any way utilized broadly as a screening test [26]. Despite limitations, population screening can be beneficial for improving general health.

4. CLINICAL PRACTICES

Genetic counselors are professionals having expert training, expertise in genetics along with counseling skills. All medical care specialists are likely to engage with genomic medication which is an integral part of genetic counseling. Experts will progressively be approached to impart and deal with the outcomes from genomic testing. It is plausible that as genomic medication becomes standard, certain jobs that are, as of now, considered as basic genetic counseling practice, may turn out to be essential for other clinicians' jobs. There exist equal chances that genetic counseling becomes an additional job responsibility of every clinician [28]. A referral from a clinical geneticist or other specialist is required for genetic counseling. However, in some cases, it might not be possible to confirm a certain diagnosis and, therefore, the patient is given information about possible differential diagnoses and any potential risk estimates. Generally, genetic counseling is recommended for inherited (germline) mutations, not for somatic changes.

Before a specialist sees a patient, s/he should have done complete research work based on information provided [29]. An updated literature search can be conducted to get detailed information about the disease. The following online websites can help in retrieving information about various genetic conditions.

1. MedGen (www.ncbi.nlm.nih.gov/medgen)

2. GeneReviews® (www.ncbi.nlm.nih.gov/books/NBK1116/)

3. Online Mendelian Inheritance in Man (OMIM; www.ncbi.nlm.nih.gov/omim).

There are different types of screening tests. For instance, different molecular tests are utilized to analyze DNA mutations; biochemical tests are used to measure enzyme activity. For some disorders, only a blood test is sufficient for screening whereas other require much advanced techniques. Gene chips are available which can find variations in multiple genes in a single experiment of gene panel sequencing. Gene products could be analyzed for diagnosis of a genetic disorder. For example, in case of heterozygous individuals, there is a 50% reduction in normal gene product [30].

Approximately, 7000 different genetic diseases have been identified so far. Most of these are untreatable and the only choice with the parents and professionals is prevention of affected births, and disease management (syndromic) in already affected individuals. Currently, more than 100 genetic disorders can be genetically screened; however, the most screened genetic disorders are cystic fibrosis, sickle cell disease, thalassemia, Down's syndrome, Huntington's disease, Alzheimer's disease and Tay-Sachs disease [31].

Next Generation Sequencing has been very useful in cases where conventional tests fail to provide any diagnosis to patients [32]. NGS-based tests have effectively identified gene defects underlying deafness, retina degeneration, mitochondriopathies and other genetically heterogeneous disorders [33]. Individuals who are heterozygous carriers for more than one recessive gene variants can easily be identified. Therefore, genetic counselors should have sufficient knowledge of genome sequencing technologies for the interpretation of potentially causative gene variants [34].

5. ETHICAL ISSUES

Genetic counseling brings together traditional medicine with the 'new genetics' in order to deal with genetic disorder/s in terms of prevention and management. Therefore, a range of perplexing ethical issues are expected to emerge in this practice. The main agenda is to keep confidentiality, veracity and truth-telling intact with counselees [35]. In carrier screening, the results of sex-linked disorders and having a status and burden of being a carrier might be traumatic for different reasons: that the 'carriers' are also considered affected to some extent and the condition could pass to their children exclusively by them.

Genetic health professionals usually face difficult scenarios in dealing with carriers/ patients and persuading them to reveal information relevant to their relatives. Specialists cannot force a counselee to reveal their information to others against their willingness [36]. But a difficult scenario arises for the counselor if the counselee makes entirely opposite and negative decision to what has been suggested to them. For instance, consider an affected man and a woman homozygous for a recessive disorder (*e.g.*, sickle-cell anemia) are directed that all their children will be affected likewise. However, knowing the genetic consequence, they still plan children. This type of decision is called dysgenic and it results in increased number of deleterious alleles in the next generation [37]. Mostly information regarding the diseases is provided in a non-directive way to counselees, so that they may be able to take decision themselves solely on the basis of factual findings and not in the influence of counselor [34].

Ethical issues involved in screening are significantly different from those involved in clinical practice, mainly revolving around healthy individuals by facilitating them to make better choices about their health. Nevertheless, it is important that individuals should have realistic assumptions for what a screening project can convey. Although, early screening can possibly save lives or improve quality of life, it is not an entirely fool-proof procedure and involves false positive and false negative results, as discussed earlier.

Also, predictive testing in children should be deferred since they cannot grasp the potential advantages, limitations and ramifications of testing and to see what this would mean for their future. Parents should be discouraged from making decisions until the child is at least a teenage or adult who can discuss and contribute in decision making. However, genetic testing should not be carried out unless the child shows a clear phenotype. But, if an older child or teenager is concerned, or if the test outcomes would largely impact his/her life choices, genetic testing may be considered [38].

In addition to this, consanguinity is an important common practice in some populations. Families might conceal their disease carrier status due to the fear of stigmatization and the associated troubles in arranging marriage for their carrier children [39]. Other complications include patients identified with variant of uncertain significance (VUS).VUS are genetic variants identified through genetic testing whose significance to the function or health of an individual is not yet known [40]. Some counselors find it quite difficult to convey to patients that their identified genetic disorder is untreatable [41]. Also, it is quite difficult to reveal genetic information by an at-risk adult to their partner before marriage [42]. Additionally, genetic counseling in asymptomatic people may trigger an untoward psychological reaction, like extreme depression, uneasiness, or even self-destructive ideation [43]. Individuals vary in terms of disease coping strategies; some people cope by seeking information whereas, others get stressed and frightened by possible unwanted outcomes of genetic testing. Thus, when genetic screening is performed, interpretation of given "risk Fig" burden and benefit is dependent over personality characteristic of individual either optimistic or pessimist.

6. FUTURE PROSPECTS

The optimization of modern techniques to elucidate genetic basis of various rare and common disorders and to maximize clinical advantages would be a challenge for future researchers. Researchers from all domains, including academia and industry, must work to interconnect and share their research findings. This will ultimately help in getting better understanding of disease mechanisms and biochemical pathways. The establishment of International Common Disease Alliance (https://www.icda.bio), in this regard, is a step in the right direction. This project is expected to facilitate the establishment of genotype–phenotype relationship across populations. Initiatives, such as this one, for improving biological insights will lead to novel preventative and therapeutic choices. A new panel-based approach called Expanded Carrier Screening (ECS) is capable of analyzing carrier status of hundreds of genetic disorders regardless of patient's race or ethnicity [11]. The main objective of both clinical genetics and genetic counseling is to extend analysis and prediction of rare, often untreatable genetic conditions, to the prediction of common, often treatable or preventable conditions. However, sequencing the entire genome generates a huge amount of data and its interpretation requires expertise. Therefore, a lot more genetic counselors will be required who are qualified to analyze genomic sequences and interpret their outcome in terms of genetic risks, and to offer suitable advice.

CONCLUDING REMARKS

The major objective of genetic counseling is to add value to the care of patients with genetic conditions and their families and to facilitate counselees in taking complex and sometimes, life changing decisions. Hence, genetic counselors should be equipped with sufficient knowledge and techniques to maximize the outcomes of genetic counseling. To date, however, many genetic disorders are not treatable and, therefore, prevention is the only practical, and economic, solution. There is a need to establish publicly accessible platforms where genetic counselors across the globe can learn from each other by sharing experiences, building on what works in other countries and adapting it to unique circumstances in one's own home country in order to improve care for patients and their families. Together, we can be solution-driven in strategically increasing professional recognition—both within and across nations.

CONSENT FOR PUBLICATION

Not Applicable.

CONFLICT OF INTEREST

The author declares no conflict of interest, financial or otherwise.

ACKNOWLEDGEMENTS

Declared none.

REFERENCES

[1]   Urban M. Early observations of genetic diseases. Lancet 1999; 354 (Suppl.): SIV21.
[http://dx.doi.org/10.1016/S0140-6736(99)90364-1] [PMID: 10691432]

[2]   Al-Essa M, Al-Shamsan L, Rashed MS, Ozand PT. Alkaptonuria: Case report and review of the literature. Ann Saudi Med 1998; 18(5): 442-4.
[http://dx.doi.org/10.5144/0256-4947.1998.442] [PMID: 17344725]

[3]   Ward OC. Further early historical evidence of Down syndrome. Am J Med Genet 2004; 126A(2): 220-0.
[http://dx.doi.org/10.1002/ajmg.a.20452] [PMID: 15057991]

[4]   Levitas AS, Reid CS. An angel with Down syndrome in a sixteenth century Flemish Nativity painting. Am J Med Genet 2003; 116A(4): 399-405.
[http://dx.doi.org/10.1002/ajmg.a.10043] [PMID: 12522800]

[5]   Down JLH. Observations on an ethnic classification of idiots London hospital reports 1866; 3: pp. 259-62.

[6]   McCarthy P, *et al.* Facilitating the genetic counselling process. London, New York: Springer 2003.

[7]   Gardner RM, *et al.* Chromosome abnormalities and genetic counseling. OUP USA 2011.
[http://dx.doi.org/10.1093/med/9780195375336.001.0001]

[8]   Comfort N. The science of human perfection: how genes became the heart of American medicine. Yale University Press 2012.
[http://dx.doi.org/10.12987/yale/9780300169911.001.0001]

[9]   Possehl C. Sheldon Clark Reed (1910-2003). Embryo Project Encyclopedia 2017.

[10]   Reed SC. A short history of genetic counseling. Soc Biol 1974; 21(4): 332-9.
[http://dx.doi.org/10.1080/19485565.1974.9988131] [PMID: 4619717]

[11]   Rose NC, Wick M. Carrier screening for single gene disorders. in Seminars in Fetal and Neonatal Medicine 2018; pp. 78-84.
[http://dx.doi.org/10.1016/j.siny.2017.06.001]

[12]   Fraser FC. Genetic counseling. Am J Hum Genet 1974; 26(5): 636-59.
[PMID: 4609197]

[13]   Biesecker BB. Goals of genetic counseling. Clin Genet 2001; 60(5): 323-30.
[http://dx.doi.org/10.1034/j.1399-0004.2001.600501.x] [PMID: 11903329]

[14]   Clarke A. Response to: What counts as success in genetic counselling? J Med Ethics 1993; 19(1): 47-9.
[http://dx.doi.org/10.1136/jme.19.1.47] [PMID: 11643100]

[15]   Matloff ET. Practice variability in prenatal genetic counseling. J Genet Couns 1994; 3(3): 215-31.
[http://dx.doi.org/10.1007/BF01412228] [PMID: 24234008]

[16]   Moharem-Elgamal S, Sammut E, Stuart G. Genetic Counseling in Inherited Cardiomyopathies. JACC Case Rep 2020; 2(3): 392-5.
[http://dx.doi.org/10.1016/j.jaccas.2020.02.007] [PMID: 34317249]

[17]   Hsia Y. Genetic Counseling: Facts, Values and Norms, *NY: Alan R. Liss, Inc., for the National Foundation—March of Dimes.* BD: OAS 1979; XV(2): 169-86.

[18]   Charrow R. Protection of human subjects: is expansive regulation counter-productive. Nw UL Rev 2007; 101: 707.

[19]   Beauchamp KA, Johansen Taber KA, Muzzey D. Clinical impact and cost-effectiveness of a 176-condition expanded carrier screen. Genet Med 2019; 21(9): 1948-57.
[http://dx.doi.org/10.1038/s41436-019-0455-8] [PMID: 30760891]

[20]   Fraser FC. Genetic counseling. Am J Hum Genet 1974; 26(5): 636-59.
[PMID: 4609197]

[21]   Ashiotis T, Zachariadis Z, Sofroniadou K, Loukopoulos D, Stamatoyannopoulos G. Thalassaemia in Cyprus. BMJ 1973; 2(5857): 38-42.
[http://dx.doi.org/10.1136/bmj.2.5857.38] [PMID: 4695698]

[22]   Bozkurt G. Results from the north cyprus thalassemia prevention program. Hemoglobin 2007; 31(2): 257-64.
[http://dx.doi.org/10.1080/03630260701297204] [PMID: 17486509]

[23]   Baig SM, Din MA, Hassan H, *et al.* Prevention of β-thalassemia in a large Pakistani family through

cascade testing. Community Genet 2008; 11(1): 68-70.
[PMID: 18196920]

[24]   Allen AB, Leary MR. Self-Compassion, stress, and coping. Soc Personal Psychol Compass 2010; 4(2): 107-18.
[http://dx.doi.org/10.1111/j.1751-9004.2009.00246.x] [PMID: 20686629]

[25]   Austin JC, Smith GN, Honer WG. The genomic era and perceptions of psychotic disorders: Genetic risk estimation, associations with reproductive decisions and views about predictive testing. Am J Med Genet B Neuropsychiatr Genet 2006; 141B(8): 926-8.
[http://dx.doi.org/10.1002/ajmg.b.30372] [PMID: 16958030]

[26]   Zhou XH. Effect of verification bias on positive and negative predictive values. Stat Med 1994; 13(17): 1737-45.
[http://dx.doi.org/10.1002/sim.4780131705] [PMID: 7997707]

[27]   Parikh R, Mathai A, Parikh S, Chandra Sekhar G, Thomas R. Understanding and using sensitivity, specificity and predictive values. Indian J Ophthalmol 2008; 56(1): 45-50.
[http://dx.doi.org/10.4103/0301-4738.37595] [PMID: 18158403]

[28]   Kelly T E. Clinical genetics and genetic counseling. 1980.

[29]   Rosenberg RN, Pascual JM. Rosenberg's Molecular and Genetic Basis of Neurological and Psychiatric Disease. Academic press 2020; 1.

[30]   Katsanis SH, Katsanis N. Molecular genetic testing and the future of clinical genomics. Nat Rev Genet 2013; 14(6): 415-26.
[http://dx.doi.org/10.1038/nrg3493] [PMID: 23681062]

[31]   Amberger JS, Bocchini CA, Schiettecatte F, Scott AF, Hamosh A. OMIM.org: Online Mendelian Inheritance in Man (OMIM®), an online catalog of human genes and genetic disorders. Nucleic Acids Res 2015; 43(D1): D789-98.
[http://dx.doi.org/10.1093/nar/gku1205] [PMID: 25428349]

[32]   Yang Y, Muzny DM, Reid JG, *et al.* Clinical whole-exome sequencing for the diagnosis of mendelian disorders. N Engl J Med 2013; 369(16): 1502-11.
[http://dx.doi.org/10.1056/NEJMoa1306555] [PMID: 24088041]

[33]   Yohe S, Hauge A, Bunjer K, *et al.* Clinical validation of targeted next-generation sequencing for inherited disorders. Arch Pathol Lab Med 2015; 139(2): 204-10.
[http://dx.doi.org/10.5858/arpa.2013-0625-OA] [PMID: 25611102]

[34]   Cummings S. Genetic Counseling. Genetic Diagnosis of Endocrine Disorders. Elsevier 2010; pp. 293-302.
[http://dx.doi.org/10.1016/B978-0-12-374430-2.00026-2]

[35]   Epstein CJ. Who should do genetic counseling, and under what circumstances? Birth Defects Orig Artic Ser 1973; 9(4): 39-48.
[PMID: 4712459]

[36]   Clarke A, Richards M, Kerzin-Storrar L, *et al.* Genetic professionals' reports of nondisclosure of genetic risk information within families. Eur J Hum Genet 2005; 13(5): 556-62.
[http://dx.doi.org/10.1038/sj.ejhg.5201394] [PMID: 15770225]

[37]   Yarborough M, Scott JA, Dixon LK. The role of beneficence in clinical genetics: Non-directive counseling reconsidered. Theor Med 1989; 10(2): 139-49.
[http://dx.doi.org/10.1007/BF00539879] [PMID: 2528837]

[38]   Ross LF. Predictive genetic testing for conditions that present in childhood. Kennedy Inst Ethics J 2002; 12(3): 225-44.
[http://dx.doi.org/10.1353/ken.2002.0019] [PMID: 12472077]

[39]   Shaw A, Hurst JA. 'I don't see any point in telling them': attitudes to sharing genetic information in

the family and carrier testing of relatives among British Pakistani adults referred to a genetics clinic. Ethn Health 2009; 14(2): 205-24.
[http://dx.doi.org/10.1080/13557850802071140] [PMID: 19052940]

[40]   Vos J, Jansen AM, Menko F, Van Asperen CJ, Stiggelbout AM, Tibben A. Family communication matters: The impact of telling relatives about unclassified variants and uninformative DNA-test results. Genet Med 2011; 13(4): 333-41.
[http://dx.doi.org/10.1097/GIM.0b013e318204cfed] [PMID: 21358410]

[41]   Forrest K, Simpson SA, Wilson BJ, *et al.* To tell or not to tell: barriers and facilitators in family communication about genetic risk. Clin Genet 2003; 64(4): 317-26.
[http://dx.doi.org/10.1034/j.1399-0004.2003.00142.x] [PMID: 12974737]

[42]   Keenan KF, Simpson SA, Miedzybrodzka Z, Alexander DA, Semper J. How do partners find out about the risk of Huntington's disease in couple relationships? J Genet Couns 2013; 22(3): 336-44.
[http://dx.doi.org/10.1007/s10897-012-9562-2] [PMID: 23297124]

[43]   Kessler S. Psychological aspects of genetic counseling. IX. Teaching and counseling. J Genet Couns 1997; 6(3): 287-95.
[http://dx.doi.org/10.1023/A:1025676205440] [PMID: 26142236]

CHAPTER 5

Genome-Wide Association Studies (GWAS)

Hafiza Noor Ul Ayan[1,2] and **Muhammad Tariq**[1,*]

[1] *National Institute for Biotechnology and Genetic Engineering College, Pakistan Institute of Engineering and Applied Sciences (NIBGE-C, PIEAS), Faisalabad, Pakistan*

[2] *Institute for Cardiogenetic, University of Lubeck, Lubeck, Germany*

Abstract: Genome-wide association studies (GWAS) are designed to find associations between genomic variants and a phenotype, usually a complex multifactorial disease. The idea for association studies in a large cohort was floated after linkage analysis, which proved extremely successful in the identification of causative genes for rare disorders, but it did not come up to expectations in the case of common complex disorders where causative alleles are less frequently aggregated in families. Ever since their advent in 2005, GWAS have transformed gene identification ventures in complex disease genetics over the past fifteen years, giving rise to several powerful associations for complex traits and disorders. Association studies are based on the "common disease common variant" hypothesis which assumes that genomic variation with low penetrance and high population frequency are involved in the causation of common complex disorders. Although GWAS, complemented with the downstream functional assessment of the variants, have been successful in identifying novel disease-causing genes and biological mechanisms, the field has also received intense criticism over the years, especially its failure in tracing the so-called 'missing heritability'. Therefore, further functional studies are mandatory to precisely establish a link between risk alleles and a phenotype. This chapter broadly covers an introduction of GWAS, their successes and limitations, and various important factors affecting the design and results, followed by challenges in the post-GWAS era.

Keywords: Genome-wide Association Studies, Linkage Disequilibrium, Multifactorial Diseases, Missing Heritability, SNPs, WGS.

1. INTRODUCTION

During the last century, conventional approaches, such as linkage analysis using PCR and conventional sequencing, were extensively used to map genomic regions co-segregating with disease phenotypes. These techniques were quite successful

* **Corresponding author Muhammad Tariq**: National Institute for Biotechnology and Genetic Engineering College, Pakistan Institute of Engineering and Applied Sciences (NIBGE-C, PIEAS), Faisalabad, Pakistan;
E-mail: tariqpalai@gmail.com

Syeda Marriam Bakhtiar and Erum Dilshad (Eds.)

in identifying genes underlying Mendelian disorders (*e.g.*, cystic fibrosis). However, linkage analyses were not found very fruitful in case of complex traits and diseases (*e.g.*, cardiovascular diseases, cancer and Parkinson's disease), wherein multiple genetic variants add to the phenotype, as well as the environmental risk factors (*e.g.*, diet, smoking, alcoholism and sedentary lifestyle) which also contribute to disease picture. These disorders and individuals with these disorders are less frequently aggregated in families, thus, the corresponding causal alleles are less likely to be shared among related patients [1]. This limitation of linkage analysis necessitated novel approaches that could be applied to dissect the genetic architecture of complex multifactorial diseases in unrelated patients. This inspired Genome-wide Association Studies, popularly known as 'GWAS' in 2005 [2].

1.1. Rationale

GWAS are designed to identify genomic locations harboring variants (a marker allele; typically, a SNP) associated with disease risk [3]. It is basically a case-control study in which genotypes associated with the certain genomic variants have different frequencies among affected and phenotypically healthy individuals. GWAS are usually designed for analyzing large cohorts of unrelated individuals or nuclear families since a large number of patients with similar disease phenotype is relatively easy to collect within a population, compared to within families (a requirement for linkage analysis). Assume that causal variants are not rare, theoretical arguments support the power of GWAS in elucidating the genetic basis of multifactorial disorders [4]. Therefore, GWAS are primarily designed around the hypothesis "common disease common variant (CDCV)", which argues that complex traits underlie genetic variants with low penetrance but high population frequency [5].

Identification of the CFH gene variant, causative for age-related macular degeneration (AMD) in European population, was among the earliest success stories of GWAS, published back in 2005 [2]. This study analyzed >100,000 SNPs in 96 affected and 50 healthy individuals to discover a strong association between a common intronic variant and the disease. However, subsequent sequencing of the identified gene revealed an exonic variant that changes tyrosine at amino acid 402 by histidine (p.Y402H). The coding variant has a larger impact with a relative risk of 7.4 in homozygous patients in comparison to individuals with wild type genotype. This study, undoubtedly, emphasized the potential of GWAS to explore underlying genetics of complex disorders. Later in 2007, Welcome Trust Case Control Consortium (WTCCC) embarked on seven GWAS initiatives, simultaneously, for seven complex diseases in the UK population (type

1 and type 2 diabetes, coronary heart disease, hypertension, bipolar disorder, rheumatoid arthritis and inflammatory bowel disease) [6]. In their landmark paper, the consortium demonstrated that for reproducible discoveries using GWAS, large sample sizes, a thorough study design and rigorous criteria are a must. By 2010, GWAS had identified more than 3000 loci for over 250 diseases and phenotypes [7]. In the following 10 years, GWAS accelerated gene discovery exponentially with more than 4300 research papers from 4500 association studies implicating around 55,000 genomic loci for over 5000 diseases [7]. Most of the GWAS data are publicly available and several user-friendly data portals are accessible that help scientists to analyze GWAS data easily.

Association depends on linkage disequilibrium (LD), which is the co-segregation of a marker allele with a causal variant, by virtue of their genomic proximity, across a population [8]. LD, a correlation structure, in genomic variants is a reflection of evolution, limited population size, mutation, natural selection and recombination rate. The statistical power of associations studies depends on several factors *e.g.*, sample size, distribution of effect sizes of causal variants segregating in the population, minor allele frequency (MAF) of the variant and LD between SNP variant and as yet unknown causative variant [9].

The core objective of GWAS is to improve the understanding of disease biology to pave way for prevention or better treatment. However, in most cases, GWAS findings do not necessarily have a utility in the prevention or treatment of disease. GWAS detect variants that are associated with phenotypic differences, therefore, the association between a genomic variant and a disease phenotype does not necessarily provide direct information about the causal gene or disease mechanism. Identification of causal variant frequently requires follow up studies to narrow down the associated region. However, novel analytical methods and molecular technologies provide us with the opportunities to fill the gap between sequence and consequence [9].

GWAS, over the past decade, have successfully detected associations of thousands of SNPs with human diseases [10]. However, the associated alleles typically have high frequency in a population with a MAF >5% [11]. Moreover, an overwhelming majority of SNPs (~90%), associated with different traits, are found in the non-coding parts of the genome [12] which further complicates identification of relevant genes, causal variants and mechanisms [13]. Nonetheless, the limitations of GWAS can be partially overcome by using cohorts of small families or sporadic patients from an isolated geographical region [14] and by using whole genome sequencing (WGS). Data generated by WGS can better capture low frequency rare variants. Moreover, it facilitates capturing variants that are in strong LD with SNPs on a genotyping array. Therefore, WGS is better in imputation (the estimation of unknown alleles based on the observation of nearby alleles in high LD) to genotype rare variants with high accuracy [15]. Additionally, several simulation studies have depicted that the use of WGS for GWAS significantly increases the mapping precision of rare variants, thus making it an efficient way of identifying, as well as, fine-mapping rare variants, in a single experiment [16]. WGS based association studies are likely to increase both variant capture and precision [17].

2. BENEFITS OF GWAS

GWAS have had phenomenal success in identifying novel variants and risk loci associated with traits and diseases, respectively. Notable examples include type 2 diabetes mellitus [18], autoimmune diseases [19], coronary artery disease (CAD) [20], schizophrenia [21] and lung cancer [22]. The major finding among these is the association of CAD and myocardial infarction (MI) to 9p21.3 [23]. Wherein follow up studies identified sequences at 9p21 that act as enhancers. Two CAD risk alleles (SNPs) are present in one of these enhancers. The variants result in the disruption of binding sites for Signal Transducer and Activator of Transcription 1 (*STAT1*) [24]. It took four years to explain the function of this locus but CAD/MI GWAS findings served as the starting point for the identification of important disease pathways.

GWAS have had a pivotal role in the discovery of novel biological mechanisms, as well. Genes of unknown function or unpredicted relevance are often implicated by these studies and follow up experimental verification of such genes can identify and explain novel biological mechanisms [9]. For example, SLC16A11 gene (17p13) was associated with type 2 diabetes in a cohort of Mexican adults [25]. SLC16A11 gene variants were shown to independently diminish the function of the encoded protein by downregulating SLC16A11 expression in the liver in a dosage-dependent manner. The low expression, consequently, results in the disruption of a crucial interaction with a chaperone protein, thereby decreasing the localization of the protein to cell surface. Follow up studies identified SLC16A11 as a proton-coupled monocarboxylate transporter which, when downregulated, affects fatty acid content of the cell and, hence, lipid metabolism. The overall result is an increased risk of type 2 diabetes [26]. These findings underscore the utility of GWAS in discovering subtle associations in even larger disease cohorts.

Information extracted from GWAS findings are utilized in a wide spectrum of applications relevant to healthcare. Genomic variants implicated by GWAS can predict the risk of certain diseases in individuals, thus facilitating early screening, prevention and/or treatment. For example, a GWAS for exfoliation glaucoma found two non-synonymous SNPs in LOXL1 gene; 99% population-attributable risk of this disease is ascribed to this gene [27]. Although GWAS are not largely directly informative regarding causative gene variants or the resultant patho-mechanisms, downstream functional validation can identify novel targets and pathways for potential therapeutic intervention. GWAS for numerous diseases *e.g.*, type 2 diabetes, rheumatoid arthritis, psoriasis, osteoporosis and schizophrenia have helped identify novel drug candidates which are being evaluated in clinical trials [9].

Though primarily tailor-made for complex disorders, GWAS also have a proven utility in the identification of novel causative genes for rare diseases. On approximately one out of every five loci discovered in GWAS, there is a causative gene variant underlying a monogenic disorder [28]. On the basis of these observations, scientists hypothesized that gene variants implicated in association studies are likely to be candidates for uncovering mutations underlying rare diseases [29]. This hypothesis has been validated by studies involving resequencing of GWAS-implicated genes, thus finding several novel monogenic or oligogenic variants for complex disorders *e.g.*, genes for obesity (*SH2B1*, *NPC1* and *ADCY3*) [30 - 33] and inflammatory bowel disease (*TNFRSF6B*, *PRDM1*, *CARD9*, *IL23R* and *RNF186*) [34 - 36]. This strategy is cost-effective and has the advantage of better statistical power, which is critical in GWAS, in comparison to WES (whole-exome sequencing) and WGS (whole genome sequencing) [37].

GWAS data can be used to spot ethnic variation of complex traits. Although some risk loci vary significantly in frequency and effect size among different ethnicities, common variants, in general, are believed to be shared by different ethnic groups [38]. GWAS can help in diverse ethnic populations to explore the genetic heterogeneity in susceptibility to disease. For example, the locus 15q25 was found in a strong association with lung carcinoma in GWAS on European patients' cohort, however, in Asian population, where the frequency of this allele is very low, its association with this disorder could not be replicated [22]. In some cases, the frequency of risk variants is very high in a particular population, or ethnic group; but is either absent in other populations or ethnic groups, or is apparently absent (founder mutations). An example is the isolated Greenlandic and Samoan communities [39]. Differences in the effect size of a risk variant, among different ethnicities, is an important factor influencing the probability of its discovery, and its impact on disease burden in different populations [40]. GWAS data have several other applications as well (Table **5.1**). Generation, management and analysis of GWAS data are simple and straightforward. The success of GWAS in identifying genes involved in complex disease, can be partially credited to methodological and technological innovations that have accelerated their performance. Several algorithms are available for calling genotypes from SNP array data with high accuracy and call rate [6, 41, 42]. Algorithms have also been designed particularly for calling rare and low-frequency variants [43, 44] and for deducing structural variants and haplotypes [45, 46]. Moreover, GWAS data can be easily shared and its public availability further facilitates novel discoveries.

Table 5.1. Applications of GWAS beyond gene identification.

Applications	References
Reconstruction of population history	[47 - 50]
Determination of ancestry and population substructure	[51, 52]
Fine-scale estimation of location of birth	[53]
Estimation of SNP heritability for complex traits	[15]
Estimation of genetic correlations between traits	[54]
Mendelian randomization studies	[55]
Genome-wide assessment of linkage disequilibrium	[56]
Paternity testing	[57]
Determination of perinatal loss	[58]
Forensic analyses	[59, 60]
Determination of cryptic relatedness	[61]
Loss-of-heterozygosity and copy number variation analyses in tumors	[62]
Direct-to-consumer and clinical diagnostic genetic testing	[63]
Prenatal and pre-implantation genetic diagnosis	[64, 65]
Embryonic DNA fingerprinting	[66]
Polygenic risk scores	[67]

3. SUCCESS STORIES

Over the past 15 years, GWAS produced a wealth of new information. Here, we discuss a few examples of complex diseases to explain some of the advances which are the direct corollary of GWAS results.

3.1. Type 2 Diabetes

GWAS have been very successful in explaining the genetics of type 2 diabetes identifying more than one hundred common variant signals [68]. GWAS carried out by sequencing have shown that majority of genetic variants causing type 2 diabetes are localized at common variant sites [69]. Moreover, most of the common variant associations underlying type-2 diabetes have been replicated in major ethnic groups as well [70]. Genotyping and sequencing in diverse populations have identified more and more ethnic-specific alleles, for example, variants in PAX4 gene have high frequency and relatively large phenotypic effect in East Asians [68]. However, efforts to identify gene-gene and gene-environment interactions have not been very successful [71].

The translation of GWAS findings understanding pathophysiological mechanisms has been one of the most laborious tasks, mainly because the majority of identified variants are located in non-coding genomic regions. However, the generation of multi-omics data from multiple cell types and tissues have facilitated the translation of GWAS loci. However, the integration of multi-omics and GWAS data into computational pipelines, has great potential to facilitate the determination of regulatory impact of a locus. It is also helping in the prioritization of disease causing variant and/or gene and major tissues likely to be involved in disease pathogenesis [72]. For example, mapping of more than 1 out of every 5 loci associated with type 2 diabetes is most likely the causal variant as per computational tools [73]. Therefore, these prioritized variants and genes need to be validated *in vitro* and then *in vivo* using animal models, ultimately followed by human models. One such example includes a study validating SLC30A8 gene variant (encoding ZnT8), a protective allele associated with a lower risk of type 2 diabetes by virtue of increased glucose responsiveness and proinsulin conversion, making *SLC30A8*/ZnT8 an interesting target for treatment of diabetes [74].

3.2. Autoimmune Diseases

In recent years, the utility of GWAS has been exploited for almost all crucial immune-mediated diseases, yielding hundreds of associated loci [75]. The establishment of computational approaches for cross-disease studies have been especially useful in the identification of pleiotropic loci, which are accelerating novel gene discovery and improving our understanding of the pathogenic relatedness of immune-mediated diseases. For example, a cross-disease study investigating disorders like ankylosing spondylitis, inflammatory bowel disease, primary sclerosing cholangitis and psoriasis identified thirty novel genome-wide significant loci without any further genotyping [76]. Moreover, transethnic studies for autoimmune diseases have shown significant genetic overlap among remote populations [77]. For example, high genetic correlation has been estimated in European and East Asian populations for Crohn disease and ulcerative colitis [38]. Studies have also been conducted to make transethnic comparison of associations at shared loci and they have been quite helpful in the identification of causal variants. For example, population-specific variation in *HLA-DRB1* associations in rheumatoid arthritis has aided in defining the critical amino acids supporting that association [78].

GWAS findings have also made significant contributions to understanding biological mechanisms underlying immune-mediated diseases. For example, another cross-disease study identified novel genes involved in pathogenesis associated with methylation variation (*DNMT3A* and *DNMT3B*), bacteria-sensing genes (*TLR4*), genes affecting host microbiome (*FUT2*) and NFKB pathway genes (*NFKB1, NFKBIA* and *TNFAIP3*) [76]. GWAS have identified some extensively pleiotropic loci that contain variants associated with different diseases in different directions; the SNP rs1800693 in TNFR1 gene, for instance, is associated with multiple sclerosis and ankylosing spondylitis but in different directions [79]. This is a risk SNP for multiple sclerosis as it causes loss of transmembrane domain of receptor resulting in increased serum soluble TNF receptor [80]. However, this SNP is protective for ankylosing spondylitis as TNF inhibition is highly effective for ankylosing spondylitis and several other autoimmune diseases [80]. Several GWAS breakthroughs have encouraged targeted therapy-development programs; for example, programs targeting M1 aminopeptidase family genes (*ERAP1* and *ERAP2*) due to their associations with psoriasis, ankylosing spondylitis, inflammatory bowel disease, type 1 diabetes and Behcet's syndrome [81].

3.3. Coronary Artery Disease (CAD)

CAD (Coronary Artery Disease) and its sequelae MI (Myocardial Infarction) are among the most deadly diseases worldwide [82]. GWAS for CAD/MI have produced several successful outcomes, starting in 2007 with the discovery of 9p21 risk locus [23]. To date, GWAS have found more than 160 genome-wide significant risk loci and more than 300 loci are indicative for CAD risk [83]. Collectively, these loci explain approximately 30-40% of CAD heritability, and can potentially help in better prediction of risk for CAD and understanding of disease pathophysiology [83]. However, most of these loci represent variants with MAF greater than 5% and are associated with moderate increases in CAD risk [84]. This suggests that common variants explain far greater fraction of CAD heritability in comparison to rare variants.

GWAS for CAD/MI have not been very successful in the identification of biological mechanisms leading to disease. Although genetic associations provide a solid basis for the identification of potential therapeutic targets, and several CAD loci have been mapped to numerous pathophysiological pathways with already reported functions in disease phenotype, a number of challenges have slowed down the process of GWAS to biology. First, most of the significantly associated variants are non-coding and are difficult to be assessed functionally. Therefore, predicting their function and identifying particular targets is not easy. Second, nearly all loci, implicated in association studies, harbor multiple genes and the most probable disease-causing gene frequently needs to be defined by thorough studies. Third, only a small number of loci have candidate genes that unambiguously explain the association signals, *LDLR* and *PCSK9*; at all other loci, the underlying gene must be determined by downstream functional analysis to elucidate patho-mechanisms. Fourth, the lack of multi-omics data for CAD may partly account for this delay [85]. Moreover, a study by Nikpay *et al.* demonstrated that CAD heritability is mostly determined by regulatory SNPs found in epigenetic sites associated with transcriptional activity [86], making its functional characterization even more challenging.

4. LIMITATIONS OF GWAS

The pivotal role of GWAS in understanding the biology of complex disorders notwithstanding, this experimental design has several limitations. In GWAS, local correlation of multiple variants due to LD enables the preliminary identification of a locus, however, it does not necessarily identify causal variants and genes [87]. As already discussed, most associations are detected in non-coding regions, which makes the biological interpretation inherently challenging [73]. Performing GWAS is, therefore, only an initial step and further measures, such as multi-ethnic population resequencing, fine-mapping, functional studies or evolutionary genetic analyses, are usually required to identify causal variants and genes [88]. However, GWAS performed by WGS instead of SNP arrays can accelerate identification of causal variants because all genetic variations are ascertained. Functional characterization is, nevertheless, equally difficult irrespective of the technology employed.

GWAS are typically designed to analyze large number of individuals (tens of thousands of individuals) and even larger number of genome variants (millions of SNPs). Therefore, GWAS have to test multiple hypotheses. This is one major limitation of association studies testing. As each of the GWAS involves millions of statistical tests, the threshold P value, ought to be adjusted to keep the overall false positive rate in check [89]. This limitation is usually overcome by applying Bonferroni correction to keep the genome-wide false-positive rate at 5%, based on the hypothesis that one million independent tests are conducted for common genetic variation. As a result, traditional association studies are unable to detect all the heritability described by SNPs, since associations which fail to achieve a threshold ($P < 5 \times 10^{-8}$) are considered insignificant [90, 91]. This limitation is likely to become even more serious an issue in the future because the increasing use of WGS in GWAS will increase the genomic coverage and number of independent tests performed [92]. However, this limitation can be overcome to some extent by involving larger sample size in association studies [29]. Another solution can be to decrease the number of tests performed *e.g.*, by using gene-based [93] or pathway-based association tests [94], using linkage regions [95], prioritized candidate genes [96] or potentially damaging SNPs [40]. Moreover, the probability of true positive results can be increased by combining related biological evidence and statistically significant data [97].

Another major limitation associated with GWAS is the missing heritability. Although, GWAS have been successful at identifying association between variants and complex diseases and traits, with a few exceptions, such as age-related macular degeneration, exfoliation glaucoma and type 1 diabetes, in most cases, these genetic variants represent a very small fraction of the estimated heritability [98]. The rest of the heritability remains unexplained in most of the complex traits. This unexplained fraction of the heritability is generally referred to as "the missing heritability". There can be several reasons for this missing heritability such as some SNPs which are filtered out because they represent only a tiny fraction of the total heritability and do not reach the predefined threshold significance value [99]. This hypothesis has found support from some studies, conducted recently, suggesting that SNPs may explain only one-third to two-thirds of the total heritability in most multifactorial traits [15]. This limitation can be dealt with by using large sample sizes [9] and novel methods and study designs [100]. Moreover, to be able to explain the missing heritability, or at least some fraction of it, we still have to improve our understanding of gene-gene and gene-environment interactions [101].

GWAS have also been largely unsuccessful in discerning epistasis. Despite the fact that model organisms such as mouse, fly and yeast have demonstrated epistasis as a crucial element in the genetic architecture of complex traits, non-additive genetic effect is very difficult to assess in humans [102]. Primarily, insufficient statistical power and challenges in study designs are responsible for difficulties in the identification of major gene-gene interactions in GWAS and post-GWAS experiments [67]. Although, there is not enough evidence that epistasis has a substantial contribution to the heritability of complex human traits, the limitation can be partly overcome by increasing the sample sizes in order to detect significant interactions [9]. Moreover, recent advances such as data filtering, Bayesian methods and artificial intelligence algorithms may increase the detection of epistatic interactions in humans [103].

The success stories of GWAS, so far, represent only to a small tip of the heritability iceberg. Revealing the remainder of this 'iceberg' will take advanced, and improvised, GWAS approach and cutting-edge study designs. GWAS data are usually analyzed assuming an autosomal additive model, which is rather limiting. Integrating dominant, recessive, over dominant, multiplicative, parent-of-origin-specific and X-linked inheritance models in GWAS can potentially identify additional variants by increasing statistical power [104].

5. POST-GWAS ERA: PROSPECTS AND CHALLENGES

GWAS have played a significant role in discoveries of human genetics over the last decade or so. These have delivered on the fundamental objective of identifying associations between common genetic variations and diseases. However, only a small fraction of these statistical associations has been fully utilized to identify causal variant, molecular function of causal variant, genes affected by causal variant and how discrepancies in the regulation of causative genes lead to altered disease risk [105]. For instance, GWAS have identified more than 200 loci associated with four neurodegenerative disorders (Alzheimer's Disease, Parkinson's Disease, Amyotrophic Lateral Sclerosis and Frontotemporal dementia) and related phenotypes [10]. However, only one of these loci (SNCA locus) was investigated in detail [105]. Therefore, instead of searching for more and more GWAS loci, downstream functional analysis of already known loci might help better understand pathophysiology of disease.

Despite criticism, the present scenario suggests that GWAS will be around for a long time in future. There will be more studies with sample sizes exceeding five million participants as data from larger cohorts (*e.g.*, UK Biobank and the Million Veterans Project) will be available [12]. Such ventures are expected to yield more GWAS loci, including rare and population specific variants, and better estimate variant effect. However, according to one opinion, the initiation of even larger GWAS identifying associations with even smaller effects might eventually result in spurious findings of all genes expressed in disease associated cells as disease causing loci [106]. Nonetheless, the growing availability of GWAS data from non-European populations will further extend gene discovery and reduce health discrepancies. Eventually, the easy access to high-throughput genome-wide technologies for mapping sites of regulatory impact will increase the translation of GWAS loci into novel biological insights. These advancements, along with technological and analytical developments, will continue to revolutionize GWAS for years to come [12].

CONCLUDING REMARKS

The experimental design of GWAS, which started around fifteen years ago in 2005, has made significant progress on the way and delivered on its promise of comprehending genetics of complex diseases. Although, the low-hanging fruits have been long picked, GWAS have shown tremendous success and will continue to do so. As of today, we have cutting-edge technologies, advanced analytical tools and extensive multi-omics databases to translate the underlying biology of GWAS loci and their role in health and disease. Despite all the criticism, GWAS clearly show no signs of slowing down. However, more functional studies are required which are intended at explaining the causal genetic variants, biological mechanisms underlying observed statistical associations and disease risk.

CONSENT FOR PUBLICATION

Not Applicable.

CONFLICT OF INTEREST

The author declares no conflict of interest, financial or otherwise.

ACKNOWLEDGEMENTS

Declared none.

REFERENCES

[1]   Morris AP, Cardon LR. Genome-Wide Association Studies. in Handbook of Statistical Genomics 2019; 597-50.
        [http://dx.doi.org/10.1002/9781119487845.ch21]

[2]   Klein RJ, Zeiss C, Chew EY, *et al.* Complement factor H polymorphism in age-related macular degeneration. Science 2005; 308(5720): 385-9.
        [http://dx.doi.org/10.1126/science.1109557] [PMID: 15761122]

[3]   Edwards SL, Beesley J, French JD, Dunning AM. Beyond GWASs: illuminating the dark road from association to function. Am J Hum Genet 2013; 93(5): 779-97.
        [http://dx.doi.org/10.1016/j.ajhg.2013.10.012] [PMID: 24210251]

[4]   Risch N, Merikangas K. The future of genetic studies of complex human diseases. Science 1996; 273(5281): 1516-7.
        [http://dx.doi.org/10.1126/science.273.5281.1516] [PMID: 8801636]

[5]   Reich DE, Lander ES. On the allelic spectrum of human disease. Trends Genet 2001; 17(9): 502-10.
        [http://dx.doi.org/10.1016/S0168-9525(01)02410-6] [PMID: 11525833]

[6]   Burton P R, *et al.* Genome-wide association study of 14,000 cases of seven common diseases and 3,000 shared controls. Nature 2007; 447: 661-78.

[7]   MacArthur J, Bowler E, Cerezo M, *et al.* The new NHGRI-EBI Catalog of published genome-wide association studies (GWAS Catalog). Nucleic Acids Res 2017; 45(D1): D896-901.
        [http://dx.doi.org/10.1093/nar/gkw1133] [PMID: 27899670]

[8]   Bush WS, Moore JH. Chapter 11: Genome-wide association studies. PLOS Comput Biol 2012; 8(12): e1002822.
        [http://dx.doi.org/10.1371/journal.pcbi.1002822] [PMID: 23300413]

[9]   Visscher PM, Wray NR, Zhang Q, *et al.* 10 Years of GWAS Discovery: Biology, Function, and Translation. Am J Hum Genet 2017; 101(1): 5-22.
        [http://dx.doi.org/10.1016/j.ajhg.2017.06.005] [PMID: 28686856]

[10]   Welter D, MacArthur J, Morales J, *et al.* The NHGRI GWAS Catalog, a curated resource of SNP-trait associations. Nucleic Acids Res 2014; 42(D1): D1001-6.
[http://dx.doi.org/10.1093/nar/gkt1229] [PMID: 24316577]

[11]   Marouli E, Graff M, Medina-Gomez C, *et al.* EPIC-InterAct Consortium; CHD Exome+ Consortium; ExomeBP Consortium; T2D-Genes Consortium; GoT2D Genes Consortium; Global Lipids Genetics Consortium; ReproGen Consortium; MAGIC Investigators. Rare and low-frequency coding variants alter human adult height. Nature 2017; 542(7640): 186-90.
[http://dx.doi.org/10.1038/nature21039] [PMID: 28146470]

[12]   Loos R J F. 15 years of genome-wide association studies and no signs of slowing down. Nat Commun 2020; 11: 5900.

[13]   Lango Allen H, Estrada K, Lettre G, *et al.* Hundreds of variants clustered in genomic loci and biological pathways affect human height. Nature 2010; 467(7317): 832-8.
[http://dx.doi.org/10.1038/nature09410] [PMID: 20881960]

[14]   Panoutsopoulou K, Tachmazidou I, Zeggini E. In search of low-frequency and rare variants affecting complex traits. Hum Mol Genet 2013; 22(R1): R16-21.
[http://dx.doi.org/10.1093/hmg/ddt376] [PMID: 23922232]

[15]   Yang J, Bakshi A, Zhu Z, *et al.* LifeLines Cohort Study. Genetic variance estimation with imputed variants finds negligible missing heritability for human height and body mass index. Nat Genet 2015; 47(10): 1114-20.
[http://dx.doi.org/10.1038/ng.3390] [PMID: 26323059]

[16]   Wu Y, Zheng Z, Visscher PM, Yang J. Quantifying the mapping precision of genome-wide association studies using whole-genome sequencing data. Genome Biol 2017; 18(1): 86.
[http://dx.doi.org/10.1186/s13059-017-1216-0] [PMID: 28506277]

[17]   Höglund J, *et al.* Improved power and precision with whole genome sequencing data in genome-wide association studies of inflammatory biomarkers. Sci Rep 2019; 9(1): 16844.

[18]   Zhao W, Rasheed A, Tikkanen E, *et al.* CHD Exome+ Consortium; EPIC-CVD Consortium; EPIC-Interact Consortium; Michigan Biobank. Identification of new susceptibility loci for type 2 diabetes and shared etiological pathways with coronary heart disease. Nat Genet 2017; 49(10): 1450-7.
[http://dx.doi.org/10.1038/ng.3943] [PMID: 28869590]

[19]   Hu X, Daly M. 2012/10/01/ 2012. What have we learned from six years of GWAS in autoimmune diseases, and what is next? Curr Opin Immunol 2012; 24: 571-5.

[20]   Nikpay M, *et al.* A comprehensive 1000 Genomes–based genome-wide association meta-analysis of coronary artery disease Nat Genet 2015; 47: pp. 1121-30.

[21]   Li Z, *et al.* Genome-wide association analysis identifies 30 new susceptibility loci for schizophrenia. Nat Genet. 2017; 49: pp. 1576-83.

[22]   Bossé Y, Amos CI. A Decade of GWAS Results in Lung Cancer. Cancer Epidemiol Biomarkers Prev 2018; 27(4): 363-79.
[http://dx.doi.org/10.1158/1055-9965.EPI-16-0794] [PMID: 28615365]

[23]   Samani NJ, Erdmann J, Hall AS, *et al.* WTCCC and the Cardiogenics Consortium. Genomewide association analysis of coronary artery disease. N Engl J Med 2007; 357(5): 443-53.
[http://dx.doi.org/10.1056/NEJMoa072366] [PMID: 17634449]

[24]   Harismendy O, Notani D, Song X, *et al.* 9p21 DNA variants associated with coronary artery disease impair interferon-γ signalling response. Nature 2011; 470(7333): 264-8.
[http://dx.doi.org/10.1038/nature09753] [PMID: 21307941]

[25]   Williams AL, Jacobs SB, Moreno-Macías H, *et al.* SIGMA Type 2 Diabetes Consortium. Sequence variants in SLC16A11 are a common risk factor for type 2 diabetes in Mexico. Nature 2014; 506(7486): 97-101.

[http://dx.doi.org/10.1038/nature12828] [PMID: 24390345]

[26]   Rusu V, Hoch E, Mercader JM, *et al.* MEDIA Consortium; SIGMA T2D Consortium. Type 2 Diabetes Variants Disrupt Function of SLC16A11 through Two Distinct Mechanisms. Cell 2017; 170(1): 199-212.e20.
[http://dx.doi.org/10.1016/j.cell.2017.06.011] [PMID: 28666119]

[27]   Thorleifsson G, Magnusson KP, Sulem P, *et al.* Common sequence variants in the LOXL1 gene confer susceptibility to exfoliation glaucoma. Science 2007; 317(5843): 1397-400.
[http://dx.doi.org/10.1126/science.1146554] [PMID: 17690259]

[28]   Hirschhorn JN. Genomewide association studies--illuminating biologic pathways. N Engl J Med 2009; 360(17): 1699-701.
[http://dx.doi.org/10.1056/NEJMp0808934] [PMID: 19369661]

[29]   Speakman JR, Loos RJF, O'Rahilly S, Hirschhorn JN, Allison DB. GWAS for BMI: a treasure trove of fundamental insights into the genetic basis of obesity. Int J Obes 2018; 42(8): 1524-31.
[http://dx.doi.org/10.1038/s41366-018-0147-5] [PMID: 29980761]

[30]   Doche ME, Bochukova eg, Su HW, *et al.* Human SH2B1 mutations are associated with maladaptive behaviors and obesity. J Clin Invest 2012; 122(12): 4732-6.
[http://dx.doi.org/10.1172/JCI62696] [PMID: 23160192]

[31]   Grarup N, Moltke I, Andersen MK, *et al.* Loss-of-function variants in ADCY3 increase risk of obesity and type 2 diabetes. Nat Genet 2018; 50(2): 172-4.
[http://dx.doi.org/10.1038/s41588-017-0022-7] [PMID: 29311636]

[32]   Liu R, Zou Y, Hong J, *et al.* Rare Loss-of-Function Variants in *NPC1* Predispose to Human Obesity. Diabetes 2017; 66(4): 935-47.
[http://dx.doi.org/10.2337/db16-0877] [PMID: 28130309]

[33]   Saeed S, Bonnefond A, Tamanini F, *et al.* Loss-of-function mutations in ADCY3 cause monogenic severe obesity. Nat Genet 2018; 50(2): 175-9.
[http://dx.doi.org/10.1038/s41588-017-0023-6] [PMID: 29311637]

[34]   Beaudoin M, Goyette P, Boucher G, *et al.* Quebec IBD Genetics Consortium; NIDDK IBD Genetics Consortium; International IBD Genetics Consortium. Deep resequencing of GWAS loci identifies rare variants in CARD9, IL23R and RNF186 that are associated with ulcerative colitis. PLoS Genet 2013; 9(9): e1003723.
[http://dx.doi.org/10.1371/journal.pgen.1003723] [PMID: 24068945]

[35]   Cardinale CJ, Wei Z, Panossian S, *et al.* Targeted resequencing identifies defective variants of decoy receptor 3 in pediatric-onset inflammatory bowel disease. Genes Immun 2013; 14(7): 447-52.
[http://dx.doi.org/10.1038/gene.2013.43] [PMID: 23965943]

[36]   Ellinghaus D, Zhang H, Zeissig S, *et al.* Association between variants of PRDM1 and NDP52 and Crohn's disease, based on exome sequencing and functional studies. Gastroenterology 2013; 145(2): 339-47.
[http://dx.doi.org/10.1053/j.gastro.2013.04.040] [PMID: 23624108]

[37]   Lessard S, Manning AK, Low-Kam C, *et al.* NHLBI GO Exome Sequence Project; GOT2D; T2D-GENES; GIANT Consortium. Testing the role of predicted gene knockouts in human anthropometric trait variation. Hum Mol Genet 2016; 25(10): 2082-92.
[http://dx.doi.org/10.1093/hmg/ddw055] [PMID: 26908616]

[38]   Liu JZ, van Sommeren S, Huang H, *et al.* International Multiple Sclerosis Genetics Consortium; International IBD Genetics Consortium. Association analyses identify 38 susceptibility loci for inflammatory bowel disease and highlight shared genetic risk across populations. Nat Genet 2015; 47(9): 979-86.
[http://dx.doi.org/10.1038/ng.3359] [PMID: 26192919]

[39]   Minster RL, Hawley NL, Su CT, *et al.* A thrifty variant in CREBRF strongly influences body mass

index in Samoans. Nat Genet 2016; 48(9): 1049-54.
[http://dx.doi.org/10.1038/ng.3620] [PMID: 27455349]

[40]   Turcot V, Lu Y, Highland HM, *et al.* CHD Exome+ Consortium; EPIC-CVD Consortium; ExomeBP Consortium; Global Lipids Genetic Consortium; GoT2D Genes Consortium; EPIC InterAct Consortium; INTERVAL Study; ReproGen Consortium; T2D-Genes Consortium; MAGIC Investigators; Understanding Society Scientific Group. Protein-altering variants associated with body mass index implicate pathways that control energy intake and expenditure in obesity. Nat Genet 2018; 50(1): 26-41.
[http://dx.doi.org/10.1038/s41588-017-0011-x] [PMID: 29273807]

[41]   Korn JM, Kuruvilla FG, McCarroll SA, *et al.* Integrated genotype calling and association analysis of SNPs, common copy number polymorphisms and rare CNVs. Nat Genet 2008; 40(10): 1253-60.
[http://dx.doi.org/10.1038/ng.237] [PMID: 18776909]

[42]   Xiao Y, Segal MR, Yang YH, Yeh RF. A multi-array multi-SNP genotyping algorithm for Affymetrix SNP microarrays. Bioinformatics 2007; 23(12): 1459-67.
[http://dx.doi.org/10.1093/bioinformatics/btm131] [PMID: 17459966]

[43]   Li G, Gelernter J, Kranzler HR, Zhao H. M3: an improved SNP calling algorithm for Illumina BeadArray data. Bioinformatics 2012; 28(3): 358-65.
[http://dx.doi.org/10.1093/bioinformatics/btr673] [PMID: 22155947]

[44]   Shah TS, Liu JZ, Floyd JAB, *et al.* optiCall: a robust genotype-calling algorithm for rare, low-frequency and common variants. Bioinformatics 2012; 28(12): 1598-603.
[http://dx.doi.org/10.1093/bioinformatics/bts180] [PMID: 22500001]

[45]   Coin LJM, Asher JE, Walters RG, *et al.* cnvHap: an integrative population and haplotype–based multiplatform model of SNPs and CNVs. Nat Methods 2010; 7(7): 541-6.
[http://dx.doi.org/10.1038/nmeth.1466] [PMID: 20512141]

[46]   El-Sayed Moustafa JS, Eleftherohorinou H, de Smith AJ, *et al.* Novel association approach for variable number tandem repeats (VNTRs) identifies DOCK5 as a susceptibility gene for severe obesity. Hum Mol Genet 2012; 21(16): 3727-38.
[http://dx.doi.org/10.1093/hmg/dds187] [PMID: 22595969]

[47]   Fu Q, Posth C, Hajdinjak M, *et al.* The genetic history of ice age Europe. Nature 2016; 534(7606): 200-5.
[http://dx.doi.org/10.1038/nature17993] [PMID: 27135931]

[48]   Lazaridis I, Patterson N, Mittnik A, *et al.* Ancient human genomes suggest three ancestral populations for present-day Europeans. Nature 2014; 513(7518): 409-13.
[http://dx.doi.org/10.1038/nature13673] [PMID: 25230663]

[49]   Reich D, Patterson N, Campbell D, *et al.* Reconstructing Native American population history. Nature 2012; 488(7411): 370-4.
[http://dx.doi.org/10.1038/nature11258] [PMID: 22801491]

[50]   Reich D, Thangaraj K, Patterson N, Price AL, Singh L. Reconstructing Indian population history. Nature 2009; 461(7263): 489-94.
[http://dx.doi.org/10.1038/nature08365] [PMID: 19779445]

[51]   Jakkula E, Rehnström K, Varilo T, *et al.* The genome-wide patterns of variation expose significant substructure in a founder population. Am J Hum Genet 2008; 83(6): 787-94.
[http://dx.doi.org/10.1016/j.ajhg.2008.11.005] [PMID: 19061986]

[52]   Price AL, Butler J, Patterson N, *et al.* Discerning the ancestry of European Americans in genetic association studies. PLoS Genet 2008; 4(1): e236.
[http://dx.doi.org/10.1371/journal.pgen.0030236] [PMID: 18208327]

[53]   Hoggart CJ, O'Reilly PF, Kaakinen M, *et al.* Fine-scale estimation of location of birth from genome-wide single-nucleotide polymorphism data. Genetics 2012; 190(2): 669-77.

[http://dx.doi.org/10.1534/genetics.111.135657] [PMID: 22095078]

[54] Bulik-Sullivan B, Finucane HK, Anttila V, *et al.* ReproGen Consortium; Psychiatric Genomics Consortium; Genetic Consortium for Anorexia Nervosa of the Wellcome Trust Case Control Consortium 3. An atlas of genetic correlations across human diseases and traits. Nat Genet 2015; 47(11): 1236-41.
[http://dx.doi.org/10.1038/ng.3406] [PMID: 26414676]

[55] Ross S, Gerstein HC, Eikelboom J, Anand SS, Yusuf S, Paré G. Mendelian randomization analysis supports the causal role of dysglycaemia and diabetes in the risk of coronary artery disease. Eur Heart J 2015; 36(23): 1454-62.
[http://dx.doi.org/10.1093/eurheartj/ehv083] [PMID: 25825043]

[56] Goode EL, Jarvik GP. Assessment and implications of linkage disequilibrium in genome-wide single-nucleotide polymorphism and microsatellite panels. Genet Epidemiol 2005; 29(S1) (Suppl. 1): S72-6.
[http://dx.doi.org/10.1002/gepi.20112] [PMID: 16342185]

[57] Kerr SM, Campbell A, Murphy L, *et al.* Pedigree and genotyping quality analyses of over 10,000 DNA samples from the Generation Scotland: Scottish Family Health Study. BMC Med Genet 2013; 14(1): 38.
[http://dx.doi.org/10.1186/1471-2350-14-38] [PMID: 23521772]

[58] Rosenfeld JA, Tucker ME, Escobar LF, *et al.* Diagnostic utility of microarray testing in pregnancy loss. Ultrasound Obstet Gynecol 2015; 46(4): 478-86.
[http://dx.doi.org/10.1002/uog.14866] [PMID: 25846569]

[59] Homer N, Szelinger S, Redman M, *et al.* Resolving individuals contributing trace amounts of DNA to highly complex mixtures using high-density SNP genotyping microarrays. PLoS Genet 2008; 4(8): e1000167.
[http://dx.doi.org/10.1371/journal.pgen.1000167] [PMID: 18769715]

[60] Kling D, Welander J, Tillmar A, Skare Ø, Egeland T, Holmlund G. DNA microarray as a tool in establishing genetic relatedness—Current status and future prospects. Forensic Sci Int Genet 2012; 6(3): 322-9.
[http://dx.doi.org/10.1016/j.fsigen.2011.07.007] [PMID: 21813350]

[61] Ramstetter MD, Dyer TD, Lehman DM, *et al.* Benchmarking relatedness inference methods with genome-wide data from thousands of relatives. Genetics 2017; 207(1): 75-82.
[http://dx.doi.org/10.1534/genetics.117.1122] [PMID: 28739658]

[62] Monzon FA, Hagenkord JM, Lyons-Weiler MA, *et al.* Whole genome SNP arrays as a potential diagnostic tool for the detection of characteristic chromosomal aberrations in renal epithelial tumors. Mod Pathol 2008; 21(5): 599-608.
[http://dx.doi.org/10.1038/modpathol.2008.20] [PMID: 18246049]

[63] Katsanis SH, Katsanis N. Molecular genetic testing and the future of clinical genomics. Nat Rev Genet 2013; 14(6): 415-26.
[http://dx.doi.org/10.1038/nrg3493] [PMID: 23681062]

[64] Srebniak MI, Diderich KEM, Joosten M, *et al.* Prenatal SNP array testing in 1000 fetuses with ultrasound anomalies: causative, unexpected and susceptibility CNVs. Eur J Hum Genet 2016; 24(5): 645-51.
[http://dx.doi.org/10.1038/ejhg.2015.193] [PMID: 26328504]

[65] Treff NR, *et al.* Single nucleotide polymorphism microarray–based concurrent screening of 24-chromosome aneuploidy and unbalanced translocations in preimplantation human embryos. Fertil Steril. 2011; 95: pp. 1606-12.

[66] Treff NR, Su J, Tao X, Miller KA, Levy B, Scott RT Jr. A novel single-cell DNA fingerprinting method successfully distinguishes sibling human embryos. Fertil Steril 2010; 94(2): 477-84.
[http://dx.doi.org/10.1016/j.fertnstert.2009.03.067] [PMID: 19394599]

[67]   Liu HY, Alyass A, Abadi A, *et al.* Fine-mapping of 98 obesity loci in Mexican children. Int J Obes 2019; 43(1): 23-32.
[http://dx.doi.org/10.1038/s41366-018-0056-7] [PMID: 29769702]

[68]   Fuchsberger C, Flannick J, Teslovich TM, *et al.* The genetic architecture of type 2 diabetes. Nature 2016; 536(7614): 41-7.
[http://dx.doi.org/10.1038/nature18642] [PMID: 27398621]

[69]   Steinthorsdottir V, Thorleifsson G, Sulem P, *et al.* Identification of low-frequency and rare sequence variants associated with elevated or reduced risk of type 2 diabetes. Nat Genet 2014; 46(3): 294-8.
[http://dx.doi.org/10.1038/ng.2882] [PMID: 24464100]

[70]   Mahajan A, Go MJ, Zhang W, *et al.* DIAbetes Genetics Replication And Meta-analysis (DIAGRAM) Consortium; Asian Genetic Epidemiology Network Type 2 Diabetes (AGEN-T2D) Consortium; South Asian Type 2 Diabetes (SAT2D) Consortium; Mexican American Type 2 Diabetes (MAT2D) Consortium; Type 2 Diabetes Genetic Exploration by Nex-generation sequencing in muylti-Ethnic Samples (T2D-GENES) Consortium. Genome-wide trans-ancestry meta-analysis provides insight into the genetic architecture of type 2 diabetes susceptibility. Nat Genet 2014; 46(3): 234-44.
[http://dx.doi.org/10.1038/ng.2897] [PMID: 24509480]

[71]   Claussnitzer M, Dankel SN, Klocke B, *et al.* DIAGRAM+Consortium. Leveraging cross-species transcription factor binding site patterns: from diabetes risk loci to disease mechanisms. Cell 2014; 156(1-2): 343-58.
[http://dx.doi.org/10.1016/j.cell.2013.10.058] [PMID: 24439387]

[72]   Cano-Gamez E, Trynka G. From GWAS to Function: Using Functional Genomics to Identify the Mechanisms Underlying Complex Diseases. Front Genet 2020; 11: 424.
[http://dx.doi.org/10.3389/fgene.2020.00424] [PMID: 32477401]

[73]   Mahajan A, *et al.* Fine-mapping type 2 diabetes loci to single-variant resolution using high-density imputation and islet-specific epigenome maps . Nat Genet 2018; 50: pp. 1505-13.

[74]   Dwivedi OP, Lehtovirta M, Hastoy B, *et al.* Loss of ZnT8 function protects against diabetes by enhanced insulin secretion. Nat Genet 2019; 51(11): 1596-606.
[http://dx.doi.org/10.1038/s41588-019-0513-9] [PMID: 31676859]

[75]   Gutierrez-Arcelus M, Rich SS, Raychaudhuri S. Autoimmune diseases — connecting risk alleles with molecular traits of the immune system. Nat Rev Genet 2016; 17(3): 160-74.
[http://dx.doi.org/10.1038/nrg.2015.33] [PMID: 26907721]

[76]   Ellinghaus D, Jostins L, Spain SL, *et al.* International IBD Genetics Consortium (IIBDGC); International Genetics of Ankylosing Spondylitis Consortium (IGAS); International PSC Study Group (IPSCSG); Genetic Analysis of Psoriasis Consortium (GAPC); Psoriasis Association Genetics Extension (PAGE). Analysis of five chronic inflammatory diseases identifies 27 new associations and highlights disease-specific patterns at shared loci. Nat Genet 2016; 48(5): 510-8.
[http://dx.doi.org/10.1038/ng.3528] [PMID: 26974007]

[77]   Okada Y, Wu D, Trynka G, *et al.* RACI consortium; GARNET consortium. Genetics of rheumatoid arthritis contributes to biology and drug discovery. Nature 2014; 506(7488): 376-81.
[http://dx.doi.org/10.1038/nature12873] [PMID: 24390342]

[78]   Raychaudhuri S, Sandor C, Stahl EA, *et al.* Five amino acids in three HLA proteins explain most of the association between MHC and seropositive rheumatoid arthritis. Nat Genet 2012; 44(3): 291-6.
[http://dx.doi.org/10.1038/ng.1076] [PMID: 22286218]

[79]   Cortes A, Hadler J, Pointon JP, *et al.* International Genetics of Ankylosing Spondylitis Consortium (IGAS); Australo-Anglo-American Spondyloarthritis Consortium (TASC); Groupe Française d'Etude Génétique des Spondylarthrites (GFEGS); Nord-Trøndelag Health Study (HUNT); Spondyloarthritis Research Consortium of Canada (SPARCC); Wellcome Trust Case Control Consortium 2 (WTCCC2). Identification of multiple risk variants for ankylosing spondylitis through high-density genotyping of immune-related loci. Nat Genet 2013; 45(7): 730-8.

[http://dx.doi.org/10.1038/ng.2667] [PMID: 23749187]

[80] Gregory AP, Dendrou CA, Attfield KE, *et al.* TNF receptor 1 genetic risk mirrors outcome of anti-TNF therapy in multiple sclerosis. Nature 2012; 488(7412): 508-11.
      [http://dx.doi.org/10.1038/nature11307] [PMID: 22801493]

[81] Agrawal N, Brown MA. Genetic associations and functional characterization of M1 aminopeptidases and immune-mediated diseases. Genes Immun 2014; 15(8): 521-7.
      [http://dx.doi.org/10.1038/gene.2014.46] [PMID: 25142031]

[82] Abubakar I, *et al.* GBD 2013 Mortality and Causes of Death Collaborators. Global, regional, and national age–sex specific all-cause and cause-specific mortality for 240 causes of death, 1990–2013: a systematic analysis for the Global Burden of Disease Study 2013. Lancet 2015; 385(9963): 117-71.
      [http://dx.doi.org/10.1016/S0140-6736(14)61682-2] [PMID: 25530442]

[83] Nelson CP, Goel A, Butterworth AS, *et al.* EPIC-CVD Consortium; CARDIoGRAMplusC4D; UK Biobank CardioMetabolic Consortium CHD working group. Association analyses based on false discovery rate implicate new loci for coronary artery disease. Nat Genet 2017; 49(9): 1385-91.
      [http://dx.doi.org/10.1038/ng.3913] [PMID: 28714975]

[84] Khera AV, Kathiresan S. Genetics of coronary artery disease: discovery, biology and clinical translation. Nat Rev Genet 2017; 18(6): 331-44.
      [http://dx.doi.org/10.1038/nrg.2016.160] [PMID: 28286336]

[85] Erdmann J, Kessler T, Munoz Venegas L, Schunkert H. A decade of genome-wide association studies for coronary artery disease: the challenges ahead. Cardiovasc Res 2018; 114(9): 1241-57.
      [http://dx.doi.org/10.1093/cvr/cvy084] [PMID: 29617720]

[86] Nikpay M, Stewart AFR, McPherson R. Partitioning the heritability of coronary artery disease highlights the importance of immune-mediated processes and epigenetic sites associated with transcriptional activity. Cardiovasc Res 2017; 113(8): 973-83.
      [http://dx.doi.org/10.1093/cvr/cvx019] [PMID: 28158393]

[87] Altshuler D, Daly MJ, Lander ES. Genetic mapping in human disease. Science 2008; 322(5903): 881-8.
      [http://dx.doi.org/10.1126/science.1156409] [PMID: 18988837]

[88] Mägi R, Horikoshi M, Sofer T, *et al.* COGENT-Kidney Consortium, T2D-GENES Consortium. Trans-ethnic meta-regression of genome-wide association studies accounting for ancestry increases power for discovery and improves fine-mapping resolution. Hum Mol Genet 2017; 26(18): 3639-50.
      [http://dx.doi.org/10.1093/hmg/ddx280] [PMID: 28911207]

[89] Joo J W J, *et al.* Multiple testing correction in linear mixed models. Genome Biol 2016; 17: 62.

[90] Dudbridge F, Gusnanto A. Estimation of significance thresholds for genomewide association scans. Genet Epidemiol 2008; 32(3): 227-34.
      [http://dx.doi.org/10.1002/gepi.20297] [PMID: 18300295]

[91] Manolio TA, Collins FS, Cox NJ, *et al.* Finding the missing heritability of complex diseases. Nature 2009; 461(7265): 747-53.
      [http://dx.doi.org/10.1038/nature08494] [PMID: 19812666]

[92] Pulit SL, de With SAJ, de Bakker PIW. Resetting the bar: Statistical significance in whole-genome sequencing-based association studies of global populations. Genet Epidemiol 2017; 41(2): 145-51.
      [http://dx.doi.org/10.1002/gepi.22032] [PMID: 27990689]

[93] Hägg S, Ganna A, Van Der Laan SW, *et al.* GIANT Consortium. Gene-based meta-analysis of genome-wide association studies implicates new loci involved in obesity. Hum Mol Genet 2015; 24(23): 6849-60.
      [http://dx.doi.org/10.1093/hmg/ddv379] [PMID: 26376864]

[94] Liu YJ, Guo YF, Zhang LS, *et al.* Biological pathway-based genome-wide association analysis identified the vasoactive intestinal peptide (VIP) pathway important for obesity. Obesity (Silver

Spring) 2010; 18(12): 2339-46.
[http://dx.doi.org/10.1038/oby.2010.83] [PMID: 20379146]

[95] Johansson Å, Marroni F, Hayward C, *et al.* EUROSPAN Consortium. Linkage and genome-wide association analysis of obesity-related phenotypes: association of weight with the MGAT1 gene. Obesity (Silver Spring) 2010; 18(4): 803-8.
[http://dx.doi.org/10.1038/oby.2009.359] [PMID: 19851299]

[96] Meyre D, Delplanque J, Chèvre JC, *et al.* Genome-wide association study for early-onset and morbid adult obesity identifies three new risk loci in European populations. Nat Genet 2009; 41(2): 157-9.
[http://dx.doi.org/10.1038/ng.301] [PMID: 19151714]

[97] Ioannidis JPA. Why most published research findings are false. PLoS Med 2005; 2(8): e124.
[http://dx.doi.org/10.1371/journal.pmed.0020124] [PMID: 16060722]

[98] Manolio TA. Bringing genome-wide association findings into clinical use. Nat Rev Genet 2013; 14(8): 549-58.
[http://dx.doi.org/10.1038/nrg3523] [PMID: 23835440]

[99] Yang J, Benyamin B, McEvoy BP, *et al.* Common SNPs explain a large proportion of the heritability for human height. Nat Genet 2010; 42(7): 565-9.
[http://dx.doi.org/10.1038/ng.608] [PMID: 20562875]

[100] Paré G, Asma S, Deng WQ. Contribution of large region joint associations to complex traits genetics. PLoS Genet 2015; 11(4): e1005103.
[http://dx.doi.org/10.1371/journal.pgen.1005103] [PMID: 25856144]

[101] Aschard H, Chen J, Cornelis MC, Chibnik LB, Karlson EW, Kraft P. Inclusion of gene-gene and gene-environment interactions unlikely to dramatically improve risk prediction for complex diseases. Am J Hum Genet 2012; 90(6): 962-72.
[http://dx.doi.org/10.1016/j.ajhg.2012.04.017] [PMID: 22633398]

[102] Buchner DA, Nadeau JH. Contrasting genetic architectures in different mouse reference populations used for studying complex traits. Genome Res 2015; 25(6): 775-91.
[http://dx.doi.org/10.1101/gr.187450.114] [PMID: 25953951]

[103] Wei WH, Hemani G, Haley CS. Detecting epistasis in human complex traits. Nat Rev Genet 2014; 15(11): 722-33.
[http://dx.doi.org/10.1038/nrg3747] [PMID: 25200660]

[104] Tam V, Patel N, Turcotte M, Bossé Y, Paré G, Meyre D. Benefits and limitations of genome-wide association studies. Nat Rev Genet 2019; 20(8): 467-84.
[http://dx.doi.org/10.1038/s41576-019-0127-1] [PMID: 31068683]

[105] Gallagher MD, Chen-Plotkin AS. The Post-GWAS Era: From Association to Function. Am J Hum Genet 2018; 102(5): 717-30.
[http://dx.doi.org/10.1016/j.ajhg.2018.04.002] [PMID: 29727686]

[106] Boyle EA, Li YI, Pritchard JK. An Expanded View of Complex Traits: From Polygenic to Omnigenic. Cell 2017; 169(7): 1177-86.
[http://dx.doi.org/10.1016/j.cell.2017.05.038] [PMID: 28622505]

CHAPTER 6

Regenerative Medicine

Hajra Qayyum[1,*] and **Syeda Marriam Bakhtiar**[1]

[1] *Department of Biosciences and Bioinformatics, Capital University of Science and Technology, Islamabad*

Abstract: Regenerative medicine (RM) is defined as a replacement and revival of human cells, tissues, or organs to reinstate or reconstruct their normal physiology. RM is regarded as a solution to provide healthy substitutes for a malfunctioning/failed organ or a tissue. It is emerging as the suitable substitute for organ transplantation. Transplantation seems impractical due to the limited availability of donors as significant disparities lie between the number of patients that require transplantation and the availability of organs from the donor, so there was a gap created. Therefore, to comply with these needs, RM has emerged as a new science to create biological replacements and exploit the body's ability of regeneration to recover and sustain normal function in diseased and damaged tissues. This chapter overviews RM in terms of adopted strategies, its clinical applications in organ engineering along with inherited challenges and their plausible solutions.

Keywords: Cell-therapy, Grafting, Organ engineering, Pluripotent stem cells, Regenerative medicine, Stem cell therapy, Tissue culturing.

1. INTRODUCTION

Regenerative medicine (RM) is described as a replacement and revival of human cells, tissues, or organs to reinstate or reconstruct their normal physiology [1]. The term "regenerative medicine" was first formulated by William Haseltine in 1999 to represent an interdisciplinary field that is an amalgam of apprehensions derived from various fields. These fields included tissue engineering, cell transplantation, stem cell biology, biomechanics prosthetics, nanotechnology, and biochemistry [1, 2].

Besides normalizing congenital anomalies, RM could be employed to repair or replace different body tissues and organs damaged by aging, ailment, or a shock. To date, promising preclinical and clinical results for the treatment of chronic

* **Corresponding author Hajra Qayyum:** Faculty of Health and Life Sciences, Capital University of Science and Technology, Islamabad, Pakistan; E-mail: hajraqayyum92@gmail.com

Syeda Marriam Bakhtiar and Erum Dilshad (Eds.)

disorders and acute injuries encourage the use of RM as an effective treatment option. It can also ameliorate ailments that can affect a multitude of organ systems and also provide support in case of dermal wounds, cardiovascular diseases and traumas, cancer, and many more.

Another treatment option that can provide the solution is the grafting of healthy organs and tissue to compensate for a malfunctioning/failed organ or a tissue. However, this option seems impractical due to the limited availability of donors as there remain significant disparities between the number of patients with diseased or damaged organs that require replacement and the availability of organs to be transplanted. As the lifespan of the population progresses and the number of new cases of organ failure rises, the supply/demand ratio for the organs intensifies. Sometimes the situation gets worsens because of serious immune complications, however, these challenges can theoretically be overcome by the application of RM strategies [3]. To comply with these needs, RM emerged as a new science to create biological replacements and exploit the body's ability of regeneration to recover and sustain normal function in diseased and damaged tissues [2].

2. APPROACHES TO RM

The field of RM involves a variety of approaches which comprises the use of materials and de novo produced cells and various other combinations to replace malfunctioning tissue, effectively replacing it structurally and functionally, or to promote the process of tissue healing. While adult humans have a limited regenerative ability in comparison to lower vertebrates, the body's innate healing response may also be used to encourage regeneration [2, 3]. Three strategies are widely adopted to pursue the aim of RM [1, 2]. These strategies are:

1. Cell-based therapy

2. Use of biomaterials

3. Scaffold implantation seeded with cells

2.1. Cell-based Therapy

All human cells are derived from the same origin *i.e.*, zygote. During development, these cells progressively differentiate into more specialized cells with specific cellular functions. This ability of differentiation possessed by cells is termed "cell potency". Cell-based therapies exploit this cellular property of potency. It involves injecting novel and healthy cells into pathological tissues. The injected cells are either the pre-differentiated or the undifferentiated stem cells which can later get differentiated depending upon the underlying circumstances [1].

The pre-differentiated cells are extracted by the patient's specific tissues as they are ready to implant just by expansion. However, it is difficult to get a substantial number of these cells in vitro or *in vivo* as they lose the usual microenvironment required for proliferation. Hence, these cells are less likely to be utilized in the future even when they do not associate with rejection and noticeable inflammatory responses [1]. On the other hand, Stem Cells (SC) can proliferate extensively, with the ability of self-renewal while they keep their undifferentiated state until they are induced to differentiate into a specific cell type. SCs are divided into various types such as autologous, allogenic, and xenogeneic depending upon the source of their origin [1].

2.1.1. Adult Stem Cells

In case of histological injuries, adult stem cells (ASCs) are derived from the tissues of an adult human body, which then perform corrective functions, restoring normal tissue functioning. Among these cells, mesenchymal stem cells (MSCs) are of special importance as they have the potential to get differentiated into other cell types that are particularly required for the amelioration of ailments related to bone, cartilage, nerves, muscles, cardiovascular, blood, and gastrointestinal [1].

2.1.2. Pluripotent Stem Cell-Based Cell Therapies

Pluripotent Stem Cells (PSCs) have the potential of infinite proliferation and getting differentiated into the cells of the three germ layers. With these two attributes, PSCs become the most suitable source for cell therapies in case of different diseases and injuries. Two types of human PSCs are in clinical use: embryonic stem cells (ESCs) and induced pluripotent stem cells (iPSCs) [4].

2.1.2.1. Embryonic Stem Cells

These cells are derived from the inner most cell of an embryo during the blastocyst stage and can proliferate extensively. ESCs keep their pluripotent state intact until they are induced to get differentiate into any of the three embryogenic germ layers. Human ESCs are usually extracted from a surplus of embryos during in-vitro fertilization. Another approach to extract ESCs could be therapeutic cloning or somatic cell nuclear transfer (SCNT) which includes the transferal of the somatic cell nucleus into an oocyte [1]. Lastly, SCs can also be obtained from amniotic fluid or placenta via the process of amniocentesis. Such cells are known as amniotic fluid stem cells (AFSCs). Human ESCs have two concerns from the clinical usage point of view, the first one is the ethical issue regarding the usage of the human embryo and the other one is immune rejection after transplantation. To address these concerns, attempts are being made to produce human ESCs from a patient's own somatic cell by the nuclear transfer but such production remains technically challenged [4].

2.1.2.2. Induced Pluripotent Stem Cells

Another strategy to get analogous stem cells is through reprogramming of adult cells to get induced pluripotent stem cells (iPSCs) [1]. Induced pluripotent stem cells (iPSCs) are described as "embryonic stem-cells like" cells acquired by the reprogramming of adult somatic cells by introducing pluripotent associated genes. iPSCs have cell potency equal to ESCs and they can replace them. Moreover, similar to ESCs, iPSCs can also give rise to the three of the germ cell layers known as endoderm, mesoderm, and ectoderm [5].

2.2. Biomaterials

Biomaterials are described as any natural or synthetic substances that incorporate or integrate with the tissues of a patient during treatment. The ideal biomaterial should possess the properties of being inert, sterile, non-carcinogenic, mechanically durable, induce no inflammatory or immune response, be affordable, simple to use, and resistant to alteration by bodily tissues. They are synthesized with an objective to fulfill, complement, or replace a natural function that has been diminished or lost [2].

In cell-based tissue engineering, cells are seeded onto a scaffold made of an appropriate biomaterial. Biomaterials used in tissue engineering mimic the biological and mechanical functions of the body's native extracellular matrix (ECM) by acting as an artificial ECM. Biomaterials provide a three-dimensional space for cells to organize into new tissues with proper structure and function, and they can also allow for the transport of cells and bioactive substances (*e.g.*, cell adhesion peptides, growth factors) to specific areas in the body. Because the majority of mammalian cells are anchorage-dependent and would die in the absence of an adhesion substrate, biomaterials serve the purpose. Biomaterials also provide mechanical support against in-vivo stresses, ensuring that the pre-defined 3-dimensional structure of the tissue is preserved during development [3].

In general, three types of biomaterials have been used to engineer tissues and organs: naturally derived materials like collagen and alginate; a-cellular tissue matrices like bladder submucosa and small intestine submucosa; and synthetic polymers like polyglycolic acid (PGA), polylactic acid (PLA), and poly lactic-c-

-glycolic acid (PLGA). Although naturally derived materials and a-cellular tissue matrices have the potential advantage of biological recognition, synthetic polymers can be made reproducibly on a wide scale with regulated strength, degradation rate, and microstructures.

Recently, regenerative medicine research has concentrated on the utilization of acellular matrices and synthetic materials. Acellular tissue matrices are collagen-rich matrices created by eliminating cellular components from tissues. The matrices are frequently created by mechanical and chemical treatment of a tissue section. After implantation, the matrices breakdown slowly and are replaced and reshaped by ECM proteins generated and secreted by transplanted or ingrowing cells. Acellular tissue matrices have been shown to enable cell ingrowth and regeneration of genitourinary tissues, including the urethra and bladder, with no signs of immunogenic rejection [6].

Polyesters derived from naturally occurring alpha-hydroxy acids, including PGA, PLA, and PLGA, are commonly employed in regenerative medicine. These polymers have received FDA approval for human use in a range of applications, including sutures. PGA, PLA, and PLGA degradation products are non-toxic, natural metabolites that are removed from the body in the form of carbon dioxide and water. Because these polymers are thermoplastic, they may be easily molded into a three-dimensional scaffold with the required microstructure, gross shape, and size using a variety of processes. Electro-spinning has been used to rapidly produce very porous scaffolds in a variety of configurations. One disadvantage of synthetic polymers is their lack of biological recognition, while several organizations are working on developing synthetic scaffolds that integrate proteins or other molecules to aid with recognition [7].

2.3. Implantation of Scaffold Seeded with Cells

This approach refers to the integration of the above-discussed two approaches. One application of this strategy is the realization of bio-artificial liver attained through the process of decellularization. It involves the elimination of liver cells maintaining the structural and functional characteristics of vascular networks, permitting organ perfusion. Later, adult hepatocytes recognize the liver matrix and support physiological functions, like albumin excretion and urea synthesis. This approach paves the way for the treatment of end-stage liver diseases [1] as depicted in Fig. (**6.1**).

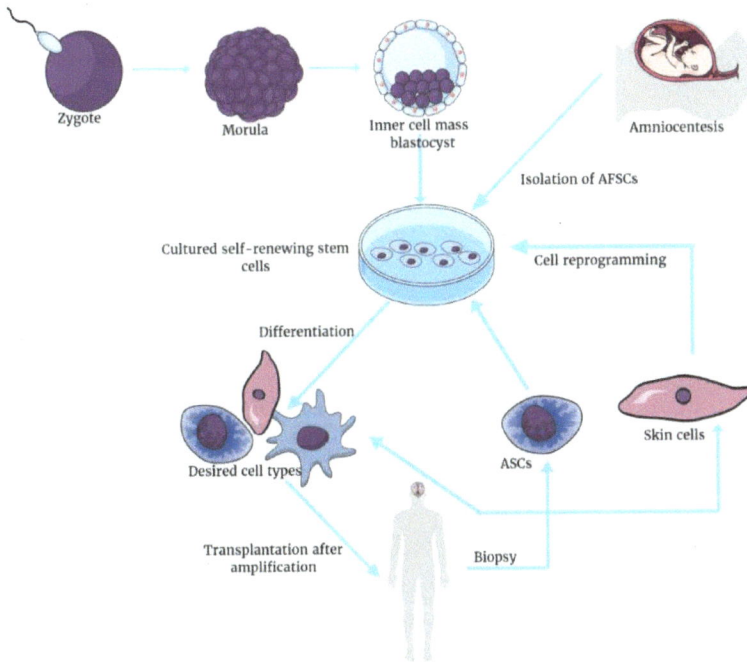

Fig. (6.1). Approaches and strategies adopted for the derivation of stem cells.

3. CLINICAL APPLICATIONS (CASE STUDIES)

Limited availability of tissue and organ has been identified as a major public health issue, due to which only a meager fraction of needy patients receive transplants. Most waiting lists for transplants do not accurately reflect the depth of the crisis because only the sick seeks such assistance. The capacity and ability to regenerate and replace damaged tissues and organs underpins the promise of regenerative medicine. Regenerative medicine has demonstrated remarkable outcomes for the regeneration and replacement of many tissues and organs such as the skin, heart, kidney, and liver, as well as the ability to fix some congenital flaws. The traditional dependence on donated tissues and organs for transplantation faces donor shortages as well as the possibility of immunological rejection of the donated body parts [8]. Some organ transplants practiced in impoverished countries suffer from transplant tourism, in which foreigners with adequate money and influence are given preference over the local population [9]. Such tactics have been denounced since they can lead to the exploitation of vulnerable persons. Despite differences in national economic strength, and hence variations in healthcare infrastructure, alleviating constraints such as a scarcity of organs and the practical challenges of collecting and storing them might increase the number of people who can receive organ transplants. As a result, techniques and technology to boost the supply of tissues and organs for transplantation must be further developed. In most circumstances, such as when people are injured in car accidents, conflicts, or natural catastrophes, tissues and organs are needed instantly for transplantation [7]. The shortage of tissues and organs not only impedes patient care but also a scientific study. The production of an infinite supply of tissues and organs is thus the most difficult task of our generation. Many initiatives have been launched to encourage organ donations and improve the utilization of donated organs. The development of laboratory-grown tissues, humanized animal organs, and bio-artificial organs is one solution. Some of these issues addressed via RM are discussed below (also see Fig. **6.2**) [3].

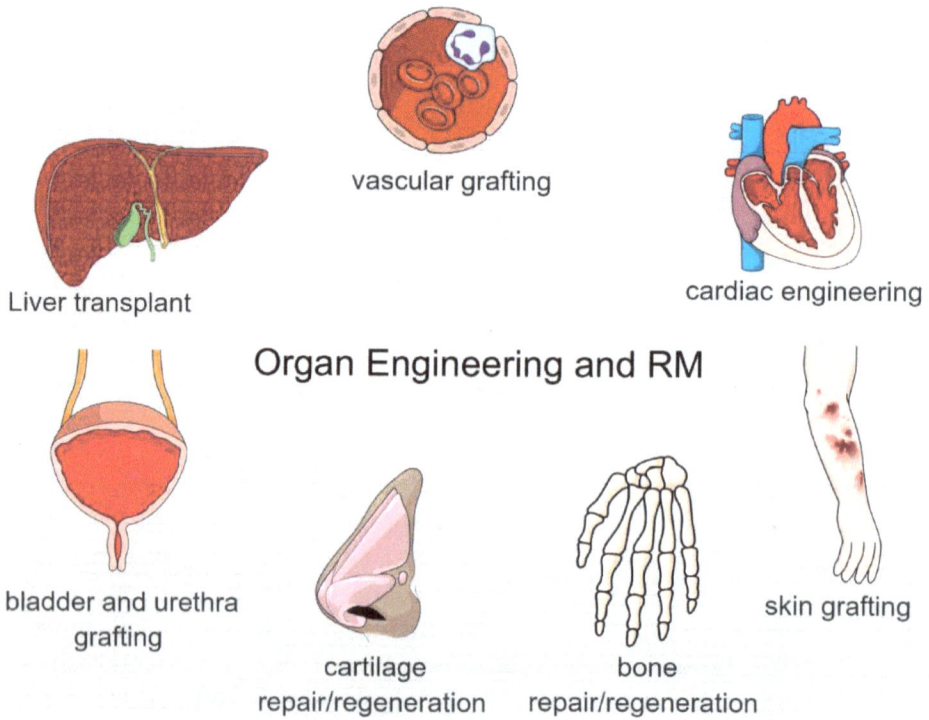

Fig. (6.2). Clinical applications of regenerative medicine in organ engineering.

3.1. Bladder and Urethra

Bladder and urethra tissues are crafted and successfully transplanted in individuals with urethral stenosis. In this case, urothelial and muscle cells are obtained by biopsy and are cultured and seeded on a biodegradable scaffold of bladder-shape after the eight weeks of initial biopsy [7]. The scaffold is then anastomosed to the stump of the native bladders with omental coverage promoting angiogenesis [10]. Clinical trials of urethral regeneration have remained successful for both animal and human beings. Woven meshes of PGA, both without or with cells, have been tested in several animal models and have been proven to restore urethras [7, 9]. Non seeded scaffolds can restore small lengths (less than 1 cm) of urethral defects; whereas cell-seeded scaffolds can successfully repair extremely big defects (up to 30 cm) to prevent the risk of stenosis and urethral stricture formation [2].

3.2. Blood Vessels

Tissue-engineered vascular grafts were created in dog and sheep models using biodegradable scaffolds seeded with autologous cells [9]. The clinical implication of this approach initiated with autologous scaffolds that were designed to replace stenosed pulmonary arteries. The success of such designed scaffolds was associated with no indication of graft blockage even months after the grafting [2, 7].

3.3. Heart

For the treatment of damaged cardiac issues through cell therapy, different types of stem cells have continuously been tested with an aim to inject them into the affected area of human heart rather than utilizing invasive surgical options. In fact, inoculation method is unsuccessful due to the risk of cell loss and absence of cell-engraftment. To repair damaged sections, newer procedures involve the use of tailored patches implanted with cells [7]. These strategies may be promising, but more research is required. Bioengineered hearts could be ideal in cases of heart failure [11]. Ott *et al.* built the first novel heart out of de-cellularized cadaveric hearts by planting the cardiac cells in a bioreactor system that was able to mimic all the required physiological conditions [9]. The designed system successfully mimicked the pumping activity of a normal heart, thus giving a new direction to the clinical research [2].

3.4. Liver

Usually in case of liver failures, cell transplantation comes as an alternate treatment to conventional transplantation. This option is supported by the underlying extraordinary regeneration potential of liver cells in an *in vivo* setting

[9]. Several methods for growing liver cells have been proposed, including identifying growth factors to promote cell proliferation, using a customized medium, and cultivating scaffolds within particular bioreactors. Perfusion decellularization has been used in recent years to grow stem cells and mature hepatocytes into the decellularized liver being tested in several animal models [2].

3.5. Skin

Skin regeneration remains a challenging process, but it holds the promise of effective treatment for injured and burned patients [12]. Generally, skin regeneration occurs through the differentiation of stem cells within the epidermis and the hair follicle. Stem cells can differentiate into keratinocytes, providing a novel perspective on the repair of many skin diseases such as severe burns, chronic leg ulcers, skin cancer, alopecia, and acne. The continuous advancement of iPS cell reprogramming technology offers a realistic method for replacing massive volumes of damaged skin with autologous cells. In contrast, the efficiency of iPS production was recently reported to be significantly increased when keratinocytes were used instead of fibroblasts [2].

3.6. Bone

Advancements in the domain of stem cell research have resulted in the evolution of cell-based treatments for repairing bone and related metabolic disorders. Despite all the advancements in orthopedic surgery, some fractures may not get healed adequately, yielding delayed union or nonunion, a longer hospital stay, and high expense [11]. Cell-based treatment for fracture healing in nonunion cases is increasingly gaining popularity. Autologous bone marrow-derived pluripotent mesenchymal stem cells (MSCs) are seeded onto 100 percent hydroxyapatite macro-porous ceramic scaffolds and utilized to treat four patients with tibia, humerus, and ulna fractures with diaphyseal segmental anomalies [2].

3.7. Cartilage Tissue

Repair and regeneration of cartilage, such as ear and joint cartilage, are nevertheless connected with limits and varying degrees of effectiveness [12]. RM proposes a new technique to build synthetic cartilage substitutes that can mimic both the physiology and anatomy of natural ears. Engineered cartilage structures could replace wounded tissues by combining appropriate cell sources with scaffolds [12].

In the treatment of knee articular cartilage defects, autologous chondrocyte implantation (ACI) has also demonstrated encouraging clinical results. Several case studies reflect positive efficacy regarding post-operative follow-up for more than ten years. By 2003, ACI had been done on over 15,000 patients worldwide, and it is now regarded as first-line therapy for anomalies larger than 2cm^2. Cultured MSCs from bone marrow have also been employed in experiments to mend injured intervertebral discs [8]. MSCs are isolated from each patient's ilium and cultured in an autogenous serum-containing medium. The collagen sponge infused with autologous MSCs is subsequently percutaneously implanted into degenerative intervertebral discs. Within two years of surgery, both patients' radiographs and computed tomography show improvements with reduced symptoms [2].

4. CHALLENGES AND FUTURE PERSPECTIVES

Despite the significant success of SCs in animal models, there still lie numerous roadblocks on the way to the clinical application of PSCs. These limitations are as follow:

4.1. Lack of Robust Lineage-Specific Differentiation Protocols

Another significant limitation is the lack of robust lineage-specific differentiation protocols for producing large numbers of purified and matured iPSC-differentiated cells. More fundamental research on reprogramming technology is required for the development of novel protocols for the production of standardized human iPSC [13]. The microRNA switch, a more recent biotechnology, is expected to facilitate the maturation and purification of iPSC differentiated cells while also reducing clonal variation. While we wait for these limitations to be overcome, it is prudent to bank iPSCs from patients suffering from specific diseases [5].

4.2. Tumorigenicity

It is due to the property of infinite proliferation of iPSCs that provides us with the multitude of human cells for transplantation. If such cells continue to proliferate in an undifferentiated state even after the transplantation, it can lead to the formation of tumors [4]. This tumorgenicity could result from the retention of undifferentiated/ immature cells in the final product, retention of activated reprogramming factors in iPSCs, or the genetic mutations that arose during cell culturing [14]. iPSCs can also become the source of teratomas and malignant tumors such as neuroblastoma and follicular carcinoma if the transplanted organ gets contaminated with undifferentiated iPSCs. Though the protocols of iPSC extraction are continuously getting optimized, the risk of contamination stills remains a big hurdle. In this regard, integration of the fine-tuned assays with "omic" approaches customized as per the genetic makeup of every individual could be seen as the only solution [10].

4.3. Immune Rejection

Undifferentiated iPSCs have been reported to elicit immune rejection even in syngeneic recipients however, differentiated iPSCs do not [4]. This observation implies that differentiated iPSCs are less immunogenic when compared with undifferentiated cells. However, immune rejection differs among various cell types such as autologous iPSC-derived retinal epithelial cells showed no immunogenic rejection when transplanted in one of the patients with muscular degeneration [15]. In some cases, allogeneic cell therapy requires immunosuppression, consistent use of which can cause higher risks of kidney failures, inflammations, and tumors. In such cases, strategies such as inactivation of major histocompatibility complex (MHC) class I and II and overexpression of CD47 in iPSCs should be adopted to evade the immune rejection especially when it comes to mismatched allogeneic recipients [16].

4.4. Heterogeneity

The heterogeneous nature of the cell population and the differentiation potential of iPSCs are significant limitations. Though PSCs are pluripotent and can proliferate indefinitely, all PSC cell lines are not homogeneous and differ in morphology, growth rate, and their tendency to differentiate into several cell lineages. Heterogeneity has been reported in both human ESCs and iPSCs and has genetic and epigenetic causes (Fig. **6.3**). There is a vivid difference in the expression levels of lineages specific genes among various cell lines. The variation could be the consequence of genetic as well as the epigenetic factors and can make different lines suitable for different purposes such as some are ideal for pancreatic differentiation and some for cardiomyocyte generation [4]. This heterogeneity can evolve within a cell-lineage during the long-term culturing, especially when PSC cell-line is yielded from a single cell [17]. To reduce this difference, protocols for the detection, reduction and monitoring of heterogeneity trials including human PSCs need to be established. Because the CRISPR-Cas9 system can improve the disease phenotype of differentiated cells, it is hoped that it can be used to address this limitation [18].

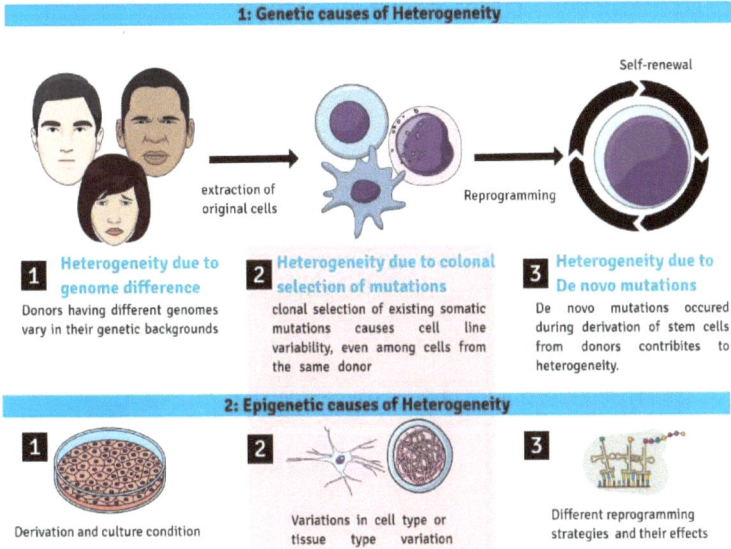

Fig. (6.3). Causes of heterogeneity in PSCs.

CONCLUDING REMARKS

RM has proved itself to be an unprecedented option in clinical settings but its potential is yet to be fully exploited. It is still facing multiple challenges which require more time and efforts before RM can operate at its full. One critical factor is heterogeneity which is decreasing the reproducibility of the research. On the other hand, eliminating complete heterogeneity can lead to elimination of pluripotency as well. Immune rejection and tumorigenicity are also affecting its effectiveness and need to be taken into account. Furthermore, adopted strategies for derivation of the PSCs also need to be optimized. All the limitations must be taken into account by the researchers and clinicians before planning their study and using RM as a treatment option.

CONSENT FOR PUBLICATION

Not applicable.

CONFLICT OF INTEREST

The authors declare no conflict of interest, financial or otherwise.

ACKNOWLEDGEMENTS

Declared none.

REFERENCES

[1]   Sampogna G, Guraya SY, Forgione A. Regenerative medicine: Historical roots and potential strategies in modern medicine. J Microsc Ultrastruct 2015; 3(3): 101-7.
[http://dx.doi.org/10.1016/j.jmau.2015.05.002] [PMID: 30023189]

[2]   Bioengineer J, Sci B, Badra S, Williams JK, Carolina N. Bioengineering. Biomed Sci 2012.
[http://dx.doi.org/10.4172/2155-9538.S2-008]

[3]   Mao AS, Mooney DJ. Regenerative medicine : Current therapies and future directions 2015; vol. 112: p. 47.
[http://dx.doi.org/10.1073/pnas.1508520112]

[4]   Yamanaka S. Pluripotent Stem Cell-Based Cell Therapy—Promise and Challenges. Cell Stem Cell 2020; 27(4): 523-31.
[http://dx.doi.org/10.1016/j.stem.2020.09.014] [PMID: 33007237]

[5]   Omole AE, Omotuyi A, Fakoya J. Ten years of progress and promise of induced pluripotent stem cells : historical origins , characteristics , mechanisms , limitations , and potential applications 2018; pp. 1-47.
[http://dx.doi.org/10.7717/peerj.4370]

[6]   Dzobo K, *et al.* Review article advances in regenerative medicine and tissue engineering. Innovation and Transformation of Medicine 2018; 2018.
[http://dx.doi.org/10.1155/2018/2495848] [PMID: 30154861]

[7]   Atala A, Forest W, Medicine R. Regenerative medicine strategies. J Pediatr Surg 2012; 47(1): 17-28.
[http://dx.doi.org/10.1016/j.jpedsurg.2011.10.013] [PMID: 22244387]

[8]   Jessop ZM, Al-sabah A, Francis WR, Whitaker IS. Transforming healthcare through regenerative medicine 2020; pp. 1-6.
[http://dx.doi.org/10.1186/s12916-016-0669-4]

[9]   Colombo F, Sampogna G, Cocozza G, Guraya SY, Forgione A. Ac ce pt cr t. J Microsc Ultrastruct 2016.
[http://dx.doi.org/10.1016/j.jmau.2016.05.002] [PMID: 30023231]

[10]   Karanika S, Karantanos T, Li L, Corn P G, Timothy C. and Therapeutic Implications 2015; vol. 34(22): 2815-22.

[11]   Stoltz J, *et al.* Stem Cells and Regenerative Medicine : Myth or Reality of the 21th Century 2015.

[12]   Han F, Wang J, Ding L, *et al.* Tissue Engineering and Regenerative Medicine: Achievements, Future, and Sustainability in Asia. Front Bioeng Biotechnol 2020; 8(March): 83.
[http://dx.doi.org/10.3389/fbioe.2020.00083] [PMID: 32266221]

[13]   Abo-al-ela HG. Research in Veterinary Science Regenerative medicine : Current and future hypothetical research directions. Res Vet Sci 2020; 135: 555-6.
[http://dx.doi.org/10.1016/j.rvsc.2020.11.004]

[14]   Scho H, Edge L. Conversations iPS Cells 10 Years Later 2016.
[http://dx.doi.org/10.1016/j.cell.2016.08.043]

[15]   Rose LF, Wolf EJ, Brindle T, *et al.* The convergence of regenerative medicine and rehabilitation: federal perspectives. NPJ Regen Med 2018; 3(1): 19.
[http://dx.doi.org/10.1038/s41536-018-0056-1] [PMID: 30323950]

[16]   Doss M X, Sachinidis A. cells Current Challenges of iPSC-Based Disease Modeling and Therapeutic

Implications.
[http://dx.doi.org/10.3390/cells8050403]

[17]   European Academies Science Advisory Council (EASAC), and (EASAC), Challenges and potential in regenerative medicine. 2020.

[18]   Hayashi Y, Ohnuma K, Furue MK. Pluripotent Stem Cell Heterogeneity. Adv Exp Med Biol 2019; 1123: 71-94.
[http://dx.doi.org/10.1007/978-3-030-11096-3_6] [PMID: 31016596]

CHAPTER 7

Emerging OMICS and Genetic Disease

Muhammad Jawad Hassan[1,*], **Muhammad Faheem**[1] and **Sabba Mehmood**[1]

[1] *Department of Biological Sciences, National University of Medical Sciences, Rawalpindi, Pakistan*

Abstract: Multiomics also described as integrative omics is an analytical approach that combines data from multiple 'omics' approaches including genomics, transcriptomics, proteomics, metabolomics, epigenomics, metagenomics and Meta transcriptomics to answer the complex biological processes involved in rare genetic disorders. This omics approach is particularly helpful since it identifies biomarkers of disease progression and treatment progress by collective characterization and quantification of pools of biological molecules within and among the various types of cells to better understand and categorize the Mendelian and non- Mendelian forms of rare diseases. As compared to studies of a single omics type, multi-omics offers the opportunity to understand the flow of information that underlies the disease. A range of omics software and databases, for example WikiPathways, MixOmics, MONGKIE, GalaxyP, GalaxyM, CrossPlatform Commander, and iCluster are used for multi-omics data exploration and integration in rare disease analysis. Recent advances in the field of genetics and translational research have opened new treatment avenues for patients. The innovation in the next generation sequencing and RNA sequencing has improved the ability from diagnostics to detection of molecular alterations like gene mutations in specific disease types. In this chapter, we provide an overview of such omics technologies and focus on methods for their integration across multiple omics layers. The scrupulous understanding of rare genetic disorders and their treatment at the molecular level led to the concept of a personalized approach, which is one of the most significant advancements in modern research which enable researchers to better comprehend the flow of knowledge which underpins genetic diseases.

Keywords: Genomics, Metabolomics, Multiomics, Proteomics.

1. INTRODUCTION TO OMICS AND GENETIC DISEASE

Rare diseases do not mean very "rare" as 8000 types of rare diseases have been described. An estimated 262.9–446.2 million people are living with a rare disease globally (Global Genes. RARE Diseases: Facts and Statistics [Available: https://globalgenes.org/rare-diseases-facts-statistics/). Rare disease classification

---

[*] **Corresponding author Muhammad Jawad Hassan:** Department of Biological Sciences, National University of Medical Sciences, Rawalpindi, Pakistan; E-mail: jawad.hassan@numspak.edu.pk

Syeda Marriam Bakhtiar and Erum Dilshad (Eds.)

and definition vary globally; in Europe, it is any disease with an incidence of less than one in 2000 (RARE DISEASES - a major unmet medical need. Luxembourg: European Commission, 2017), in the United States (US), they are conditions affecting fewer than 200,000 people (Global Genes. RARE Diseases: Facts and Statistics- Available at: https://globalgenes.org/rare-diseases-facts-statistics/], and in China, they define it as a disorder prevalent in less than one in 500,000 within the population [1]. Numerous common issues faced by patients ranked under the 'rare' umbrella. However, the problems faced by patients and the disease burden imposed on the country's population remain the same, as obtaining a diagnosis, suitable medical care and access to support services is always a great challenge for patients with a rare disease. Next-generation sequencing techniques have increased the chances of identification of causative mutation in these patients as compared to single gene testing alone, with a significant increase in diagnostic rates, and it is believed that "integrated multi-omic analysis" may further increase this diagnostic yield. On the other hand, "multi-omic" approach aids the explanation of genotypic and phenotypic heterogeneity, which is not possible with single omic analyses.

2. ADVANCED TECHNIQUES IN "OMICS"

The recent advancement in technology has revolutionized many fields of research. "OMICS" study that includes genomics, transcriptomics, metabolomics and proteomics, has also gained the attention with potential to analyse the molecular data at a higher pace. The adopted advanced high-throughput techniques for "OMICS" data are now often incorporated in the routine biological research. The newly advanced techniques help us to analyse and generate tera- to penta-bytes data files on a routine basis. These big-datasets lead to the understanding of biological systems and solving biological question. In this chapter, we are discussing the applications of these techniques in different biological research.

2.1. Emerging Omics Techniques: Genomics and Transcriptomics

2.1.1. Genomics

The first discipline of OMICS that appears at first is genomics, which deals with the study of entire genomes unlike genetics which focuses on single genes or individual variants. Genomics has been utilized in different facets of research and clinical applications which range from diagnostics, pharmaceuticals, pharmacogenomics, disease prevention, gene therapy, and developmental biology to comparative and evolutionary genomics. The Whole Genome Sequencing (WGS) data generation initiated with the Human Genome project (HGP), which was initiated in 1990 and completed in 2003. With time, the genome sequencing technology has evolved which transformed the DNA sequencing industry. During the start of the 21st century, completion of WGS of a single haploid human genome took many years with spending of more than 3 billion dollars [2]. The advancement in the sequencing technology over the period of time has improved. These days, WGS is as cheap as a few thousand dollars with some days of work. Advance NEXT Generation Sequencing (NGS) techniques like nanopore (*e.g.* MinION), SMRT (single molecule real-time; *e.g.* sequel system) and Semiconductor (*e.g.* Ion S5 sequencer) are the keys for reducing the cost and time [3 - 5].

Unlike the traditional Sanger sequencing technology, the NGS methods are more popular and in use these days. The most frequently used NGS to date is sequencing by synthesis (SBS) method. These methods utilize a solid support which contains micro wells where the sequencing reactions occur. The individual DNA molecules which have to be sequenced are distributed in these micro wells or linked to a solid support. The DNA fragment sequence is identified while its complementary strand is being synthesized, thus, each of the sequenced DNA fragment serves as a template. The nucleotides in the reaction are labelled or upon incorporation identified *via* chemical reaction, which can be detected or imaged.

Roche 454 pyro sequencing was the first SBS based NGS technology developed in 1996 that was introduced in the market (1999) for genomics purposes. This technology was based on the detection of pyrophosphate (PPi) as a by-product upon insertion of a nucleotide. The PPi released is converted into ATP by the enzyme present in the reaction. This ATP is utilized as a substrate by luciferase-catalysed reaction to emit light [6]. The 454-sequencing technology was generally utilized for genomics especially metagenomics samples, since it has long read lengths of up to 600-800 nt which typically can be achieved with high throughput of 25 million bases with 99% or more accuracy in a 4 hrs reaction run, thus facilitating genome assembly.

Since, there are multiple complicated steps involved, so there are error chances while reading homopolymer sequences longer than 6bp, thus, pyrosequencing was replaced by Illumina sequencing which has become industrial standard. Illumina sequencing also supports a range of procedures which include exome and targeted sequencing, genomic sequencing, metagenomics, Chromatin immunoprecipitation sequencing and RNA sequencing. Illumina technology was first established by Solexa and Lynx Therapeutics. In this technique, genome is chopped into DNA fragments, and combined with designed adapters (forked adapters) at the both ends of DNA fragments [7]. This technique sequencing is known as "bridge amplification" wherein the DNA fragments have a length of about 500bp ligated with adapters. The adapters are linked on a solid support (Flow cell) where the amplification takes place by incorporation of dyed-nucleotides which are imaged to record the sequence [8]. There are repetitive rounds of amplification to produce clonal "clusters" consisting of around 1000 copies of each oligonucleotide fragment. Each glass slide supports millions of such similar cluster reactions. The dyed-nucleotides similarly function as terminators of synthesis in every reaction that are cleared post detection for the next synthesis round. Fluorescent detection in illumina increases the speed of detection due to direct imaging, in comparison to camera-based imaging [8].

Ion Torrent™ is another SBS technique used in genomics sold by Thermo-Fisher. This technique converts directly the nucleotide sequence in the digital data on a semiconductor chip [3]. In the DNA synthesis reaction, once an accurate nucleotide is inserted in the DNA growing chain, a hydrogen ion is discharged, which alters the pH. Such pH fluctuation causes the voltage change which is recorded by the ion sensor. In the reaction cell, each of four nucleotides is passed at a time, and voltage change is recorded on the incorporation of appropriate nucleotide.

PacBio sequencing which is also known as SMRT (Single Molecule Real Time) sequencing, allows big fragments to be sequenced ranging from 30-50 kb or even longer. The SMRT technology includes a DNA polymerase with bound DNA (to be sequenced) at the bottom of a well (zero-mode waveguide (ZMV) in SMRT flow cell). The light energy is guided by ZMV chamber, and when a labelled nucleotide (phospho-linked fluorophore) is incorporated in the growing DNA, different fluorescence is recorded for each nucleotide. The latest PacBio instrument (the Sequel) carries 1million of ZMVs which can generate around ~ 365,000 reads (average read 10-15kb and 7.6 Gb of output) [9].

2.1.2. Transcriptomics

Omics that deals with the entire set of ribonucleic acids (RNA) transcripts (Transcriptome) in a cell is known as transcriptomics [10]. The initial efforts to study transcriptome started in early 1990s, with time the technology has advanced since late 1990s when transcriptomics became very familiar discipline. There are various technological advances that have transformed the discipline. There are two main existing techniques in transcriptomics: Microarrays, that quantify RNAs which are already determined, and RNA sequencing, that use high-throughput sequencing that capture all the sequences.

Over the time, many microarrays were developed that cover identified genes in both model and organisms. Technological advancement also uplifted the design and manufacturing of microarrays which has improved the specificity of probes with capability to test many genes in a single array. Innovations in the fluorescence detected improved sensitivity and measuring accuracy for low abundance transcripts [11, 12].

RNA sequencing (RNA-seq) allows to quantify the whole RNA expression profile of a sample. In RNA-seq, the isolated RNAs are first amplified into complementary DNA (cDNA). The cDNA molecules are then fragmented and added with adapter at both ends and then sequenced in parallel fashion. The short reads are then assembled and aligned to reconstruct the RNA sequences based on overlapped sequences of the short reads. The reconstruction is an easy process based on the availability of a reference genome [13]. Though, RNA-seq can also be performed with no reference genome, which is known as "*de novo* RNA-seq". The RNA-seq also measures the levels of RNA expression more precisely than the microarray technology [13].

Unlike DNA, which has a fixed number of genes, the quantity of RNAs varies in cell types. Therefore, RNA sequencing aims to not only identify but moreover quantify the transcripts in the samples. Whereas, there have been obstacles in accurate measurement of the RNAs quantity in the desired sample. Different technologies that are used for RNA-seq are 454 (Roche), SOLiD (Thermo Fisher Scientific), Illumina, PacBio and Ion Torrent (Thermo Fisher Scientific). The typical read length for these technologies varies as Illumina (50-300bp), 454 (700bp), Ion Torrent (400bp), SOLiD (50bp) and PacBio (10,000bp).

2.2. Emerging Omics Techniques: Proteomics and Metabolomics

2.2.1. Proteomics

Proteomics aims at the global study of proteins which are made-up of merely 22 genetically-encoded amino acids. Proteome is the complete set of proteins carried by an organism. Proteomics not only deals with the total protein number but also their functional and structural aspects as well. This approach facilitates to comprehend the complex nature of an organism. Currently, proteomics techniques allow a large-scale, high throughput identification, detection, and functional studies of proteome. Proteomics is practically complex because it involves analysis and classification of total protein signature of a genome.

Unlike genomics, proteomics is more complex as its level of expression varies. Its expression is not only dependent on the respective mRNA levels but also on translational regulation and control. Therefore, the proteomics data is considered authentic for characterization of a biological system [14]. Techniques which are utilized in proteomics can be overviewed based on the purpose of the analysis that includes, purification techniques, analytical techniques, characterization, structural analysis, and quantification and sequence analysis.

The conventional protein purification techniques are chromatographic approaches. Three of the most commonly used chromatographic techniques are Ion Exchange Chromatography (IEC), affinity chromatography and Size Exclusion Chromatography (SEC). IEC is the purification tool which separates proteins based on their net charge carried by its amino acids. Based on the comparative net charge, proteins are separated using different charged mediums [15]. Affinity chromatography uses a reversible interaction between the proteins to be purified and ligand of the chromatographic matrix [16]. SEC separates proteins based on their molecular size. Proteins are applied to pass through a porous carrier medium with distinct size porosity, based on permeation; proteins get separated according to their sizes [17].

Most commonly used analytical techniques in proteomic studies are ELISA, western blot and protein microarrays. Enzyme-linked immunosorbent assay (ELISA) is a highly delicate technique and broadly used in diagnostics. This assay uses antibodies or antigen linked to a solid support and an enzyme-conjugated antibody is used for detection. The enzyme activity is measured to detect the corresponding antibody or antigen in the sample under investigation [18]. Western blot is another analytical technique used for the detection of low abundance of proteins. This technique separates proteins using electrophoresis; proteins are transferred to a nitrocellulose membrane and precise detection is performed with enzyme-linked antibodies [19]. Protein microarray is a high-throughput technique to detect proteins at a large scale, their activities, interactions and function. This technique uses a glass slide, beads or membrane to immobilize the proteins and detect them with probes [20].

The techniques utilized in proteomics for proteins characterization are gel-based approaches and mass spectrometry. Sodium dodecyl sulphate-polyacrylamide gel electrophoresis (SDS-PAGE) is a common protein resolving technique. This technique separates protein on the basis of their sizes that facilitates the molecular weight approximation. During SDS-PAGE, proteins are denatured and SDS gives a positive charge to protein masking their intrinsic charges. In a constant electric field, SDS-interacting proteins will migrate towards the anode and each with a different speed which is dependent on their mass. This allows proteins to separate on a gel based on their masses [21]. Two-dimensional gel electrophoresis (2D-PAGE) which is another gel-based technique that separates proteins based on their charge and mass. Proteins are separated based on their charges in the first dimension and the second dimension is used to separate on the basis of their mass [22].

Mass-spectrometry (MS) is a potent analytical technique which is used for quantification of known and identify unknown samples under investigation. The detection process in MS involves ionization of the sample followed by separation of ions based on the m/z ratio in the presence of magnetic or electric fields and finally detection of the ions with a particular m/z value [23]. Edman sequencing is a technique used to determine the sequence of amino acids in proteins. It was established by Pehr Edman in 1950. This method relies on chemical reactions which eliminate and identify amino acids which are present at N-terminal of polypeptide chain of protein. Edman sequencing has a significant role in the development of therapeutic proteins as well as quality assurance in biopharmaceutics [24].

Quantitative techniques ICAT, SILAC and iTRAQ are advanced methods for proteomics quantification. The ICAT is a method that uses isotopic labelling where chemical labelling reagents are utilized for proteins quantification. ICAT has increased the proteins range which can be analysed and allows sequence identification and precise quantification of proteins from a complex mixture. ICAT reagents include affinity tags for labelled isotopes isolation, reactive groups and isotopically coded linker [25]. Stable Isotopic Labeling with Amino Acids in Cell Culture (SILAC) is a MS-based method for quantitative proteomics which relies on labelling of entire cellular proteome. The metabolic labelling with "light" or "heavy" form of amino acids is performed during cell culture, which are identified by MS. A variety of studies are facilitated *via* SILAC which include gene expression, post-translational modifications and cellular signalling [26]. Isobaric tag for relative and absolute quantitation (iTRAQ) is a multiplex protein labeling approach used for quantitative proteomics based on tandem MS. This method is based on protein labeling with isobaric tags (4-plex and 8-plex) for absolute and relative quantification. It is based on labelling of N-terminus and side chain amine groups of protein, fractionated *via* liquid chromatography and final analysis by MS [27].

Understanding the protein structure is a key to comprehend its function. Once the structure for a protein is solved then its underlying mechanism can be studied in details like mechanisms of enzyme for instance. Structures are also important for drug design, vaccine design, protein-protein and protein-ligand interaction studies. Two of the widely used techniques for protein structure studies are X-ray crystallography and Nuclear Magnetic Resonance (NMR) spectroscopy. NMR spectroscopy has a main role in the structure determination and protein dynamics and other biological molecules. Structural determination *via* NMR spectroscopy includes different phases and each uses a distinct set of highly specific techniques. Sample preparation takes place at first followed by measurements which are interpreted to solve the structure [28]. X-ray crystallography uses a highly purified protein sample which is crystallized. These protein crystals are diffracted with X-rays to obtain diffraction patterns which are processed to get the crystal packing symmetry information. This information is processed to obtain the protein three-dimensional structure [29].

2.2.2. Metabolomics

Metabolomics deals with the study of metabolism at the global level. The word "metabolome" was first used by Oliver and colleagues in 1998, while their pioneer work was on yeast metabolism [30]. Metabolomics is an advancing field that widely quantifies and identifies endogenous and exogenous low molecular weight small molecule (<1 kDa), metabolites of a biological system in a high-throughput approach [31]. Metabolomics helps to analyze substances of system biology like urine, blood, and feces, and later studies small molecule metabolites of different metabolic pathway products and matrices [32]. Different methods involved in metabolomics approaches include NMR, chromatography and mass spectrometry [33]. Capillary electrophoresis, as founded by Soga, is becoming more famous as a separation technique for charged metabolites before mass spectral analysis [34].

The principle of NMR relies on energy absorption and re-emission of by some atom nuclei, which are influenced by external magnetic field [35]. NMR can quantify and identify a huge range of compounds with detection range in the order of μM or nM [35, 36]. The NMR method uses different spectrums like carbon spectrum ($_{13}C$ NMR), a hydrogen spectrum ($_1H$ NMR), or phosphorus spectrum ($_{31}P$ NMR), amongst which $_1H$ NMR is the most commonly used method [37 - 39]. MS allows analysis in low concentrations, that can range from pico- or attomole [3, 5, 34]. Various types of MS instruments perform tandem MS or MS/MS, that is a precise mass technique allowing structural elucidation [40, 41]. Compared to NMR, the metabolite detectability in MS depends on its ionization efficiency that is influenced by sample composition. Usually, NMR requires a minimal sample volume of 30-600 μl, while for MS analysis, a few microliters are sufficient. Moreover, MS has a greater resolution but the dynamics range is lower that NMR [42]. MS is also coupled with chromatographic separation techniques which is less evident for NMR [43]. Normally, one of the mentioned techniques is utilized in metabolomics, but the combination of MS and NMR can improve the metabolites' identification process [43, 44].

3. OMICS AND DIAGNOSIS OF GENETIC DISEASES

3.1. Back To The Future

Until the human genome was not sequenced, scientists relied on slow progressing and effort intensive techniques for the mapping and isolation of disease associated genes. For instance, in 1970s, the effort to isolate the genes for Huntington's disease began and until 1993 it was not successful. With the advent of human genome sequencing, karyotyping became possible which allowed precise location of every gene in a definite position and to understand genomic regions which differ from one person to another referred to as "polymorphic regions" especially single nucleotide polymorphisms (SNP's) became of special interest to every researcher, which spread throughout the genome with the rate of 1 SNP per 1000 base pairs [45, 46]. These polymorphisms show a strong link with disease associated genes so researchers began to work on developing a method through which millions of disease-related SNPs from the entire genome can be studied simultaneously.

The huge cohort of thousands of patients can be evaluated and facilitated to map hundreds of genomic rare and common variants responsible for disease predisposition by assistance of fine quality map of human genome along with high-throughput genotyping and statistical tools. Even then researchers were unable to address many questions related to very complex disorders, so they blended genomics with other omics techniques including epigenomics, transcriptomics, proteomics, metabolomics and microbiomics [47]. Omics approach to clarify many concepts including the genetic variation in coding regions of the gene is responsible for causing Mendelian disorders in general and common disorders resulting from changes in gene regulation. Depending on the environment and genetic background, the same genetic variants often contribute to different final outcomes. Taken together, integration of different omics data types provides a rationale for the development of systematic biology techniques to pinpoint the associated molecular patterns of the disease [48]. Each discrete part of omics data on its own provides different aspects including differences in disease association. Such data typically helps to develop genetic markers which can be tested during molecular studies of the disease; it promotes better insight into biological processes and pathways that can act as treatment targets during disease progression.

Nature of the disease is another important aspect in designing multiomic studies as only few etiological factors are involved in simple diseases originating from single gene variants which play a deterministic role in disease onset and development, whereas disease progression and severity of numerous disorders are influenced by "modifier genes" or environmental factors. For instance, the most obvious cause of cystic fibrosis is the mutation in a single chloride channel, which gives clues to consider the function of this gene [49, 50]. However, the etiology of very complex disorder is not focused on a single factor, rather it can be an outcome of a combination of multiple factors which converge to a phenotypically similar state. Along with that, complex disorders appear over the time and may involve genetic or environmental factors, so in the absence of an obvious deterministic aspect that prompts the disorder, single layer of data is always associated with other information provided through multilayered data which cumulatively manifests the causative effect in the biological cascade [51]. Therefore, detailed mechanistic insight into coordinated layers of omics data at multiple time points is needed to address the complex disorder.

3.2. Advances In Omics Technologies For Disease Diagnosis (examples)

High-throughput sequencing and cost-effective massive parallel technologies have revolutionized the diagnosis of diseases in clinical research and clinical practice. Techniques like mass spectroscopy, genome and exome sequencing are already in use for the diagnosis of rare diseases, to notify cancer progression and treatment and to create a predictive animal model for diseases in healthy individuals. Genome-wide association studies (GWAS) for instance have been used to identify disease loci however, in most of the time, a causative variant or a gene is not identified [52, 53]. Here, the integration of other omics data can be helpful for understanding the pathophysiology of the disease. On other hand, data generated by the experiments which are more proximal to individual's phenotype are not often comprehensive and are very expensive like proteomics so challenge remains open to find out a causative origin of diseases. Except rare disorders, no single technique is sufficient to explain the complexity behind the different molecular cascades leading to human diseases [54]. Ideally, there is a need for a holistic approach by combining different techniques to fix all the puzzles for disease diagnosis, interpretation of all molecular events and to clarify roadmap towards clinical care and therapeutics.

Multi-omics datasets such as transcriptomics, genomics, metabolomics proteomics and microbiomics present new information and provide an understanding of diseases but also elucidate challenges. Precisely, a new set of statistical methods and analytical tools are needed for merging contrasting omics data sets, as well as standardized quality control metrics. Moreover, omics data must deal with the challenges for interpretation of molecular cascades, their cross networks for a better guide to clinical care and therapeutics. Each type of data individually cannot capture the entire biological complexity of the human disorder but each dataset plays a crucial role in advancing clinical practice. Furthermore, the integration of multiomic techniques gives a holistic view of disease etiology and molecular processes that have begun to enable personalized medicine at a surprisingly comprehensive molecular level.

3.3. Mendelian Disorders

Mendelian disorders are the one which resulted from a mutation in a single gene which runs in families and can be autosomal or sex-linked, and can be inherited in either recessive or dominant fashion. Although polygenic disorders are more frequent than monogenic but still, they provide a major contribution toward understanding the genetic disease etiology and mechanism. These disorders include prominent developmental delay, intellectual disability, ectodermal dysplasia, neuromuscular disorders and structural abnormalities and collectively accounted in 10% of the children [55].

Different techniques used to detect above mentioned disorders include chromosomal microarray analysis (CMA), which is mostly recommended as the very first test for children born with dysmorphism, autism spectrum disorders, multiple congenital diseases, and intellectual/ developmental disabilities. Even though CMA is very effective than conventional karyotyping, but still the diagnosis yield for these group of disorders is about 20% only. Other congenital anomalies are due to insertions, deletions, translocations, and point mutations which disrupt the gene, which cannot be predicted by using CMA. Gross parallel sequencing of the entire genome or particular regions can be merged simultaneously to detect such genomic variations, but in big data analysis, cost and time consumption remains a challenge to the researchers for parallel sequencing data interpretation. With the advent of whole exome sequencing, this challenge has been partially addressed but still not sufficient for incidental findings [56]. Targeted gene panels overcome the time/ cost-related and gene diagnosis yield challenges. They also provides efficient data analysis and highthroughput without the need for specialized expertise and computing infrastructure for genetic disease diagnosis.

In addition, the integration of omics with RNA sequencing (RNA-seq) or network analyses provides additional information and facilitates in prioritizing the most likely causative variant. During analysis of a patient with an uncharacterized disorder, DNA sequence analysis is used along with array comparative genomic hybridization (aCGH) that is useful for the identification of most likely casual mutations, however, evidence exists for unsuspecting variants' pathogenicity including synonymous and intronic variants that affect splicing patterns, deletion of a non-coding exon and upstream region that give rise to an ablated expression of a transcript provided through RNA-seq [57].

3.4. Non-mendelian/common Disorders

Non-Mendelian disorders are complex than Mendelian disorders and are multifactorial in which disease progression and severity of disorder are influenced by "modifier genes" and environmental factors. Recently, researchers have developed multi omic approaches to better understand complex disorders with more accuracy. For instance, to study molecular pathways involved in age-related diseases, integrated transcriptomics, epigenomics, glycomics and metabolomics have been studied along with network and enrichment analysis which identified several modules and novel molecular networks related to discrete aspects of aging [57]. Similarly, gene expression studies on the liver and adipose tissues through bioenergetics measurements in the mitochondria and cell lines and the microarray followed by GWAS by integrated various omic datasets help to study the gene-gene, gene-phenotype links and embedded gene co-expression network modeling for understanding complex disorders like non-alcoholic fatty liver disease, autoimmune, kidney, urinary, infectious diseases and cancer [58 - 60]. For instance, cancer cell line panels are available for predicting the potential molecular mechanism dysregulation. These panels are co-operated with the analysis of transcriptome, small transcriptome (miRNAs) and proteomes which gives a holistic picture to study related pathways and disease progression [61]. It also facilitates in the identification of different sub group carcinomas with distinct molecular features.

Moreover, omics approaches facilitate rapid hypothesis generation, for example a group of scientists worked on the rejection of kidney transplant and they validated the importance of calreticulin as a major protein to tubular atrophy and human interstitial fibrosis. Likewise, H1N1 influenza viral infections are extensively studied through integrated omic techniques including metabolomics, proteomics and lipidomics and they found pro-inflammatory lipid precursors related to viral pathogenicity [62]. Likewise, common diseases such as obesity, autism, schizophrenia and diabetes are complex disorders with genetic and environmental etiology. Thousands of the gene loci have been reported for these human disorders, however finding the most authentic causative gene is still a major task [63, 64]. To overcome this limitation, various methods have been developed to analyze multiple omics datasets including enrichment analysis and networks. Taken together, these advances in omics highlight the identification of common molecular factors involved in infections and immune functions and also a significant role of complex disease diagnostics and prognostic in the future.

4. OMICS DATABASES

Integration of disease and healthy OMICS datasets is essential for a comprehensive understanding of biological processes taking place in humans. Big data omics has revolutionized our approach and improved our concepts of biological processes. There are several tools, software and databases available for multi-omics datasets; we tried to summarize these in Table **7.1**.

Usually, the term integrated omics is used for integration of two datasets or when the only genome level data is integrated. We have shown a list of important tools and databases for OMICS in Table **7.1**. This approach facilitates the finding of novel biological factors.

Table 7.1. List of important tools and databases for OMICS.

Name	Function	Websites	References
WikiPathways	Collage of pathways amenable to automated and manual workflows for mapping of genes, proteins, and metabolites	http://wikipathways.org/	[65]
MixOmics	Provides a wide range of linear multivariate methods for data exploration, integration, dimension reduction and visualization of biological data sets	http://mixomics.org/	[66]
MONGKIE	Multi-layered omics data such as somatic mutations, copy number variations, and gene expression data	http://yjjang.github.io/mongkie/	[67]
GalaxyP, GalaxyM	Development of a complete suite for integrated omics analysis, proteomics informed by transcriptomics analysis available to the typical bench scientist	https://usegalaxy.org/	[68]
CrossPlatform Commander	Detection of novel biomarkers, their ranking and annotation with existing knowledge using corresponding Transcriptomics and Proteomics data sets	http://www.ruhr-uni-bochum.de/mpc/software/ xplatcomm/index.html. en	[69]

(Table 1) cont.....

Name	Function	Websites	References
PhenoLink	Phenotype links to a multitude of ~omics data, *e.g.*, gene presence/absence (determined by *e.g.*: CGH or next- generation sequencing), gene expression (determined by *e.g.*: microarrays or RNA-Seq), or metabolite abundance (determined by *e.g.*: GC-MS)	http://bamics2.cmbi.ru.nl/websoftware/phenolink/	[70]
Paintomics	Integrated visual analysis of transcriptomics and metabolomics data	http://www.paintomics.org	[71]
iCluster	Detection of novel biomarkers, their ranking and annotation with existing knowledge using corresponding Transcriptomics and Proteomics data sets	https://www.mskcc.org/departments/ epidemiology-biostatistics/biostatistics/icluster	[72]
MapMap	Visualize and map gene expression, metabolite or other data, displays large datasets in diagrams of metabolic pathways	https://mapman.gabipd.org/	[73]

5. OMICS: GENETIC DISEASE MANAGEMENT AND THERAPEUTICS

Nature of disease is a significant factor to consider when designing a multi-omic analysis. Simple diseases with mutations in a single gene have little etiological influences, and these factors usually show a deterministic function in disease growth, but the incidence or progression of certain diseases is influenced by "modifier genes" or environmental factors. A single chloride channel mutation is the most common cause of cystic fibrosis, allowing disease-related research to concentrate on this gene's function [49]. Thus, focused omics activities at particular time points, based on immediate molecular changes caused by the causative factor, can provide enough information to aid in the development of new therapeutic strategies.

Complex diseases have a much more complicated etiology that is not based on a single cause. A number of factors can unite to produce phenotypically similar states. Since reactive effects normally outnumber causative effects in the absence of a strong deterministic factor which causes the disease, findings from a single layer of data are often associative [47]. Furthermore, since most common, complex diseases evolve over time and include both environmental and genetic factors, complete mechanistic understanding would necessitate the collection of organized sets of many omics data at multiple time points from a variety of disease-relevant tissues [74].

Multi-omics studies, as compared to studies of a single omics kind, enable researchers to better comprehend the flow of knowledge which underpins the genetic disease. Researchers may use multi-omics to gain a better idea of how knowledge flows from the original cause of disease (genetic, environmental, or developmental) to the functional effects or related interactions [51]. These advantages of integrated omics will significantly aid in the management of genetic diseases and future therapeutic approaches.

6. CHALLENGES AND OPPORTUNITIES

6.1. Reference Populations and Phenotyping

Bits of knowledge acquired from omics to deal with a sickness are for the most part similar. We think about omics information from healthy and infected people and expect that this distinction is able to identify the illness. Notwithstanding, in complex aggregates both "health" and "sickness" bunches are heterogeneous concerning many perplexing components, for example, populace structure, cell type variation, gender differences, and other obscure variables. One system to defeat heterogeneity related to any human populace is the "reductionist methodology", which expects to coordinate intently as potential groups of patients and controls to outnumber a large number of ecological variables from this examination [47]. Interestingly, an integrative omics method regularly depends on a "comprehensive" evaluation that endeavors to question an adequately huge number of people and link the numerous sources of inconstancy with factual models. The distinctions in the illness and a healthy body are then contrasted with distinguished factors which have a bigger involvement in the disease. Accordingly, omics examines the assortment of enormous datasets that precisely identify fluctuation in health controls. Assortment of such information is now achievable through multi omics.

The OMICS methodologies, and the most noteworthy test have the capacity to incorporate various changes in the foundation models, instead of investigating age, sex, time, and populace explicit examples. Accordingly, we anticipate the future use of omics innovations, especially in the sex explicitness setting, to fill significant gaps in our knowledge and lead to the advancement of more instructive models of a natural setting of sickness [75]. Sex is one of the significant factors of organic capacity, and most sicknesses display some degree of sex dimorphism. Accordingly, any customized treatment plan should consider sex.

CONCLUDING REMARKS

At present, no single methodology exists for handling, dissecting and deciphering all information from various Omics methods. The requirement for multimodal information blend systems and improvement of reproducible, highthroughput, easy to use and successful structures should be aimed for to make this discipline progress. Every standard living being model and a non-standard model creature present various difficulties because of the uniqueness of metabolites, quality articulation predisposition, epigenetic regulations and cell-type particularity of a given omics datasets. Also, with the fast headway of advancements for transcriptomics, genomics metabolomics, and proteomics, the local area needs to accept difficulties presented by these complex datasets to normalize test quality, investigation pipelines, information examination of pipelines and information designs for public information accessibility. Besides, as devices develop, they should become easy to understand, interoperable and viable for computationally serious investigations. Coordinated omics is not only an arrangement of apparatuses, however a durable worldview for natural translation of multi-omics datasets which will possibly uncover new experiences into fundamental science, just as wellbeing and infection.

CONSENT FOR PUBLICATION

Not applicable.

CONFLICT OF INTEREST

The author declares no conflict of interest, financial or otherwise.

ACKNOWLEDGEMENTS

Declared none.

REFERENCES

[1]   He J, Kang Q, Hu J, Song P, Jin C. China has officially released its first national list of rare diseases. Intractable Rare Dis Res 2018; 7(2): 145-7.

[http://dx.doi.org/10.5582/irdr.2018.01056] [PMID: 29862160]

[2]   Venter JC, Adams MD, Myers EW, *et al.* The sequence of the human genome. Science 2001; 291(5507): 1304-51.
        [http://dx.doi.org/10.1126/science.1058040] [PMID: 11181995]

[3]   Rothberg JM, Hinz W, Rearick TM, *et al.* An integrated semiconductor device enabling non-optical genome sequencing. Nature 2011; 475(7356): 348-52.
        [http://dx.doi.org/10.1038/nature10242] [PMID: 21776081]

[4]   Eid J, Fehr A, Gray J, *et al.* Real-time DNA sequencing from single polymerase molecules. Science 2009; 323(5910): 133-8.
        [http://dx.doi.org/10.1126/science.1162986] [PMID: 19023044]

[5]   Kasianowicz JJ, Brandin E, Branton D, Deamer DW. Characterization of individual polynucleotide molecules using a membrane channel. Proc Natl Acad Sci USA 1996; 93(24): 13770-3.
        [http://dx.doi.org/10.1073/pnas.93.24.13770] [PMID: 8943010]

[6]   Siqueira JF Jr, Fouad AF, Rôças IN. Pyrosequencing as a tool for better understanding of human microbiomes. J Oral Microbiol 2012; 4(1): 10743.
        [http://dx.doi.org/10.3402/jom.v4i0.10743] [PMID: 22279602]

[7]   Bentley DR, Balasubramanian S, Swerdlow HP, *et al.* Accurate whole human genome sequencing using reversible terminator chemistry. Nature 2008; 456(7218): 53-9.
        [http://dx.doi.org/10.1038/nature07517] [PMID: 18987734]

[8]   Buermans HPJ, den Dunnen JT. Next generation sequencing technology: Advances and applications. Biochim Biophys Acta Mol Basis Dis 2014; 1842(10): 1932-41.
        [http://dx.doi.org/10.1016/j.bbadis.2014.06.015] [PMID: 24995601]

[9]   Rhoads A, Au KF. Pacbio sequencing and its applications. Genomics Proteomics Bioinformatics 2015; 13(5): 278-89.
        [http://dx.doi.org/10.1016/j.gpb.2015.08.002] [PMID: 26542840]

[10]   Berg JM, Tymoczko JL, Stryer L. Biochemistry. 2002.

[11]   Pozhitkov AE, Tautz D, Noble PA. Oligonucleotide microarrays: widely applied poorly understood. Brief Funct Genomics Proteomics 2007; 6(2): 141-8.
        [http://dx.doi.org/10.1093/bfgp/elm014] [PMID: 17644526]

[12]   McLachlan GJ, Do K-A, Ambroise C. Analyzing microarray gene expression data. Hoboken, NJ, USA: John Wiley & Sons, Inc. 2004.
        [http://dx.doi.org/10.1002/047172842X]

[13]   Wang Z, Gerstein M, Snyder M. RNA-Seq: a revolutionary tool for transcriptomics. Nat Rev Genet 2009; 10(1): 57-63.
        [http://dx.doi.org/10.1038/nrg2484] [PMID: 19015660]

[14]   Cox J, Mann M. Is proteomics the new genomics? Cell 2007; 130(3): 395-8.
        [http://dx.doi.org/10.1016/j.cell.2007.07.032] [PMID: 17693247]

[15]   Jungbauer A, Hahn R. Ion-Exchange Chromatography. Methods Enzymol 2009; 463: 349-71.
        [http://dx.doi.org/10.1016/S0076-6879(09)63022-6] [PMID: 19892182]

[16]   Hage DS, Anguizola JA, Bi C, *et al.* Pharmaceutical and biomedical applications of affinity chromatography: Recent trends and developments. J Pharm Biomed Anal 2012; 69: 93-105.
        [http://dx.doi.org/10.1016/j.jpba.2012.01.004] [PMID: 22305083]

[17]   Voedisch B, Thie H. Size Exclusion Chromatography. In: Kontermann R, Dübel S, Eds. Antibody Engineering. Berlin, Heidelberg: Springer Berlin Heidelberg 2010; pp. 607-12.
        [http://dx.doi.org/10.1007/978-3-642-01144-3_38]

[18]   Lequin RM. Enzyme immunoassay (EIA)/enzyme-linked immunosorbent assay (ELISA). Clin Chem 2005; 51(12): 2415-8.

[http://dx.doi.org/10.1373/clinchem.2005.051532] [PMID: 16179424]

[19]   Kurien B, Scofield R. Western blotting. Methods 2006; 38(4): 283-93.
       [http://dx.doi.org/10.1016/j.ymeth.2005.11.007] [PMID: 16483794]

[20]   James P. Chips for proteomics: a new tool or just hype? BioTechniques 2002; 4-10.
       [http://dx.doi.org/10.2144/dec02james]

[21]   Nowakowski AB, Wobig WJ, Petering DH. Native SDS-PAGE: high resolution electrophoretic
       separation of proteins with retention of native properties including bound metal ions. Metallomics
       2014; 6(5): 1068-78.
       [http://dx.doi.org/10.1039/C4MT00033A] [PMID: 24686569]

[22]   Issaq HJ, Veenstra TD. Two-dimensional polyacrylamide gel electrophoresis (2D-PAGE): advances
       and perspectives. Biotechniques 2008; 44(5): 697-700, 700.
       [http://dx.doi.org/10.2144/000112823] [PMID: 18474047]

[23]   Zhang Y, Fonslow BR, Shan B, Baek MC, Yates JR III. Protein analysis by shotgun/bottom-up
       proteomics. Chem Rev 2013; 113(4): 2343-94.
       [http://dx.doi.org/10.1021/cr3003533] [PMID: 23438204]

[24]   Doucet A, Overall CM. Amino-Terminal Oriented Mass Spectrometry of Substrates (ATOMS) N-
       terminal sequencing of proteins and proteolytic cleavage sites by quantitative mass spectrometry.
       Methods Enzymol 2011; 501: 275-93.
       [http://dx.doi.org/10.1016/B978-0-12-385950-1.00013-4] [PMID: 22078539]

[25]   Shiio Y, Aebersold R. Quantitative proteome analysis using isotope-coded affinity tags and mass
       spectrometry. Nat Protoc 2006; 1(1): 139-45.
       [http://dx.doi.org/10.1038/nprot.2006.22] [PMID: 17406225]

[26]   Ong SE, Mann M. Stable isotope labeling by amino acids in cell culture for quantitative proteomics.
       Methods Mol Biol 2007; 359: 37-52.
       [http://dx.doi.org/10.1007/978-1-59745-255-7_3] [PMID: 17484109]

[27]   Wiese S, Reidegeld KA, Meyer HE, Warscheid B. Protein labeling by iTRAQ: A new tool for
       quantitative mass spectrometry in proteome research. Proteomics 2007; 7(3): 340-50.
       [http://dx.doi.org/10.1002/pmic.200600422] [PMID: 17177251]

[28]   Cavalli A, Salvatella X, Dobson CM, Vendruscolo M. Protein structure determination from NMR
       chemical shifts. Proc Natl Acad Sci USA 2007; 104(23): 9615-20.
       [http://dx.doi.org/10.1073/pnas.0610313104] [PMID: 17535901]

[29]   Ameh ES. A review of basic crystallography and x-ray diffraction applications. Int J Adv Manuf
       Technol 2019; 105(7-8): 3289-302.
       [http://dx.doi.org/10.1007/s00170-019-04508-1]

[30]   Oliver S, Winson MK, Kell DB, Baganz F. Systematic functional analysis of the yeast genome. Trends
       Biotechnol 1998; 16(9): 373-8.
       [http://dx.doi.org/10.1016/S0167-7799(98)01214-1] [PMID: 9744112]

[31]   Nalbantoglu S. Metabolomics: basic principles and strategies In: Nalbantoglu S, Amri H, Eds.
       Molecular Medicine. IntechOpen 2019.
       [http://dx.doi.org/10.5772/intechopen.88563]

[32]   Ju R, Liu X, Zheng F, et al. Removal of false positive features to generate authentic peak table for
       high-resolution mass spectrometry-based metabolomics study. Anal Chim Acta 2019; 1067: 79-87.
       [http://dx.doi.org/10.1016/j.aca.2019.04.011] [PMID: 31047152]

[33]   Wu X, Sun X, Zhao C, et al. Exploring the pharmacological effects and potential targets of
       paeoniflorin on the endometriosis of cold coagulation and blood stasis model rats by ultra-performance
       liquid chromatography tandem mass spectrometry with a pattern recognition approach. RSC Advances
       2019; 9(36): 20796-805.
       [http://dx.doi.org/10.1039/C9RA03525G] [PMID: 35515565]

[34]   Soga T, Ohashi Y, Ueno Y, Naraoka H, Tomita M, Nishioka T. Quantitative metabolome analysis using capillary electrophoresis mass spectrometry. J Proteome Res 2003; 2(5): 488-94.
[http://dx.doi.org/10.1021/pr034020m] [PMID: 14582645]

[35]   Agin A, Heintz D, Ruhland E, *et al.* Metabolomics – an overview. From basic principles to potential biomarkers (part 1). Med Nucl (Paris) 2016; 40(1): 4-10.
[http://dx.doi.org/10.1016/j.mednuc.2015.12.006]

[36]   Puig-Castellví F, Alfonso I, Tauler R. Untargeted assignment and automatic integration of [1] H NMR metabolomic datasets using a multivariate curve resolution approach. Anal Chim Acta 2017; 964: 55-66.
[http://dx.doi.org/10.1016/j.aca.2017.02.010] [PMID: 28351639]

[37]   Zhang A, Ma Z, Sun H, *et al.* High-Throughput Metabolomics Evaluate the Efficacy of Total Lignans From Acanthophanax Senticosus Stem Against Ovariectomized Osteoporosis Rat. Front Pharmacol 2019; 10: 553.
[http://dx.doi.org/10.3389/fphar.2019.00553] [PMID: 31191306]

[38]   Zhang A, Sun H, Wang P, Wang X. Salivary proteomics in biomedical research. Clin Chim Acta 2013; 415: 261-5.
[http://dx.doi.org/10.1016/j.cca.2012.11.001] [PMID: 23146870]

[39]   Larive CK, Barding GA Jr, Dinges MM. NMR spectroscopy for metabolomics and metabolic profiling. Anal Chem 2015; 87(1): 133-46.
[http://dx.doi.org/10.1021/ac504075g] [PMID: 25375201]

[40]   Jacob M, Malkawi A, Albast N, *et al.* A targeted metabolomics approach for clinical diagnosis of inborn errors of metabolism. Anal Chim Acta 2018; 1025: 141-53.
[http://dx.doi.org/10.1016/j.aca.2018.03.058] [PMID: 29801603]

[41]   Baldwin MA. Mass spectrometers for the analysis of biomolecules Biological Mass Spectrometry. Elsevier 2005; Vol. 402: pp. 3-48.
[http://dx.doi.org/10.1016/S0076-6879(05)02001-X]

[42]   Marshall DD, Powers R. Beyond the paradigm: Combining mass spectrometry and nuclear magnetic resonance for metabolomics. Prog Nucl Magn Reson Spectrosc 2017; 100: 1-16.
[http://dx.doi.org/10.1016/j.pnmrs.2017.01.001] [PMID: 28552170]

[43]   Kim HK, Choi YH, Verpoorte R. NMR-based plant metabolomics: where do we stand, where do we go? Trends Biotechnol 2011; 29(6): 267-75.
[http://dx.doi.org/10.1016/j.tibtech.2011.02.001] [PMID: 21435731]

[44]   Markley JL, Brüschweiler R, Edison AS, *et al.* The future of NMR-based metabolomics. Curr Opin Biotechnol 2017; 43: 34-40.
[http://dx.doi.org/10.1016/j.copbio.2016.08.001] [PMID: 27580257]

[45]   Chial H. Rare Genetic Disorders: Learning About Genetic Disease Through Gene Mapping, SNPs, and Microarray Data. Nature Education 2008; 1(1): 192.

[46]   LaFramboise T. Single nucleotide polymorphism arrays: a decade of biological, computational and technological advances. Nucleic Acids Res 2009; 37(13): 4181-93.
[http://dx.doi.org/10.1093/nar/gkp552] [PMID: 19570852]

[47]   Hasin Y, Seldin M, Lusis A. Multi-omics approaches to disease. Genome Biol 2017; 18(1): 83.
[http://dx.doi.org/10.1186/s13059-017-1215-1] [PMID: 28476144]

[48]   Antonarakis SE, Beckmann JS. Mendelian disorders deserve more attention. Nat Rev Genet 2006; 7(4): 277-82.
[http://dx.doi.org/10.1038/nrg1826] [PMID: 16534515]

[49]   Welsh MJ, Smith AE. Molecular mechanisms of CFTR chloride channel dysfunction in cystic fibrosis. Cell 1993; 73(7): 1251-4.

[http://dx.doi.org/10.1016/0092-8674(93)90353-R] [PMID: 7686820]

[50] Karczewski KJ, Snyder MP. Integrative omics for health and disease. Nat Rev Genet 2018; 19(5): 299-310.
[http://dx.doi.org/10.1038/nrg.2018.4] [PMID: 29479082]

[51] Civelek M, Lusis AJ. Systems genetics approaches to understand complex traits. Nat Rev Genet 2014; 15(1): 34-48.
[http://dx.doi.org/10.1038/nrg3575] [PMID: 24296534]

[52] Begum F, Ghosh D, Tseng GC, Feingold E. Comprehensive literature review and statistical considerations for GWAS meta-analysis. Nucleic Acids Res 2012; 40(9): 3777-84.
[http://dx.doi.org/10.1093/nar/gkr1255] [PMID: 22241776]

[53] Manolio TA. Genomewide association studies and assessment of the risk of disease. N Engl J Med 2010; 363(2): 166-76.
[http://dx.doi.org/10.1056/NEJMra0905980] [PMID: 20647212]

[54] Ki CS. Recent Advances in the Clinical Application of Next-Generation Sequencing. Pediatr Gastroenterol Hepatol Nutr 2021; 24(1): 1-6.
[http://dx.doi.org/10.5223/pghn.2021.24.1.1] [PMID: 33505888]

[55] Badano JL, Katsanis N. Beyond Mendel: an evolving view of human genetic disease transmission. Nat Rev Genet 2002; 3(10): 779-89.
[http://dx.doi.org/10.1038/nrg910] [PMID: 12360236]

[56] Misra BB, Langefeld CD, Olivier M, Cox LA. Integrated omics: tools, advances, and future approaches. J Mol Endocrinol 2018; JME-18-0055.
[PMID: 30006342]

[57] Kudryashova KS, Burka K, Kulaga AY, Vorobyeva NS, Kennedy BK. Aging Biomarkers: From Functional Tests to Multi-Omics Approaches. Proteomics 2020; 20(5-6): 1900408.
[http://dx.doi.org/10.1002/pmic.201900408] [PMID: 32084299]

[58] Eddy S, Mariani LH, Kretzler M. Integrated multi-omics approaches to improve classification of chronic kidney disease. Nat Rev Nephrol 2020; 16(11): 657-68.
[http://dx.doi.org/10.1038/s41581-020-0286-5] [PMID: 32424281]

[59] Rebollar EA, Antwis RE, Becker MH, *et al.* Using "Omics" and Integrated Multi-Omics Approaches to Guide Probiotic Selection to Mitigate Chytridiomycosis and Other Emerging Infectious Diseases. Front Microbiol 2016; 7: 68.
[http://dx.doi.org/10.3389/fmicb.2016.00068] [PMID: 26870025]

[60] Turanli B, Karagoz K, Gulfidan G, Sinha R, Mardinoglu A, Arga KY. A Network-Based Cancer Drug Discovery: From Integrated Multi-Omics Approaches to Precision Medicine. Curr Pharm Des 2019; 24(32): 3778-90.
[http://dx.doi.org/10.2174/1381612824666181106095959] [PMID: 30398107]

[61] Chakraborty S, Hosen MI, Ahmed M, Shekhar HU. Onco-Multi-OMICS Approach: A New Frontier in Cancer Research. BioMed Res Int 2018; 2018: 1-14.
[http://dx.doi.org/10.1155/2018/9836256] [PMID: 30402498]

[62] Lim ECP, Brett M, Lai AHM, *et al.* Next-generation sequencing using a pre-designed gene panel for the molecular diagnosis of congenital disorders in pediatric patients. Hum Genomics 2015; 9(1): 33.
[http://dx.doi.org/10.1186/s40246-015-0055-x] [PMID: 26666243]

[63] Liu G, Dong C, Liu L. Integrated Multiple "-omics" Data Reveal Subtypes of Hepatocellular Carcinoma. PLoS One 2016; 11(11): e0165457.
[http://dx.doi.org/10.1371/journal.pone.0165457] [PMID: 27806083]

[64] Tisoncik-Go J, Gasper DJ, Kyle JE, *et al.* Integrated Omics Analysis of Pathogenic Host Responses during Pandemic H1N1 Influenza Virus Infection: The Crucial Role of Lipid Metabolism. Cell Host Microbe 2016; 19(2): 254-66.

[http://dx.doi.org/10.1016/j.chom.2016.01.002] [PMID: 26867183]

[65]   Slenter DN, Kutmon M, Hanspers K, *et al.* WikiPathways: a multifaceted pathway database bridging metabolomics to other omics research. Nucleic Acids Res 2018; 46(D1): D661-7.
[http://dx.doi.org/10.1093/nar/gkx1064] [PMID: 29136241]

[66]   Rohart F, Gautier B, Singh A, Lê Cao KA. mixOmics: An R package for 'omics feature selection and multiple data integration. PLOS Comput Biol 2017; 13(11): e1005752.
[http://dx.doi.org/10.1371/journal.pcbi.1005752] [PMID: 29099853]

[67]   Jang Y, Yu N, Seo J, Kim S, Lee S. MONGKIE: an integrated tool for network analysis and visualization for multi-omics data. Biol Direct 2016; 11(1): 10.
[http://dx.doi.org/10.1186/s13062-016-0112-y] [PMID: 26987515]

[68]   Davidson RL, Weber RJM, Liu H, Sharma-Oates A, Viant MR. Galaxy-M: a Galaxy workflow for processing and analyzing direct infusion and liquid chromatography mass spectrometry-based metabolomics data. Gigascience 2016; 5(1): 10.
[http://dx.doi.org/10.1186/s13742-016-0115-8] [PMID: 26913198]

[69]   Kohl M, Megger D A, Trippler M, *et al.* A practical data processing workflow for multi-OMICS projects Biochim Biophys Acta 2014; 1844(1): 52-62.
[http://dx.doi.org/10.1016/j.bbapap.2013.02.029]

[70]   Bayjanov JR, Molenaar D, Tzeneva V, Siezen RJ, van Hijum SAFT. PhenoLink - a web-tool for linking phenotype to ~omics data for bacteria: application to gene-trait matching for Lactobacillus plantarum strains. BMC Genomics 2012; 13(1): 170.
[http://dx.doi.org/10.1186/1471-2164-13-170] [PMID: 22559291]

[71]   García-Alcalde F, García-López F, Dopazo J, Conesa A. Paintomics: a web based tool for the joint visualization of transcriptomics and metabolomics data. Bioinformatics 2011; 27(1): 137-9.
[http://dx.doi.org/10.1093/bioinformatics/btq594] [PMID: 21098431]

[72]   Shen R, Olshen AB, Ladanyi M. Integrative clustering of multiple genomic data types using a joint latent variable model with application to breast and lung cancer subtype analysis. Bioinformatics 2009; 25(22): 2906-12.
[http://dx.doi.org/10.1093/bioinformatics/btp543] [PMID: 19759197]

[73]   Thimm O, Bläsing O, Gibon Y, *et al.* mapman: a user-driven tool to display genomics data sets onto diagrams of metabolic pathways and other biological processes. Plant J 2004; 37(6): 914-39.
[http://dx.doi.org/10.1111/j.1365-313X.2004.02016.x] [PMID: 14996223]

[74]   Gibson G. *A primer of human genetics.* 2015.

[75]   Arnold AP, van Nas A, Lusis AJ. Systems biology asks new questions about sex differences. Trends Endocrinol Metab 2009; 20(10): 471-6.
[http://dx.doi.org/10.1016/j.tem.2009.06.007] [PMID: 19783453]

CHAPTER 8

Integrated Bioinformatics and Computational Biology Approaches: Applications in Diagnosis and Therapeutics

Fatima Shahid[1], **Shifa Tariq Ashraf**[1], **Hayeqa Shahwar Awan**[1], **Amina Basheer**[1] and **Amjad Ali**[1,*]

[1] *Department of Industrial Biotechnology, Atta-ur-Rahman School of Applied Biosciences (ASAB), National University of Sciences and Technology (NUST), Islamabad, Pakistan*

Abstract: The advent of bioinformatics and integrated biology approaches has given rise to new avenues of diagnostic and therapeutic regimes. Living systems have been explored to identify disease-associated biomarkers that facilitate the early diagnosis of perilous medical conditions. Likewise, gene networks are pondered upon to obtain better insights into biochemical systems that can assist in the prediction and testing of the effects of various interactions within the systems. Genomics and proteomics-based approaches are being explored to facilitate the early diagnosis of cancers, shifting the paradigm towards noninvasive diagnostic alternatives. Bioinformatics has also fueled pharmacogenomics and pharmacogenetics-based strategies that have in turn contributed to the development of personalized medications. Similarly, the reverse vaccinology approach has emerged as a prominent option to combat deadly pathogens that were otherwise unrestrainable. This chapter highlights the fruits of integrated bioinformatics in diagnosing and treating detrimental conditions.

Keywords: Integrated bioinformatics, Precision medicine, Computational diagnostic tools, *In silico* Therapeutics, Reverse vaccinology.

1. INTRODUCTION

Bioinformatics and computational biology are integrative fields that apply *in silico* methods to explore the large assembly of biological data, for instance, genetic sequences, protein samples, and cell populations to devise advanced predictions. These computational methods include mathematical modelling, simulation, and analytical methods. Computational models can be constructed for

---
[*] **Corresponding author Amjad Ali**: Department of Industrial Biotechnology, Atta-ur-Rahman School of Applied Biosciences (ASAB), National University of Sciences and Technology (NUST), Islamabad, Pakistan; E-mail: Amjad_uni@gmail.com

Syeda Marriam Bakhtiar and Erum Dilshad (Eds.)

the potent diagnosis of disease progression and in response to therapeutics at a personalized level.

1.1. Exploration of Disease-Associated Biomarkers

Biomarkers are the distinct characteristics that are evaluated and serve as indicators of biological, pharmacological, as well as pathogenic processes in response to therapeutic interventions or exposure. Biomarkers are used as a tool for the prediction of disease severity, and drug response, as well as in the drug development process [1]. For instance, the detection of specific autoantibodies in the patient's blood is a potential biomarker used to detect autoimmune diseases. For rheumatoid arthritis (RA), rheumatoid factors are considered predominant diagnostic biomarkers. Hence, for detection purposes, anti-citrullinated protein/peptide antibodies (ACPAs) formed against the patient's own body citrullinated proteins are considered. These ACPAs can be detected at early stages as potential biomarkers in the blood, before the onset of symptoms associated with RA. Therefore, these biomarkers can be helpful in the prognosis of RA [2].

Biomarkers have been discovered through different high-throughput techniques to comprehend transcriptomics such as microarray, gene expression data, and genomics strategies that include genome sequencing, genome annotation, along with proteomics techniques and metabolomics frameworks which comprise mass spectrometry and nuclear magnetic resonance imaging, respectively. Proteins, peptides, genetic markers, and/or histological data have the potential to act as biomarkers. Generally, a genetic biomarker is a single gene or a collection of genes [3, 4]. Some of these have been described as follows:

Human Epithelial-growth Factor (HER2) is a protein receptor present on the cells of the human body. In colorectal cancer tumors, HER2 gene and its receptors are overexpressed by 3-4% while in the case of breast tumors, it is overexpressed up to 20-30%. Therefore, this gene is used as a predictive and prognostic marker in case of both cancers [5]. Likewise, carbohydrate antigen125 (CA125) is a high molecular weight glycoprotein which serves as a serum biomarker. In patients with epithelial ovarian cancer, the expression of CA125 increases as compared to a normal state. Moreover, by overexpression of this CA125 different signaling pathways including P13K/AKT and ERK pathways are stimulated. Similarly, Human Epididymis protein 4 (HE4) is another protein coded by the WFD2 gene that acts as a protease inhibitor, and overexpression of this protein in ovarian cancer has been observed that can, in turn, irritate EFGR and MAPK signaling pathways. Due to these significant roles, HE4 was approved by the Food and Drug Administration (FDA) as a monitoring biomarker in women with epithelial ovarian cancers. In contrast to HE4, the concentration of ApoA1 is decreased in the serum of patients with ovarian cancer and can serve as a potential biomarker. Likewise, BRCA1, BRCA2, and p53 are genetic biomarkers that are attributed to breast cancer. However, the BRCA1 gene, located on chromosome 17q12-21 is pondered upon and hypermethylation of BRCA1 was found to be involved in both ovarian as well as breast tumors. Moreover, p53 is another potential biomarker that is a tumor suppressor gene and reportedly 50% cases of ovarian cancer have a mutation in this gene [6].

Similarly, glycated Haemoglobin (HbA1c) is a traditional biomarker for the diagnosis of diabetes and pre-diabetes. Fructosamine (FA) is a keto-amine that is formed by the glycosylation of total serum proteins majorly albumin. When the concentration of glucose is high, the concentration of FA increases. Hence, FA can serve as another biomarker for the screening of diabetes. Similarly, HDL-C, another biomarker of diabetes is a major lipoprotein that is associated with insulin secretion. If the concentration of HDL-C is lower, it will eventually lead to the development of diabetes from the pre-diabetic state [7]. Moreover, Alzheimer's disease is the most common neurodegenerative disorder and in the United States, it is the 6th leading cause of death [8]. Some biomarkers associated with Alzheimer's are cerebrospinal fluid (CSF), amyloid β, phosphorylated tau, and tau proteins [9].

1.2. Computational Models as Tools to Identify Key Biomarkers

Biomarkers are the driving force for the prognosis, diagnosis, and treatment of a disease and are identified by different computational and bioinformatics tools that are curated. Resultantly, these tools can help scientists in the early diagnosis and treatment of a disease [3].

The advent of DNA microarray technology has aided in the transition from systematic methods to biological discovery; these transitions have already started to have a deep impact on biological research, medicine, and pharmacology. The quantitative data about the complete cell transcription profile pledges to become an effective way of studying the basic biology, disease diagnosis, drug development facilitation, and modify therapeutics to specific pathologies. These data can help generate the database containing living processes information [10].

Researchers have worked on survival related gene network modules [11]. In a study, a deep learning-based risk stratification model was developed for lung cancer by choosing an illustrative gene from survival-related network modules. Similarly, a new computational model was presented, based on SimRank and density-based clustering recommender model for prediction of miRNA-associated diseases (SRM-DAP) [12]. Another sample-specific method was provided that establishes an indicator with individual specified Dynamical Network Biomarkers (DNB) which are used for early detection of the pre-disease state of a specific sample. For example in case of influenza A, 144 genes were selected as DNB based on microarray data [12]. Similarly, another method was used for establishing a pathway network of the phenotype of a gene. It initially constructed a network of the biological pathway, and then the GeneRank algorithm was employed for the selection of disease-associated pathways [12]. Signal Transduction Networks (STNs) that regulate basic cellular processes, for instance cell growth, cell cycle, inflammation, and cell death processes are interrupted by diseases. These computational and mathematical models allow the systemized assessment of STNs disruptions and adaptive feedback via *in silico* simulations. STNs are changed in any disease thus provide an attractive approach to discover or even become the latest biomarker [13, 14].

The resulting potent biomarkers are important in the development of new and improved therapeutics and diagnostics. There are several different methods through which problems of this nature are addressed [15]. Two main groups in which these methods are divided are based on filtering methods and those groups are wrapper or model-based approaches [16].

Generally, filtering methods are used as pre-processing steps, and the choice of feature is independent of machine learning algorithms and features are selected based on their scores in different statistical tests. In wrapper methods, subsets of the feature are used to train models by using these features. A study held by W. Pan *et al.* compared different filtering methods, and highlighted the pros, and cons of using two different methods. He suggested that although the filtering method is robust as compared to the wrapper method but it considers each gene as an individual gene and the correlation between the genes is not considered. Hence, filtering methods are not able to rank genes among the significant genes. Therefore, wrapping methods are more accurate even though filtering methods are mostly applied [16, 17]. Another study carried out by Li and Yang *et al.* has compared the overall functioning of Support Vector Machine (SVM) and Ridge Regression (RR) for the gene expression datasets' classification and examination of the impact of recursive processes that are involved in the classification accuracy. They emphasized that the ridge regression (RR) has the best performance and the wrapper methods are advantageous over the filtering method [18].

1.3. Annotation of Disease Associated Mutations

Disease-associated mutations are generally missense mutations that can occur in the coding regions of a gene and alter the amino acids of proteins. Disease-associated point mutations are accessible from databases such as the Human gene mutations database (HGMD), Online Database of Mendelian Inheritance in Man (OMIM), and HGVBase. In recent times, there have been numerous public and commercial projects for assembling and interpreting human genomic variations. The aim of these projects is to provide a perception of how a genotype is linked with the disease and how it will influence our response to the drug. These projects comprise the human genome annotation, SNP Consortium, as well as many gene-specific databases. The automated annotation approaches based on evolutionary and structural parameters, can lead to the understanding of the molecular basis of diseases. More than 4,000,000 mutations have been identified and with over 20,000 variations have been annotated with a phenotype and we are facing challenges because of several uncharacterized mutations [19]. There is a need for an algorithm for automatic annotation of these genes to understand how they may affect the regulation of a gene and the functions of the products of proteins. Annotation tools developed for one organism can be used to anticipate the normal or pathological condition of another organism. Cuppon and co-workers used two bioinformatics tools Polyphen and SIFT for the annotation of a single nucleotide polymorphism (SNP). For analysis of SNPs, several tools have been developed by The National Cancer Institute as part of its Cancer Genome Anatomy Project's Genetic Annotation Initiative (CGAP-GAI) and genome resources are UCSC's GoldenPath Genome Browser and HapMap consortium [20, 21].

1.4. Identification of Epigenetic Drivers

Epigenetics deal with the heritable alterations in gene expression or gene activity without alteration in the DNA sequences. Epigenetic processes are crucial for the functioning of many organisms. These processes include methylation, phosphorylation, ubiquitination, acetylation, and sumolyation. DNA methylation plays a major role in silencing of tumor suppressor genes, hence altering various cellular processes, signal transduction, cell cycle checkpoints, and apoptosis. Different epigenetic drivers bring about genetic alterations. For example, *hMLH1* genes are involved in DNA repair mechanism. It has been reported that four types of primary colorectal cancers possess methylation of the *hMLH1* gene showing microsatellite instability and in sporadic colorectal cancer, epigenetic inactivation of this gene is a general method of mismatch repair gene inactivation. It has been reported that in almost every type of cancer, there is hypermethylation of CpG islands promotors (CGI) which is a key mechanism of silencing of tumor suppressor genes (TSGs) in cancerous cells [22].

The inactivation of the gene that is involved in the repair of double strands break and the epigenetic errors present in mitotic genes are epigenetic drivers of genetic alterations. Similarly, *CHFR* genes play a major role in mitotic checkpoints and DNA methylation inactivates these genes in different malignancies, such as in breast and colorectal cancer [23].

2. ROLE OF SYSTEMS BIOINFORMATICS (NETWORK-BASED METHODS FOR HUMAN DISEASE GENE PREDICTION)

In recent times, the union of classical bioinformatics and systems biology has given birth to a relatively new approach called Systems Bioinformatics. The core focus is to assimilate information across various levels using a top-down approach that's data-driven along with a bottom-up approach, known as bioinformatics and systems biology, respectively. The dawn of technologies revolving around "omics" has provided a platform for the rise of Systems Bioinformatics. These technologies cover a wide range of information covering fields like proteomics, transcriptomics, and genomics, all the way to metagenomics, pharmacogenomics, metabolomics and epigenomics. This approach studies the properties of the system collectively rather than summing up the properties derived from individual components of the system. This leads to the most important method in Systems Bioinformatics *i.e.* Multiple networks construction that represents each omics level and their integration in a network that is layered and exchanges information between and within those layers [24]. Hence, we will discuss in the following few headings how Systems Bioinformatics plays a significant role in the enhancement of diagnostics and therapeutics to pave way to precision medicine.

2.1. Systems Modelling and Simulation

Gene networks are complex biochemical systems, and in order to predict and test the validity of their behaviors, the effects of various interactions (such as dynamic, simultaneous and multiple) within the system components need to be described that are otherwise too complex to infer spontaneously. Simulation of developed mathematical models is significant to explore these gene networks due to their complex nature. Mathematical models can be further used to investigate these complex systems, to define the underlying system components and their behaviors based on data retrieved from experiments and predict behavior responses to a given perturbation based on the description of the basic fundamentals of their function [25].

Complex gene networks are generally described by two types of models, 'quantitative' and logical [26, 27]. In quantitative models, differential equations are used to define the dynamic interactions present in a network that are non-linear in nature, while on the other hand, the latter uses the Boolean approach to define the network dynamics qualitatively. Quantitative models are rather an accurate representation of information that can easily be compared with time-dependent experimental data. But they highly depend on the information of the kinetic parameters and mechanistic details and, so, their application to a well-characterized molecular network is limited to small sized networks. However, qualitative logical models do not depend on any such knowledge and can be applied to networks with a known structure on a large scale, but they can only provide limited information, since quantitative predictions cannot be provided through this approach, nor can they assist in selecting improved alternative behaviors. To summarize, each approach has its pros and cons and a recent study suggests that combining the two approaches might prove to be ideal to deal with the challenges in systems biology [26].

In diagnostics and pharmacology, mathematical models are absolutely essential. For instance, a study developed mathematical models of the blood coagulation network, which were spatio-temporal in nature to assist diagnostics, therapeutics and drug development [28]. Mathematical models are further applied to the exploration of drug combinations by developing models of drug targeted pathways [29]. Systems biology when coupled with conventional bioinformatics can strengthen and complement each other in diagnostics and therapeutics where tangible predictions are vital [25]. Another study revealed the significance of how mathematical modelling can be combined with high-throughput data in developing personalized cancer treatments [30]. In systems biology, to optimize the estimation and validation of parameters, multi-omics data can be integrated and can be used in constraint-based modelling as a constraint [31].

2.2. Network-Based Diagnostics and Therapeutics

One of the most significant hallmarks of Systems Bioinformatics is the use of computational diagnostics by detecting important molecular biomarkers. Several recent advanced studies that have addressed the computational diagnostic issues, have used such networks to describe cellular systems by the analysis of genes, proteins, complexes, and isoforms, simultaneously. In current molecular diagnostics research, an example of such successful combination of Systems Bioinformatics, is an online database called MelGene. This database is a highly comprehensive tool that has frequently updated group of data collected from various genetic association studies in cutaneous melanoma, including meta-analysis results of all suitable polymorphisms [32]. The resultant network connections that are proposed by the tool, highlight new loci that are associated with the risk of cutaneous melanoma. Numerous recent studies show how proteomics data that is interpreted using network-based approaches can propose additional significant insights into the dynamics and mechanics of protein assemblies, and henceforth into the mechanisms of the system at the molecular level. Additionally, these approaches based on networks can be used in the reconstruction of a disease perturbed network model on a cellular level that shows the interactions of differentially expressed proteins that have been identified in cellular pathways associated with targeted pathophysiology. An example is of a study held by Shirasaki *et al.* [33] where they used a coupled technique by combining affinity purification to Mass spectrometry (MS) in order to explore the protein expression profile of Huntington's disease.

Furthermore, the identification of several cellular pathways that have been altered under various physiological conditions has been made easy through the development of various network-based approaches, which can further enhance the discovery of key biomarkers. For instance, functional enrichment analysis of KEGG pathways or GO biological processes [33] of proteins that are differentially expressed can be achieved using free license tools such as, Gene Set Enrichment Analysis (GSEA) [34], Protein ANalysis THrough Evolutionary Relationships (PANTHER) [35] and Database for Annotation, Visualization and Integrated Discovery (DAVID) [36] as well as other tools such as Ingenuity Pathway Analysis and MetaCore [37]. Several other tools pave the path for the application of Systems Bioinformatics in the discovery of essential biomarkers. A successful example of such a tool is GWAB, which makes use of computational approaches and systems methods to enhance and boost association signals that are weak for GWAS, which stands a common problem when this type of data is analyzed. This tool operates by integrating data that is publicly available in the form of p-values (GWAS statistics) for Single Nucleotide Polymorphisms (SNPs) along with reference genes for a disease under study [38].

2.3. Tools/ Data Bases Used in Diagnosis and Treatment Regimens

There are several tools that are presently available, which can aid in the application of systems Bioinformatics in drug discovery. Tools such as C(2) Maps [39], SDTNBI [40], PROMISCUOUS [41] and Chem2Bio2RDF [42] are a few examples that collectively provide integrated pharmacology and systems databases drug-target prediction, chemo-informatics analysis, drug repositioning analysis, and networks of disease-gene-drug connectivity relationships. A list of tools and databases that adopt Systems Bioinformatics approaches can be seen in Table **8.1**.

2.4. Contribution of Bioinformatics in Cancer Diagnostics and Therapeutics

Genomics and proteomics are used in combination with bioinformatics to obtain the finest medical benefits. Proteomics can be further divided into functional and expression subgroups. The former deals with interaction between proteins, their association with nucleic acids or their existences as parts of complexes while the latter explores the differential protein expression that varies from tissue to tissue and can be useful in the diagnosis and treatment of cancer. Hence this field shows a promise to minimize cancer associated death rate [43, 44].

Table 8.1. Tools and databases for systems bioinformatics methodologies in diagnostics and therapeutics.

Tools	Link
Network- based therapeutics	-
TCM-Mesh	http://mesh.tcm.microbioinformatics.org/
SDTNBI	The program is available on request
systemsDock	http://systemsdock.unit.oist.jp/iddp/home/index
BindingDB	https://www.bindingdb.org/bind/index.jsp
NFFinder	http://nffinder.cnb.csic.es/
NutriChem	http://sbb.hku.hk/services/NutriChem-2.0/FoodDisease.php
TIMMA-R	https://cran.r-project.org/web/packages/timma/
Network-based diagnostics	
GWAB	http://www.inetbio.org/gwab/
Netter	https://github.com/JRuyssinck/netter
MetaNetVar	https://github.com/NCBI-Hackathons/Network_SNPs
NetDecoder	http://netdecoder.hms.harvard.edu/
MUFFINN	http://www.inetbio.org/muffinn/
HitWalker2	https://github.com/biodev/HitWalker2

Protein arrays promise to assist the medical professionals in diagnosing cancer by avoiding invasive procedures. Bioinformatics have revolutionaries' plasma-based diagnostics techniques and they now require lesser time and give consistent results. To practice an oncoproteomics driven diagnosis, proteome profiles and MS analysis have been used. The process is comprised of protein isolation, separation, purification, 2 dimensional (2D) electrophoresis, image analysis identification and characterization of proteins and finally functional analysis [43]. For instance, researchers obtained serum samples from individuals suffering from breast and ovarian cancers. Using 2D electrophoresis and matrix assisted laser desorption/ionization (MALDI) and analysis of time of flight (TOF) techniques, the serum samples were evaluated. It was reported that two biomarkers from these thermostable serum samples namely clusterin and alpha-1-acid glycoprotein were evidently decreased in case of breast cancer. On the other hand, transthyretin was found to be present in reduced quantity in ovarian cancer patients. This study clearly highlighted the efficacy of proteome profiling and 2D electrophoresis in cancer diagnostics [45]. Examining tumor profiles may assist in differentiating between malignant and benign cases. Another research based on SELDI(Surface-enhanced-laser desorption/ionization) MS provided useful information about alpha heptoglobin being a potential biomarker for the detection of ovarian cancer [46]. Stathmin, a protein involved in remodeling of microtubules that form the cytoskeleton, has been reportedly linked to leukemia in children by using proteome profiling. Certain post translational modifications including phosphorylation that hindered cytoskeleton formation, were highlighted in cancer patients. This was not possible with simple microarrays [47]. Genomics and proteomics have facilitated the comparison between normal cell stathmin and cancer cell levels of stathmin. Experiments have been directed to control the over expression by using duplex mir20 backbone shRNA^{STMN1} and post treatment genomic and proteomic evaluations to analyze the degree of damage done to the tumor [48].

Moreover, Chromatin immunoprecipitation assay (CHiP) has been used to determine the connection of BRCA1 with BP1. Bioinformatics based studies established their relation to be inverse in nature, pointing out the role of BP1 in suggesting BRAC1 and behaving as a promising target for cancer therapy [49].

Researchers have tried to develop therapeutic strategies to counter cancer but the problem of cancer drug resistance prevails. Genomics has assisted in solving this issues as scientists are now able to study the underlying mechanisms at genome level that participate in drug resistance mechanisms and can make efforts to dodge them [50].

Systems bioinformatics has emerged as a potent tool to better understand epigenomics, pharmacogenomics and metabolomics. The designed frameworks are applied to systems and their associated data to acquire enhanced computational knowledge regarding diagnostics and therapeutics that contribute largely towards precision medicine [51]. For instance, it has been found that tumor growth factor beta and matrix metallo-proteinase 9 are involved in the progression of hepato-cellular carcinoma. Systems bioinformatics based analysis using Petri net models and biological regulatory networks elucidated that these work in a feedback loop and their associated changes were recognized in both, normal and diseased states. This information can be used for both, diagnostic as well as therapeutic purposes [52].

Moreover, to device a therapy, the place of malfunction needs to be pinpointed. Using Boolean logic gates, pathways are modeled and their relative interactions are studied. All the failures that could possibly occur in the pathway are estimated. This is followed by designing of specific drugs to counter these faults and the efficacy of the administered drugs are also evaluated computationally. Hence, suitable drugs to revert the system to a non-cancer state have been explored [53].

Clearly, the human genome project and allied sequencing of the human genome have enabled precise exploration of disease mechanisms at genomic level. The recent developments in the field of cancer drug development include the probing of new alterations by genomic means and offering protection of personal data at preliminary stages of research. Also, the tumors are classified at molecular level and their libraries are publicly available along with potent inhibitor data. Novel screening is done at molecular level and the National Institute of Health funds the research and facilities the trials [54].

3. APPLICATION IN PRECISION MEDICINE AND PHARMACOGENOMICS

3.1. Pharmacogenomics and Pharmacogenetics in Personalized Medicine

Pharmacogenomics is an indication of personalized medication. It refers to a change in perspective from the outlook; 'one-drug fits-all' to 'the correct medication for the perfect patient at the perfect time and in the optimum quantity'. This does not imply that every patient will be dealt uniquely in contrast to any other patient. Instead, patients are segregated into cohorts based on their genetics and different markers that assist in prediction of the progression of disease and results of therapy [55]. During the past twenty years, investigation of human genetics has been powered by frontline sequencing technologies, prompting a more profound comprehension of the connection between human wellbeing and genetic variation [56].

Precision medicine has broad applications in the field of genetics. For instance, some of the emerging applications include, conforming the selection of drugs, pharmacogenomics-informed pharmacotherapy, and administering drugs according to the genetic features of the patient [57]. Precision medicine deals with genetic variations and genetic analysis in relation to the metabolism of drugs. For instance, advanced cancer treatment regimens are the fruits of precision medicine. Various drugs are being developed and marketed that have the potential to target explicit subcellular locations and cell signaling in order to fit with a patient's genetic layout [58]. As the sequencing technologies advance, they will be integrated into a collection of clinical situations. Integrating pharmacogenomic profiles of patients will unquestionably elevate the fluency by which practitioners can suggest medication [59].

Moreover, pharmacogenomics possesses a couple of significant roles in precision medicine. Firstly, it assists pharmaceutical companies in the progression of drugs along with their discovery. Secondly, it guides the general physicians to pick the perfect drug for their patients on the basis of their genetic variations, to circumvent adverse drug reactions, and ensuring maximum drug efficacy by prescribing the accurate dosage. Pharmacogenomics promises that people can be given personalized medications. This can be done by considering information related to an individual's atmosphere, food intake, age, routine, and present physical health, as well as pharmacogenetic testing [60].

3.2. Pharmacogenomics and Pharmacogenetics in Drug Development

The terminologies pharmacogenetics and pharmacogenomics are used to characterize the association between an individual's several genetic variants and the drug responses generated on those variants [61]. Two major principles are in focus when pharmacogenetics comes to light: pharmacokinetics and pharmacodynamics [62]. To effectively create customized medication routines for patients, comprehension of pharmacogenomics, pharmacokinetics and pharmacodynamics is significant. Each medication being introduced in the body experiences the cycle of absorption, distribution, metabolism, and excretion (ADME). Pharmacokinetics is the collection of all of these cycles, which decides the amount of the medication that needs to arrive at the site of activity for an effective therapeutic result [60].

The pharmacological influence of a drug on the purposed biologic pathway is depicted by pharmacodynamics [62]. The drug in turn induces biochemical and physiological changes in an individual's body. The activity of the drug and the impact it has on the body is termed as pharmacodynamics. It decides how accurately the destined cells, for example, neurons or heart tissue, react to the medication [60]. Briefly, pharmacodynamics is what the medication does to the patient, while pharmacokinetics is how the patient reacts to a drug. A difference in pharmacodynamics or pharmacokinetics can cause a possibility of toxic responses or fluctuating drug efficacy [62].

The drug company regulates the complex balance amid the pharmacodynamics pharmacokinetics to achieve the maximum projected effect the drug has to offer and the minimal possible disadvantageous reactions the patient might receive. However, the inborn genetic polymorphism an individual possesses can lead to an alteration in the harmony of pharmacodynamics and pharmacokinetics, subsequently causing a modification in the way the drug and the body cooperate with each other [60]. Pharmacokinetics related issues are linked to 40% of drug evolution failures [63]. There are over 170 genes that are suspected to play a part in drug distribution, out of which over half are identified as polymorphic [64]. The odds of failure of a drug in preclinical and clinical setting due to the lack of efficacy have been minimized, by the selection of an appropriate target picked by pharmacogenomic approaches [65].

For the drug to act, it is essential to recognize the promising target as the first step in the cycle of drug discovery. An enzyme in an imperative pathway, any transporter, receptor(s), any protein in the transduction of a signal or a protein that has been fashioned in a pathological state can be a potent target. When the human genome was sequenced, the amount of drug targets was calculated to be about 8000, out of the 8000, 4990 could be worked upon –for antibodies 2329 and for drug proteins 794 2329:antibodies and 749:drug proteins [66]. Drugs founded on targets displaying extensive polymorphisms can have disparities in their outcome [67]. In case such a drug is administered continuously, it can lead to imprecise results in the preclinical and clinical settings. To avoid this situation, the targets must be categorized on the basis of pharmacogenetic analysis employing proteomics and selection of appropriate drug compounds is required [68].

Notably, the implementation of pharmacogenomics and Pharmacogenetics fundamentals in the drug advancement process has decreased the drug quantity, escalated the pace of absorption and the drug targeting has increased exceptionally [69].

3.3. Pharmacogenomics in Establishment of Drug Application Guidelines

As a component of the drug development process, the food and drug authority, FDA, has listed some guidelines that are to be fulfilled by the pharmaceutical industries for the submission of pharmacogenetic data [70]. Composed in 2009, the Clinical Pharmacogenetics Implementation Consortium (CPIC) had set strategies on drug treatment on the basis of pharmacogenetic material. Since March of 2017, CPIC has formulated 36 strategies which are publicly available [71].

As the majority of the pharmacogenetic test results are not scientifically grounded, such examinations cannot be utilized by the FDA for regulatory choices. At present, the submission of pharmacogenetic information has been made obligatory by the FDA for particular cases and supports intentional submission for other particular cases. Rules have been established relating to when a total pharmacogenetic report should be submitted and when a truncated report should be submitted. Moreover, there are discrete rules for submitting pharmacogenetic information regarding investigational new medication applications and unaccepted and accepted advertising applications. As per the

FDA's opinion, the integration of pharmacogenetic data is beneficial for all areas of research, however the drug industries have a dispute among themselves regarding this issue [72].

The FDA requires an acknowledged pharmacogenetic test as a legitimate biomarker for construction of regulatory decisions. In order to be accepted as a legitimate biomarker, a pharmacogenetic test must possess well rooted attributes and a reliable scientific structure. For instance, the enzymes responsible for drug metabolism can serve as substantial biomarkers for pharmacogenetic tests associated with the evaluation of safety and efficacy of a drug. Typically, reduced dosage of warfarin is required by the patients who possess allele variant of CYP2C9 and VKORC1 gene, in comparison to the patients having normal wild type alleles. Incorporation of pharmacogenetic data has been done in the warfarin drug label as this is a credible biomarker [73 - 75].

Submission of a thorough report of the pharmacogenetic data has been made mandatory by the FDA, in case these outcomes have been utilized in animal model-based studies for making decisions, for choosing the subjects, to abide by the drug safety in the clinical trials, as well as for dose variation or its alteration. If the sponsor utilizes the pharmacogenetic analysis results to evaluate/assess the efficacy, selection of dosage, safety and the procedure followed in the clinical trials, they need to submit the complete data. A truncated report of the pharmacogenetic analysis has to be proposed to the FDA in case the test is a credible biomarker for the drug and the sponsor does not utilize the pharmacogenetic analysis results to uphold the outcomes of the trial. There's no obligation for the submission of data in case where the pharmacogenetic analysis has been done for research or exploratory study since they cannot be treated as credible biomarkers. Nonetheless, the voluntary proposition of such experimental pharmacogenetic analysis data is encouraged by the FDA [68].

Both FDA along with the sponsor are facilitated by submission of pharmacogenetic analysis. This helps FDA to notice and judge the pharmacogenetic fundamentals and ultimately decrease the needless lag in evaluating the forthcoming submissions where pharmacogenetic examination is an essential element of the drug augmentation. Additionally, the sponsors get in touch with the FDA experts indifferently, debate over scientific statistics and get their associative speculation. The pharmacogenetic evaluation can be used by the sponsor to endorse the efficacy and safety of the drug product [76].

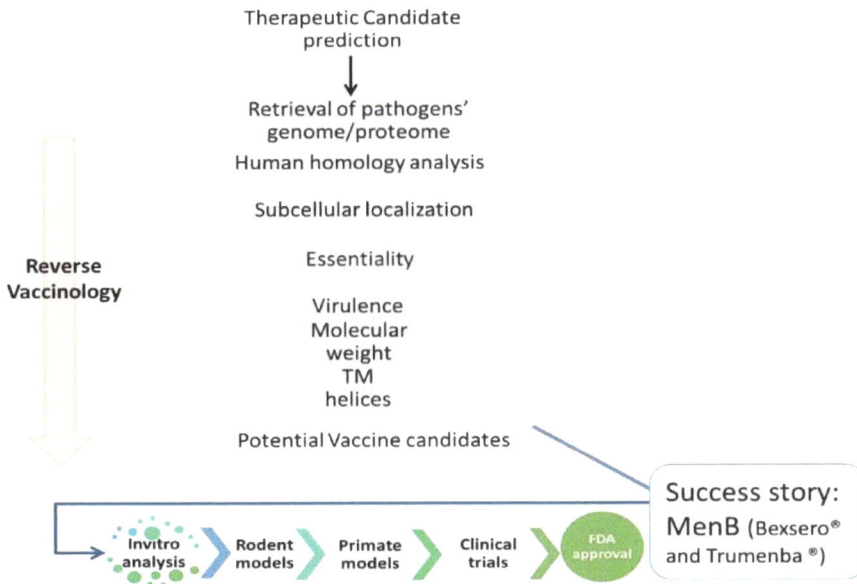

Fig. (8.1). The reverse vaccinology workflow followed by *in vitro* analysis

Recently, FDA has begun to emphasize on preparing genetic catalogs for new medications and drugs, and has issued polices for refreshing product tags for various current treatment regimes, like for, 6-mercaptopurine and the blood thinner warfarin. Currently, approximately 140 drugs have pharmacogenetic data in their concerned FDA product label. Pharmacogenetics data in product labels goes from boxed indications, the most significant level of caution, to statistics in the clinical pharmacology segment [60].

4. REVERSE VACCINOLOGY-A PROGRESSIVE STEP TOWARDS THERAPEUTIC INNOVATION

The availability of whole genome sequences of bacteria, viruses as well as parasites have enabled us to apply reverse vaccinology-based strategies to avoid their infections.

The approach differs from conventional vaccinology as it reduces the time of vaccine development and is economically feasible [77]. It has also been amalgamated with pan genomics to enable drug target identification against pathogens [78]. The strategy is based on genomic mining and spotting those genes or proteins of the pathogen that are not present in the human host or resemble those of the gut flora. This step is followed by checking the subcellular localization of proteins as these slightly differ in case of vaccine and drug targets. The bacterial essential and virulent proteins are picked and filters like the presence of lower molecule weight (>110 kDa) and lesser transmembrane helices are applied. Finally the filtered candidates are annotated and can be used as vaccine candidates to obtain specific antigenic and immunogenic epitopes for vaccine development or as drug targets to develop efficacious drugs [79, 80]. This workflow has been briefly described in Fig. (**8.1**) [77, 81].

Moreover, certain pipelines have been developed to speed up the process of vaccine development through reverse vaccinology. Some examples of these include Vaxign, VacSol, PanRV and Tepitool [82 - 85].

A prominent successful example of reverse vaccinology approach is the development of Group B meningococcus (MenB) vaccine that has ended a long quest for putative therapy against this pathogen. The surface exposed proteins (SEPs) of this bacterium were known to confer protective immunity. Genome screening resulted in 600 novel genes encoding for SEPs. *Escherichia coli* expression vector system was used to express 350 of these. These were later purified and used to immunize mouse models. The sera obtained from these model animals was analyzed by using ELISA and FACS techniques. As a result, 85 SEPs among which 25 had the potential to express bactericidal activity were discovered over a short period of 18 months. These assisted the researchers with apt knowledge to develop MenB vaccine [81].

Similarly, malarial parasite is a difficult pathogen to tackle due to the presence of a hand full of antigens that vary at different points of the parasite's life cycle. Gaining better insights into the genome of *Plasmodium falciparum* and obtaining potential vaccine candidates is another important fruit of reverse vaccinology. These identified candidates can be joined to potent adjuvants to develop a formulation that can confer protective immunity [86].

Moreover, there is no possible way to cultivate hepatitis C virus in lab settings. Hence the experiments to curb it could not possibly proceed swiftly. Using genome sequencing, recombinant protein expression studies are now possible that have vastly upgraded the diagnostic regime. Envelope proteins have been obtained using genomic analysis that when administered to chimpanzees, have conferred immunity against the virus [87].

The ongoing corona virus pandemic has changed the norms around the world. Several efforts have been directed to counter this virus. Reverse vaccinology strategies have also been employed. Economically feasible chimeric vaccines that promise lesser side effects and higher efficacy have been predicted. However, further wet lab investigations in this regard are required to support the claimed therapeutic benefits [88 - 90].

CONCLUDING REMARKS

Integrated Bioinformatics has surfaced as an aspiring field and holds a promise to revolutionize the field of medicine in the coming years. Diseases are quite complex and heterogeneous at molecular levels and are controlled by a number of variable factors. These can be genetic, epigenetic factors or may be controlled by external stimuli like environment or drugs. While it currently seems impossible to replace the conventional diagnostic and therapeutic approaches, better knowledge of the living systems may assist clinicians to come up with improved strategies to target complex diseases. Computational biology-based diagnostics as well as therapeutics can putatively aid in timely detection and prevention of diseases.

CONSENT FOR PUBLICATION

Not applicable.

CONFLICT OF INTEREST

The author declares no conflict of interest, financial or otherwise.

ACKNOWLEDGEMENTS

Declared none.

REFERENCES

[1]   Strimbu K, Tavel JA. What are biomarkers? Curr Opin HIV AIDS 2010; 5(6): 463-6.
       [http://dx.doi.org/10.1097/COH.0b013e32833ed177] [PMID: 20978388]

[2]   Nakken B, Papp G, Bosnes V, Zeher M, Nagy G, Szodoray P. Biomarkers for rheumatoid arthritis: From molecular processes to diagnostic applications-current concepts and future perspectives. Immunol Lett 2017; 189: 13-8.
       [http://dx.doi.org/10.1016/j.imlet.2017.05.010] [PMID: 28526580]

[3]   Azuaje F. Bioinformatics and biomarker discovery. Wiley Online Library 2010; 1: 19.

[4]   Ballman KV. Biomarker: Predictive or Prognostic? J Clin Oncol 2015; 33(33): 3968-71.
       [http://dx.doi.org/10.1200/JCO.2015.63.3651] [PMID: 26392104]

[5]   Cooke T, Reeves J, Lanigan A, Stanton P. HER2 as a prognostic and predictive marker for breast cancer. Ann Oncol 2001; 12 (Suppl. 1): S23-8.
       [http://dx.doi.org/10.1093/annonc/12.suppl_1.S23] [PMID: 11521717]

[6]   Arjmand M, Zahedi A. Clinical biomarkers for detection of ovarian cancer. J Mol Cancer 2019; 2(1): 3-7.

[7]   Dorcely B, Katz K, Jagannathan R, *et al.* Novel biomarkers for prediabetes, diabetes, and associated

complications. Diabetes Metab Syndr Obes 2017; 10: 345-61.
[http://dx.doi.org/10.2147/DMSO.S100074] [PMID: 28860833]

[8]   Tejada-Vera B. Mortality from Alzheimer's disease in the United States: data for 2000 and 2010: US Department of Health and Human Services. Centers for Disease Control and 2013.

[9]   Sharma N, Singh AN. Exploring biomarkers for Alzheimer's disease. J Clin Diagn Res 2016; 10(7): KE01-6.
[PMID: 27630867]

[10] Young RA. Biomedical discovery with DNA arrays. 2000; 102(1): 9-15.

[11] Choi H, Na KJ. Integrative analysis of imaging and transcriptomic data of the immune landscape associated with tumor metabolism in lung adenocarcinoma: Clinical and prognostic implications. Theranostics 2018; 8(7): 1956-65.
[http://dx.doi.org/10.7150/thno.23767] [PMID: 29556367]

[12] Cai Y, Huang T, Yang J. Applications of Bioinformatics and Systems Biology in Precision Medicine and Immunooncology. Hindawi 2018.
[http://dx.doi.org/10.1155/2018/1427978]

[13] Nagarajan N, Yapp EK, Le NQK, Kamaraj B, Al-Subaie AM, Yeh H-Y. Application of Computational Biology and Artificial Intelligence Technologies in Cancer Precision Drug Discovery. Biomed Res Int 2019; 2019: 8427042.
[http://dx.doi.org/10.1155/2019/8427042]

[14] Kolch W, Fey D. Personalized computational models as biomarkers. J Pers Med 2017; 7(3): 9.
[http://dx.doi.org/10.3390/jpm7030009] [PMID: 28862657]

[15] Wang Y, Tetko IV, Hall MA, *et al.* Gene selection from microarray data for cancer classification—a machine learning approach. Comput Biol Chem 2005; 29(1): 37-46.
[http://dx.doi.org/10.1016/j.compbiolchem.2004.11.001] [PMID: 15680584]

[16] Inza I, Larrañaga P, Blanco R, Cerrolaza AJ. Filter versus wrapper gene selection approaches in DNA microarray domains. Artif Intell Med 2004; 31(2): 91-103.
[http://dx.doi.org/10.1016/j.artmed.2004.01.007] [PMID: 15219288]

[17] Pan W. A comparative review of statistical methods for discovering differentially expressed genes in replicated microarray experiments. Bioinformatics 2002; 18(4): 546-54.
[http://dx.doi.org/10.1093/bioinformatics/18.4.546] [PMID: 12016052]

[18] Li F, Yang Y. Analysis of recursive gene selection approaches from microarray data. Bioinformatics 2005; 21(19): 3741-7.
[http://dx.doi.org/10.1093/bioinformatics/bti618] [PMID: 16118263]

[19] Mooney SD, Klein TE. The functional importance of disease-associated mutation. BMC Bioinformatics 2002; 3(1): 24.
[http://dx.doi.org/10.1186/1471-2105-3-24] [PMID: 12220483]

[20] Mooney S. Bioinformatics approaches and resources for single nucleotide polymorphism functional analysis. Brief Bioinform 2005; 6(1): 44-56.
[http://dx.doi.org/10.1093/bib/6.1.44] [PMID: 15826356]

[21] Gao M, Zhou H, Skolnick J. Insights into disease-associated mutations in the human proteome through protein structural analysis. Structure 2015; 23(7): 1362-9.
[http://dx.doi.org/10.1016/j.str.2015.03.028] [PMID: 26027735]

[22] Chatterjee A, Rodger EJ, Eccles MR, Eds. Epigenetic drivers of tumourigenesis and cancer metastasis Seminars in cancer biology. Elsevier 2018.

[23] Toyota M, Suzuki H. Epigenetic drivers of genetic alterations. Advances in genetics. Elsevier 2010; pp. 309-23.

[24] Ostrowski J, Wyrwicz LS. Integrating genomics, proteomics and bioinformatics in translational studies

of molecular medicine. Expert Rev Mol Diagn 2009; 9(6): 623-30.
[http://dx.doi.org/10.1586/erm.09.41] [PMID: 19732006]

[25]   Kitano H. Computational systems biology. Nature 2002; 420(6912): 206-10.
[http://dx.doi.org/10.1038/nature01254] [PMID: 12432404]

[26]   Le Novère N. Quantitative and logic modelling of molecular and gene networks. Nat Rev Genet 2015; 16(3): 146-58.
[http://dx.doi.org/10.1038/nrg3885] [PMID: 25645874]

[27]   Samaga R, Klamt S. Modeling approaches for qualitative and semi-quantitative analysis of cellular signaling networks. Cell Commun Signal 2013; 11(1): 43.
[http://dx.doi.org/10.1186/1478-811X-11-43] [PMID: 23803171]

[28]   Huang L, Jiang Y, Chen Y. Predicting drug combination index and simulating the network-regulation dynamics by mathematical modeling of drug-targeted EGFR-ERK signaling pathway. Sci Rep 2017; 7(1): 40752.
[http://dx.doi.org/10.1038/srep40752] [PMID: 28102344]

[29]   Ram PT, Mendelsohn J, Mills GB. Bioinformatics and systems biology. Mol Oncol 2012; 6(2): 147-54.
[http://dx.doi.org/10.1016/j.molonc.2012.01.008] [PMID: 22377422]

[30]   Vijayakumar S, Conway M, Lió P, Angione C. Seeing the wood for the trees: a forest of methods for optimization and omic-network integration in metabolic modelling. Brief Bioinform 2018; 19(6): 1218-35.
[PMID: 28575143]

[31]   Antonopoulou K, Stefanaki I, Lill CM, *et al.* Updated field synopsis and systematic meta-analyses of genetic association studies in cutaneous melanoma: the MelGene database. J Invest Dermatol 2015; 135(4): 1074-9.
[http://dx.doi.org/10.1038/jid.2014.491] [PMID: 25407435]

[32]   Shirasaki DI, Greiner ER, Al-Ramahi I, *et al.* Network organization of the huntingtin proteomic interactome in mammalian brain. Neuron 2012; 75(1): 41-57.
[http://dx.doi.org/10.1016/j.neuron.2012.05.024] [PMID: 22794259]

[33]   Kanehisa M, Goto S, Sato Y, Furumichi M, Tanabe M. KEGG for integration and interpretation of large-scale molecular data sets. Nucleic Acids Res 2012; 40(D1): D109-14.
[http://dx.doi.org/10.1093/nar/gkr988] [PMID: 22080510]

[34]   Subramanian A, Tamayo P, Mootha VK, *et al.* Gene set enrichment analysis: A knowledge-based approach for interpreting genome-wide expression profiles. Proc Natl Acad Sci USA 2005; 102(43): 15545-50.
[http://dx.doi.org/10.1073/pnas.0506580102] [PMID: 16199517]

[35]   Mi H, Lazareva-Ulitsky B, Loo R, *et al.* The PANTHER database of protein families, subfamilies, functions and pathways. Nucleic Acids Res 2004; 33(Database issue) (Suppl. 1): D284-8.
[http://dx.doi.org/10.1093/nar/gki078] [PMID: 15608197]

[36]   Huang DW, Sherman BT, Lempicki RA. Systematic and integrative analysis of large gene lists using DAVID bioinformatics resources. Nat Protoc 2009; 4(1): 44-57.
[http://dx.doi.org/10.1038/nprot.2008.211] [PMID: 19131956]

[37]   Ekins S, Nikolsky Y, Bugrim A, Kirillov E, Nikolskaya T. Pathway mapping tools for analysis of high content data. High Content Screening 2007; pp. 319-50.

[38]   Shim JE, Bang C, Yang S, *et al.* GWAB: a web server for the network-based boosting of human genome-wide association data. Nucleic Acids Res 2017; 45(W1): W154-61.
[http://dx.doi.org/10.1093/nar/gkx284] [PMID: 28449091]

[39]   Huang H, Wu X, Pandey R, *et al.* C2Maps: a network pharmacology database with comprehensive disease-gene-drug connectivity relationships. BMC Genomics 2012; 13(S6) (Suppl. 6): S17.

[http://dx.doi.org/10.1186/1471-2164-13-S6-S17] [PMID: 23134618]

[40] Wu Z, Cheng F, Li J, Li W, Liu G, Tang Y. SDTNBI: an integrated network and chemoinformatics tool for systematic prediction of drug-target interactions and drug repositioning. Brief Bioinform 2017; 18(2): 333-47.
[PMID: 26944082]

[41] von Eichborn J, Murgueitio MS, Dunkel M, Koerner S, Bourne PE, Preissner R. PROMISCUOUS: a database for network-based drug-repositioning. Nucleic Acids Res 2011; 39(Database) (Suppl. 1): D1060-6.
[http://dx.doi.org/10.1093/nar/gkq1037] [PMID: 21071407]

[42] Chen B, Dong X, Jiao D, *et al.* Chem2Bio2RDF: a semantic framework for linking and data mining chemogenomic and systems chemical biology data. BMC Bioinformatics 2010; 11(1): 255.
[http://dx.doi.org/10.1186/1471-2105-11-255] [PMID: 20478034]

[43] Joshi S, Tiwari AK, Mondal B, Sharma A. Oncoproteomics. Clin Chim Acta 2011; 412(3-4): 217-26.
[http://dx.doi.org/10.1016/j.cca.2010.10.002] [PMID: 20955692]

[44] Cho WCS, Cheng CHK. Oncoproteomics: current trends and future perspectives. Expert Rev Proteomics 2007; 4(3): 401-10.
[http://dx.doi.org/10.1586/14789450.4.3.401] [PMID: 17552924]

[45] Goufman EI, Moshkovskii SA, Tikhonova OV, *et al.* Two-dimensional electrophoretic proteome study of serum thermostable fraction from patients with various tumor conditions. Biochemistry (Mosc) 2006; 71(4): 354-60.
[http://dx.doi.org/10.1134/S000629790604002X] [PMID: 16615854]

[46] Ye B, Cramer DW, Skates SJ, *et al.* Haptoglobin-α subunit as potential serum biomarker in ovarian cancer: identification and characterization using proteomic profiling and mass spectrometry. Clin Cancer Res 2003; 9(8): 2904-11.
[PMID: 12912935]

[47] Tan HT, Wu W, Ng YZ, *et al.* Proteomic analysis of colorectal cancer metastasis: stathmin-1 revealed as a player in cancer cell migration and prognostic marker. J Proteome Res 2012; 11(2): 1433-45.
[http://dx.doi.org/10.1021/pr2010956] [PMID: 22181002]

[48] Rana S, Maples PB, Senzer N, Nemunaitis J. Stathmin 1: a novel therapeutic target for anticancer activity. Expert Rev Anticancer Ther 2008; 8(9): 1461-70.
[http://dx.doi.org/10.1586/14737140.8.9.1461] [PMID: 18759697]

[49] Kluk BJ, Fu Y, Formolo TA, *et al.* BP1, an isoform of DLX4 homeoprotein, negatively regulates BRCA1 in sporadic breast cancer. Int J Biol Sci 2010; 6(5): 513-24.
[http://dx.doi.org/10.7150/ijbs.6.513] [PMID: 20877436]

[50] Joana Dinis , Marta Gromicho , Celia Martins , Antonio Laires , Jose Rueff , Rueff J. Genomics and cancer drug resistance. Curr Pharm Biotechnol 2012; 13(5): 651-73.
[http://dx.doi.org/10.2174/138920112799857549] [PMID: 22122479]

[51] Oulas A, Minadakis G, Zachariou M, Sokratous K, Bourdakou MM, Spyrou GM. Systems Bioinformatics: increasing precision of computational diagnostics and therapeutics through network-based approaches. Brief Bioinform 2019; 20(3): 806-24.
[http://dx.doi.org/10.1093/bib/bbx151] [PMID: 29186305]

[52] Tariq Ashraf S, Obaid A, Tariq Saeed M, *et al.* Formal model of the interplay between TGF-β1 and MMP-9 and their dynamics in hepatocellular carcinoma. Math Biosci Eng 2019; 16(5): 3285-310.
[http://dx.doi.org/10.3934/mbe.2019164] [PMID: 31499614]

[53] Layek R, Datta A, Bittner M, Dougherty ER. Cancer therapy design based on pathway logic. Bioinformatics 2011; 27(4): 548-55.
[http://dx.doi.org/10.1093/bioinformatics/btq703] [PMID: 21193523]

[54] Strausberg RL, Simpson AJG, Old LJ, Riggins GJ. Oncogenomics and the development of new cancer

therapies. Nature 2004; 429(6990): 469-74.
[http://dx.doi.org/10.1038/nature02627] [PMID: 15164073]

[55]   Sadée W, Dai Z. Pharmacogenetics/genomics and personalized medicine. Hum Mol Genet 2005; 14 (Suppl. 2): R207-14.
[http://dx.doi.org/10.1093/hmg/ddi261] [PMID: 16244319]

[56]   van der Wouden CH, Böhringer S, Cecchin E, *et al.* Generating evidence for precision medicine: considerations made by the Ubiquitous Pharmacogenomics Consortium when designing and operationalizing the PREPARE study. Pharmacogenet Genomics 2020; 30(6): 131-44.
[http://dx.doi.org/10.1097/FPC.0000000000000405] [PMID: 32317559]

[57]   Cecchin E, Stocco G. Pharmacogenomics and Personalized Medicine. Genes (Basel) 2020; 11(6): 679.
[http://dx.doi.org/10.3390/genes11060679] [PMID: 32580376]

[58]   Friedman AA, Letai A, Fisher DE, Flaherty KT. Precision medicine for cancer with next-generation functional diagnostics. Nat Rev Cancer 2015; 15(12): 747-56.
[http://dx.doi.org/10.1038/nrc4015] [PMID: 26536825]

[59]   Kaye AD, Mahakian T, Kaye AJ, *et al.* Pharmacogenomics, precision medicine, and implications for anesthesia care. Baillieres Best Pract Res Clin Anaesthesiol 2018; 32(2): 61-81.
[http://dx.doi.org/10.1016/j.bpa.2018.07.001] [PMID: 30322465]

[60]   Chandra R. The role of pharmacogenomics in precision medicine. CONTINUING EDUCATION 2017.

[61]   Mooney SD. Progress towards the integration of pharmacogenomics in practice. Hum Genet 2015; 134(5): 459-65.
[http://dx.doi.org/10.1007/s00439-014-1484-7] [PMID: 25238897]

[62]   Johnson JA. Pharmacogenetics: potential for individualized drug therapy through genetics. Trends Genet 2003; 19(11): 660-6.
[http://dx.doi.org/10.1016/j.tig.2003.09.008] [PMID: 14585618]

[63]   Hugo K. The Drug Discovery Process. Wiley Handbook of Current and Emerging Drug Therapies 2006.
[http://dx.doi.org/10.1002/9780470041000.cedt001]

[64]   Grech G, Grossman I. Preventive and Predictive Genetics: Towards Personalised Medicine. Springer International Publishing 2015.
[http://dx.doi.org/10.1007/978-3-319-15344-5]

[65]   Rao M, Gorey S. Pharmacogenomics and modern therapy. Indian J Pharm Sci 2007; 69(2): 167.
[http://dx.doi.org/10.4103/0250-474X.33138]

[66]   Burgess J, Golden J. Cracking the druggable genome. Bio-IT World 2002.

[67]   Durham LK, Webb S, Milos P, Clary C, Seymour A. The serotonin transporter polymorphism, 5HTTLPR, is associated with a faster response time to sertraline in an elderly population with major depressive disorder. Psychopharmacology (Berl) 2004; 174(4): 525-9.
[http://dx.doi.org/10.1007/s00213-003-1562-3] [PMID: 12955294]

[68]   Adithan C, Surendiran A, Pradhan SC. Role of pharmacogenomics in drug discovery and development. Indian J Pharmacol 2008; 40(4): 137-43.
[http://dx.doi.org/10.4103/0253-7613.43158] [PMID: 20040945]

[69]   Ojha A, Joshi T. A review on the role of pharmacogenomics in drug discovery and development. Int J Pharm Sci Res 2016; 7(9): 3587.

[70]   Guidance for industry. Pharmacogenomic data submission 2005.

[71]   Saito Y, Stamp L, Caudle K, Hershfield M, McDonagh E, Callaghan J, *et al.* CPIC: clinical pharmacogenetics implementation consortium of the pharmacogenomics research network. Clin Pharmacol Ther 2016; 99(1): 36-7.

[http://dx.doi.org/10.1002/cpt.161] [PMID: 26094938]

[72] Little S. The impact of FDA guidance on pharmacogenomic data submissions on drug development. IDrugs 2005; 8(8): 648-50.
[PMID: 16044373]

[73] Gage BF, Lesko LJ. Pharmacogenetics of warfarin: regulatory, scientific, and clinical issues. J Thromb Thrombolysis 2008; 25(1): 45-51.
[http://dx.doi.org/10.1007/s11239-007-0104-y] [PMID: 17906972]

[74] Lee SY, Kim JS, Kim JW. A case of intolerance to warfarin dosing in an intermediate metabolizer of CYP2C9. Yonsei Med J 2005; 46(6): 843-6.
[http://dx.doi.org/10.3349/ymj.2005.46.6.843] [PMID: 16385662]

[75] Lee SY, Nam MH, Kim JS, Kim JW. A case report of a patient carrying CYP2C9*3/4 genotype with extremely low warfarin dose requirement. J Korean Med Sci 2007; 22(3): 557-9.
[http://dx.doi.org/10.3346/jkms.2007.22.3.557] [PMID: 17596671]

[76] Bullock P. Pharmacogenetics and its impact on drug development. Drug Benefit Trends 1999; 11(1): 53-4.

[77] Rappuoli R. Reverse vaccinology. Curr Opin Microbiol 2000; 3(5): 445-50.
[http://dx.doi.org/10.1016/S1369-5274(00)00119-3] [PMID: 11050440]

[78] Naz A, Obaid A, Shahid F, Dar HA, Naz K, Ullah N, *et al.* Reverse vaccinology and drug target identification through pan-genomics. Pan-genomics: Applications, Challenges, and Future Prospects. Elsevier 2020; pp. 317-33.
[http://dx.doi.org/10.1016/B978-0-12-817076-2.00016-0]

[79] Shahid F, Ashraf ST, Ali A. Reverse vaccinology approach to potential vaccine candidates against Acinetobacter baumannii Acinetobacter baumannii. Springer 2019; pp. 329-36.

[80] Rappuoli R. Reverse vaccinology, a genome-based approach to vaccine development. Vaccine 2001; 19(17-19): 2688-91.
[http://dx.doi.org/10.1016/S0264-410X(00)00554-5] [PMID: 11257410]

[81] Pizza M, Scarlato V, Masignani V, *et al.* Identification of vaccine candidates against serogroup B meningococcus by whole-genome sequencing. Science 2000; 287(5459): 1816-20.
[http://dx.doi.org/10.1126/science.287.5459.1816] [PMID: 10710308]

[82] He Y, Xiang Z, Mobley HL. Vaxign: the first web-based vaccine design program for reverse vaccinology and applications for vaccine development J Biomed Biotechnol 2010; 29: 75-05.
[http://dx.doi.org/10.1155/2010/297505]

[83] Rizwan M, Naz A, Ahmad J, *et al.* VacSol: a high throughput in silico pipeline to predict potential therapeutic targets in prokaryotic pathogens using subtractive reverse vaccinology. BMC Bioinformatics 2017; 18(1): 106.
[http://dx.doi.org/10.1186/s12859-017-1540-0] [PMID: 28193166]

[84] Naz K, Naz A, Ashraf ST, *et al.* PanRV: Pangenome-reverse vaccinology approach for identifications of potential vaccine candidates in microbial pangenome. BMC Bioinformatics 2019; 20(1): 123.
[http://dx.doi.org/10.1186/s12859-019-2713-9] [PMID: 30871454]

[85] Paul S, Sidney J, Sette A, Peters B. TepiTool: a pipeline for computational prediction of T cell epitope candidates Current protocols in immunology 2016; 114(1): 1-9.
[http://dx.doi.org/10.1002/cpim.12]

[86] Hoffman SL, Rogers WO, Carucci DJ, Venter JC. From genomics to vaccines: Malaria as a model system. Nat Med 1998; 4(12): 1351-3.
[http://dx.doi.org/10.1038/3934] [PMID: 9846563]

[87] Choo Q, Kuo G. Vaccination of chimpanzees against infection by the hepatitis C virus. Proceedings of the National Academy of Sciences 1994; 1294-8.

[88]   Enayatkhani M, Hasaniazad M, Faezi S, Guklani H, Davoodian P, Ahmadi N, *et al.* Reverse vaccinology approach to design a novel multi-epitope vaccine candidate against COVID-19: an in silico study. J Biomol Struct Dyn 2020; 1-16.
[PMID: 32295479]

[89]   Naz A, Shahid F, Butt TT, Awan FM, Ali A, Malik A. Designing multi-epitope vaccines to combat emerging coronavirus disease 2019 (COVID-19) by employing immuno-informatics approach. Front Immunol 2020; 11: 1663.
[http://dx.doi.org/10.3389/fimmu.2020.01663] [PMID: 32754160]

[90]   Zaheer T, Waseem M, Waqar W, *et al.* Anti-COVID-19 multi-epitope vaccine designs employing global viral genome sequences. Peer J 2020; 8: e9541.
[http://dx.doi.org/10.7717/peerj.9541] [PMID: 32832263]

CHAPTER 9

Multi-omics Data Integration: Applications in Systems Genomics

Anam Naz[1,*], Ammara Siddique[2], Aqsa Ikram[1], Bisma Rauff[5], Huma Tariq[3] and **Sajjad Ahmed[4]**

[1] *Institute of Molecular Biology and Biotechnology (IMBB), The University of Lahore (UOL), Lahore, Pakistan*

[2] *Atta-ur-Rahman School of Applied Biosciences (ASAB), National University of Sciences and Technology (NUST), Islamabad, Pakistan*

[3] *Department of Zoology, Hazara University, Manshera, Pakistan*

[4] *Department of Health and Biological Sciences, Abasyn University, Peshawar, Pakistan*

[5] *Department of Biomedical Engineering, University of Engineering and Technology (UET), Lahore, Narowal Campus, Pakistan*

Abstract: Interpretation of molecular differences and intricacy at multiple stages, for instance proteome, genome, epigenome, metabolome, and transcriptome is needed for a thorough understanding of disease and human health. Biology has been reliant on data produced at these stages, which is collectively referred to as multi-omics data, after the emergence of sequencing techniques. Among all the aspects of biology, rapid development in high-throughput data initiation has enabled to carry out research on multi-omics systems biology. Metabolomics, proteomics, and transcriptomics data can provide answers to the targeted biological queries about the expression of metabolites, proteins, and transcripts, independently. A concise summary of multi-omics data sources, challenges in datasets integration, and visualization portals is also discussed.

Keywords: Genomics, Metabolomics, Proteomics, Transcriptomics, Omics.

1. INTRODUCTION

The approach of systematic multi-omics integration can methodically annotate, model, and assimilate such considerable sets of data. Multi-omics data availability has modernized the domain of biology and medicine by generating opportunities for different methods of an integrated system. Analysis of clinical and multi-omics data has acquired the lead in deriving productive understandings of cellular functions. Multi-omics data integration provides necessary information regarding

* **Corresponding author Anum Naz**: Institute of Molecular Biology and Biotechnology, University of Lahore, Lahore, Pakistan; E-mail: anam.naz@imbb.uol.edu.pk

Syeda Marriam Bakhtiar and Erum Dilshad (Eds.)

biomolecules from respective layers and appears to be capable of understanding complex biology holistically as well as systematically [1]. Integrated approaches link the exclusive omics data, either in a simultaneous or sequential way, in order to comprehend the interaction of molecules [2]. They are helpful in evaluating data flowing towards different levels and therefore assist in linking genotype to phenotype variance. Integrative approaches are capable of studying the biological processes holistically, hence improving predictive accuracy and disease phenotype prognostics and therefore can ultimately help in improved therapy and inhibition [3].

In order to analyze the multifaceted biological methods, integrative methodology should be adopted which links multiomics data for highlighting the functions and interconnections of engaged biomolecules. With the advancement in highthroughput practices and accessibility of multiomics data, numerous promising methods and tools have been established for data analysis, interpretation, and integration. Multiomics integration approach has been reviewed and comprehensively reviewed in studies related to animals [4], humans [5] microbes [6], and their combinations [7]. In contrast, multiomics integration in plants is difficult owing to metabolic assortment, poor annotation of large genomes, and occurrence of various symbionts having complex networks for interaction. Several inclusive analyses are present particularly on plant multiomics integration and their practical use in precision plant breeding, green systems biology, and other biological and biotechnological applications [8]. Moreover, the development of highthroughput techniques and considerable multiomics data ahead of broad data biology might remain vast, and possibly troublesome for the inexperienced investigators. Omics data derived from inadequately categorized species are frequently feed to the software exclusive of any appropriate curation and unaware of technology's constraint, that might result in inaccurate interpretations.

The integration of data related to multi-omics draw holistic knowledge of biological methods and disorders comes with several tests. Heterogeneity in distinct omics data, considerable sets of data leading towards computation of thorough study, and absence of correct information which assists in highlighting different tool sets and software make analysis and integration of multiomics data a challenging job. Multiomics data are generated using variety of programs, and therefore formats and storage of data show considerable differences. Tools for analysis of multiomics integration require particular data, and hence individual omics data needs proper preprocessing.

1.1. Advanced Techniques in "Omics"

Advancements in omics technologies have led to tremendous success in molecular characterization of wide range of complicated human disorders for instance, cancer. Analysis of multiomics integration employing genomics, proteomics, epigenomics, and metabolomics, is attributing advancement of precision medicine in clinical setups. Several patho-mechanisms of cancer development, treatment resistance and risk factors have been revealed and the information has been used in taking right treatment decisions. The application of integrated omics analyses has been limited which has impeded the possible miraculous developments in the diagnostic and research avenues. A lot of efforts are still needed to improve the methodical infrastructure for commendable generation, evaluation, and annotation of multiomics integration data. The proper utilization of this modern approach will lessen the burden of wrong treatments against any particular molecular disease [9].

1.2. Omics-Driven Targeted Therapy

Some latest findings have potentiated the significance of omics-driven targeted treatment in patients suffering from non-small cell lung cancer. The comparison of results between patients suffering from lung adenocarcinoma who were treated by using omics driven directed therapy and individuals who received typical therapies supports this modern approach of decision making. FFT model (fast and frugal decision tree model) was established to estimate the effects of omics-based approach on the treatment of lung cancer patients. Omics-driven therapy decisions were positively related with better overall survival rate and progression free survival of the patients [10].

1.3. Meta-omics

The integrated OMIC discipline is crucial for deep understanding of a disease and thus is helpful in combating many diseases. Gut microbiome shows a significant influence on human well-being and illness and modern expansion of omics methodologies, involving shotgun metagenomics, phylogenetic microbiome profiling based on markers, metatranscriptomics, metagenomics, and metaproteomics, has led to the proficient representation of microbial communities. Modern omic methodologies provide deep taxonomic resolution of the microbial taxa, reveal the taxa specific functions and metabolic actions within an intricate microbiome. Applications of metaomics techniques to clinical samples of microbial diseases have led to the identification of disease-causing microbial species and culprit metabolites. This identification helps the development of treatment options and drugs against these diseases and pathogens. The microbiome-targeted drug discovery has investigated extensive drug-microbiome interactions and has significantly improved human health management. These drug-microbiome interactions are crucial to evaluate the patient-specific treatment response to any disease therapy thus making these techniques disparagingly imperative in the modern-day era of research on microbiome and also precision medicine [11].

1.4. Transcriptomics

The advancement in molecular biology has led to comprehensive depiction of the cellular genome and the transcriptome which indicates the comprehensive set of transcribed RNA species in a certain tissue or cell. Transcriptomics and next-generation sequencing have made it possible to attain unequaled level of information regarding phenotypic differences of cells. These differences are attributed to differential gene expression exhibited by cells in definite physiological and pathological states. The quantification and estimation of these transcriptional differences are a reward of transcriptomics [12]. The tissues are multifaceted systems composed of various cell types. Distinct microenvironments are being exhibited by different tissues which are attributed to many genetic, cellular and physiological factors. Such spatial heterogeneity is caused by differential gene expression and can also be estimated by transcriptomes quantification techniques [13].

RNA-Seq is employed to estimate the global expression of gene by fragmentation of RNA, followed by capturing, sequencing, and computational analysis. The RNA samples for sequencing are prepared and polyadenylated mRNA is measured and normalized among different groups. The gene expression is quantified and differential expression among different groups is highlighted. *Xenopus* has been used to estimate the power of high-throughput sequencing of RNA to comprehend specific patterns of expressions of genes during development [14].

1.5. Single-Dimensional Transcriptomic Assessment versus Integrated Omics

Sequencing techniques and immunological methods have been extensively employed to reveal information about cellular forms and positions at single-cell genomic, transcriptomic, epigenomic and proteomic levels. Transcriptomic evaluation delivers knowledge relating to molecular connections amid gene and the protein, making biological methods and ailments understandable. Single-dimensional transcriptomic assessment is more strengthened by the integration of transcriptome with other "omics" making multi-dimensional analysis for comprehensive understanding of cellular functions. Multi-omics integrated examination of both genome as well as transcriptome is achieved by separate /comparable extraction of genomic DNA followed by cytoplasmic mRNA. Similarly, an integrated study of transcriptomes and epigenomes is achieved by parallel/individual extraction of genomic DNA followed by mRNA. Proteomic and transcriptomic analyses can be integrated by employing processes of direct imaging, assays for proximity ligation (PLA), assays for proximity extension (PEA), and methods based on sequencing [15]. The chromatin organization and epigenetic regulation can be investigated by integration of ChIP-sequencing and RNA-sequencing datasets [16].

1.6. Rewards of Integrated Omics

Integrated and combinational analysis of 'multi-omics' datasets at single cell and population level has provided a deep understanding of the heterogeneous process of aging which is driven by interconnected molecular changes. This high-profile information of controlling prominence of gene expression in aging is being employed in devising aging interventions. Aging Atlas is a database which provides such precious information derived by high-throughput omics technologies to life science researchers around the world [17]. Epigenetic landscapes are very crucial factors in the alteration of physiologic phenotype and in the progression of abnormal phenotypes in many diseases and cancers. The methylome landscape has been delineated by high resolution multi-omics methods and oncogenic factors of esophageal squamous cell carcinoma (ESCC) have been characterized. Such epigenome profiling provides information about biomarker and target discovery [18].

2. PATHWAY PROFILING USING SYSTEM GENOMICS

A pathway profiling and genetic networks by using system biology approaches may shed light by projecting candidate proteins onto protein functional relationship systems. Gene expressions are often used as surrogate representations of pathway activation and inhibition. The use of expression signatures to compute pathway activation level has been very important to appropriately address the complexity of diseases and providing strategies of targeted therapeutics. So, pathway profiling and genetic networks help researchers gain mechanistic insight into gene, proteins and metabolic compounds lists extracted from multi-omics experiments.

The construction of pathway interaction networks using system biology has been accomplished through three distinct methods: (1) literature mining of all reported metabolites, gene, protein or biochemical interactions; (2) computational and statistical predictions grounded on available data; (3) systematic and high throughput profiling of metabolites, genes and proteins (Fig. **9.1**).

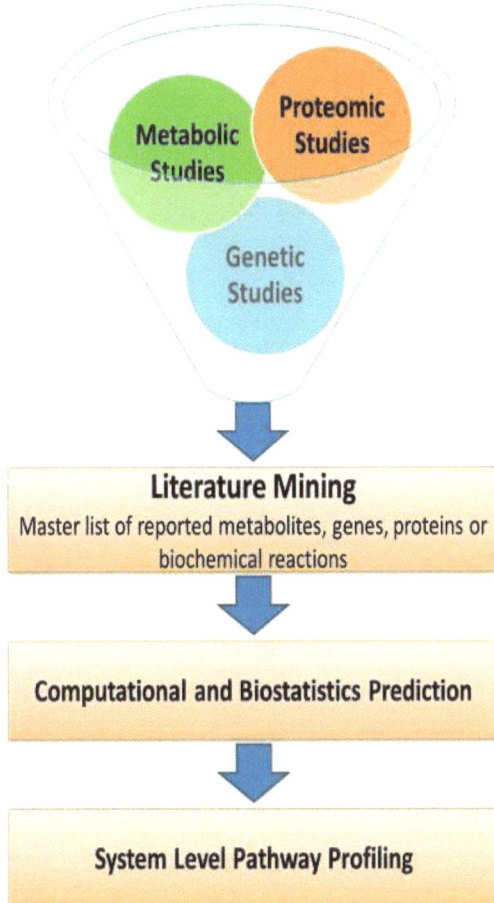

Fig. (9.1). Construction of pathway interaction networks using system biology.

3. CATEGORIES OF PATHWAY PROFILING AND GENETIC NETWORK

Pathway profiling and genetic network is a vast field of study and can be categorized into four keys, slightly overlapping categories including metabolic profiling, signaling profiling, protein interaction, and gene profiling.

3.1. Metabolic Pathway Profiling

Metabolic pathways are important to establish a difference between normal and abnormal metabolic phenotype. Amid many 'omics' technologies, metabolomics is often used to outline metabolites that are present in various biological samples and are the products of diverse metabolic pathways. The first pathogen-host interactions by using integrated genome-scale metabolic network were reported for the erythrocytes *infected with Plasmodium falciparum* infection [19]. Another analysis of the integration of metabolic network was adopted for *Mycobacterium tuberculosis* infecting alveolar macrophages [19]. A metabolic scale remodeling of the pathogen infection with 1,027 reactions and 661 genes was retrieved. The host metabolic profiling was derived from Recon1 representing 3394 reactions and about 1410 genes. This study concludes the elimination of 86 genes. In another analysis, the same pathogenic infection of macrophages was investigated by means of advanced metabolic networks and setups [20]. This metabolic pathway contained 915 genes and about 1192 reactions. Here for human metabolism reconstruction, Recon 2.2 was utilized, with 1675 associated genes and 7,785 reactions.

3.2. Signaling Pathways Profiling

Signaling pathways integrate information from one reaction of the cell to another *via* a series of protein interactions. Dysregulation of cellular processes by abnormal signaling pathways causes many common diseases, including cancers and diabetes. If used in an appropriate way, various system level approaches can help in many ways to explain the function of a gene of interest, their synthesis, regulation and potential interaction partners. In astudy, Ideker *et al.* worked on a GAL (galactose utilization), a pathway in the yeast Saccharomyces cerevisiae, implementing an integrated approach connecting molecular expressions and interactions to comprehend how various genes are regulated [21]. Steffen *et al.* adopted the same approach in assembling a large PPI network against yeast. This system, named NetSearch, enabled them to reconstruct pathways for mitogen activated protein kinases in yeast which are involved in various cellular processes. Kelley *et al.* in 2003 devised PATHBLAST, an efficient tool to align paths across multiple PPI networks. This tool enables the search for homologous paths across networks by accommodating "gaps" and "mismatches". Following this success, Shlomi *et al.* proposed QPath, which improved the results of PATHBLAST. Aided by computational tools and experimental approaches, the growth of public databases [22] for pathways [23] and Gene Ontology [24] for functional annotations enabled pathway identification methods to use these annotations for both prediction and validation of results.

3.3. Networks for Protein-Protein Interaction

Data for protein-protein interaction originates from various investigational studies engaging high-throughput screening and computational projections to categorize their possible correlations. Computational approaches were highly recognized for the prediction of protein-protein interactions. More than 38,000 experimental studies identified human protein-protein interactions comprising about 73,000 interactions [25]. Major databases employed for the curation analysis include: BioGRID [26], DIP [27], IntAct [28], and MINT [29]. These databases are frequently used sources for the data related to health sciences research. Dezső *et al.* identified genes specific for diseases on the basis of their scoring statistics and topological importance in protein pathway [30]. Goh *et al.* reported a clear difference between essential genes and disease triggering genes [31] Goñi *et al.* associated two neurodegenerative diseases in two tissues [32]. Their PPI network analysis revealed that Alzheimer's disease associated proteins are more central in the brain, whereas blood tissues are the hotspot of multiple sclerosis related proteins. System biology has also been approached to characterize important host factors critically involved in the regulation of viral infections. Farooq *et al.* 2020 screened out 1027 connections between 829 proteins. Among these, 14 are related to the viruses whereas 815 are related to human proteins.

3.4. Gene Regulatory Networks

Studies employing a gene regulatory network ended up with global interactions between human illnesses and associated genes. Disease genes have high expression levels, expression patterns which are specific for the tissues and high rate of mutation over evolutionary stretch. With this evidence, several analyses have been conducted based on omics programs at different levels to recognize and prioritize disease causing genes. Wu *et al.* employed approaches for gene classification to distinguish whether a gene can cause disease or not [33]. Nguyen and Ho used enriched analysis approach by integrating the identified genes of disease with neighboring diseased genes [34]. Franke *et al.* recommended an integrated network of genes that could be helpful in the identification of genes causing diseases [35]. Lee *et al.* investigated functional interaction of a human gene network [36]. Valentini proposed a novel technique to categorize genes as per cancer modules incorporating networks formed from distinctive functional information sources. Aerts *et al.* explained a bioinformatics method that generates diverse prioritizations for heterogeneous sources of data, which are integrated and fused on global ranking by means of order statistics. Chuang *et al.* (2007) explained a classifier based on a network for diagnosis of breast cancer. According to this process, the profiles for gene-expression of both metastatic as well as nonmetastatic subjects are superimposed upon human network for proteinprotein interaction [37]. Efroni *et al.* (2007) also presented a related report, identifying pathways correlated with datasets of cancer gene expression. Expression data was used for scoring known pathways for consistency and activity of their connections in the given sample [38].

4. DESIGNING EXPERIMENTS FOR OMICS DATA INTEGRATION

4.1. Multi-Omics Data from Genome to Phenome: Integration in Systems Genomics

The approach of Multiview learning is through the division of machine learning approaches. Basically, it deals with multi modal sets of data and, specifically, with the patterns shown by various features. This learning technique has spread rapidly. This spread is encouraged by the persistent rise of actual functions, which are on the basis of multi-view data. In computation biology, for instance, several experiments are proposed like protein expression, miRNA, and studies for genome wide association and various others for diverse sample sets. In bioinformatics/computational biology, multi-view learning methodologies/ techniques have been extensively useful because the diverse genome wide sources of data collect information about complicated biological systems. Every aspect offers a discrete feature of the similar domain and encodes diverse biologically related patterns. These kinds of integrations of these aspects/views deliver a deeper models of the underlying systems than those generated by a single aspect alone [39].

The data integration that is relevant to mRNA expression and/or protein abundance by using regulatory network systems has been studied in relevant to the expression of genes that play an important role in puberty of bovines [40].

Among the various system genomics approaches, expression quantitative trait loci (eQTL) focuses on the integration of data of genomics and transcriptomics has been used to detect the regions in genomes that are linked to the transcript levels [41]. These eQTLs could be cis- acting or trans-acting. Cis-acting eQTL is found near the gene which forms a transcript, whereas, trans-acting eQTL is found either at some distance or on the other chromosome. This represents that the pragmatic eQTL shows actually the place of a locus that controls the targeted gene expression [41].

A current multi-parental population investigation of heterogeneous stocks of mice, rats and human has found candidate genes for targets. These targeted candidate genes have been mapped to different phenotypes of diseases [42]. The investigators have applied a differential expression analysis that is followed by the eQTL approach. They have further employed a mixed model evaluation on sequences of founder animals. They have found various variants in the identified genomes' region. Though, such findings can identify different variants in genes involved in disease pathogenesis, but whether these casual genes themselves have an important function in the progression of complex phenotypes comes as a question or a challenge [43].

The questions need to be answered are that how significant eQTL is for analyses of these genetic networks which cause variation in phenotypes? and could these eQTL results gathered from transcriptomics analysis be associated to the level of proteomics? Though transcriptomics data and phenomics data do not appear to be linked, mapping the genetic variants for the expression of gene can present a meaningful system/base for investigating considerable effects of these phenotypes and associating genetic determinants to the disease [43].

Clustered regularly interspaced short palindromic repeats, CRISPR in combination with the protein, Cas protein (CRISPR/Cas) technology directs RNA into a genome of cell (the nuclease). It cuts the genome at targeted locations and the method is known as genome editing. Cong and his colleagues introduced this technology for the first time [44]. Various site-directed mutagenesis research works have been performed across different animal models and different populations [45, 46]. Site-directed editing of genome has revolutionized the quality of genome modifications that way that this technology can be acquired to the level which is comparable to zinc-finger nucleases systems and also transcription activator for instance, effector nucleases.

Fig. (**9.2**) illustrates the A) collection of multi-omics databases (proteomics, genomics, metabolomics, and transcriptomics), B) Analysis of these single layered and mutilayered muti-omics databases that include GWAS, genomic predictions, differential expression analyses *via* proteomics and metabolomics databases to network and eQTL/mQTL/pQTL analyses, C) results and validation of these analyses in system genomics and D) prospective application of these strategies in health and welfare including the selection of casual, functional and regulatory variants, biomarkers and drug target selections, improvement in diagnosis sector and better phenotype state selections and genomic predictions of disease risk.

4.2. Software and Tools Used for Integration

In this chapter, our prime focus is on the methods and tools that carry out the integration of multiomics data and also review their applications in order to understand the complicated biology of humans. Tools are selected on the basis of the below stated conditions:

1. The methodology should run an integrative phase where different sets of data are evaluated in a synchronized manner (these datasets should be in parallel integration pattern instead of sequential pattern). Platforms for instance, O-Miner and Galaxy, assist in the study of multi-omics data, although individually [47].

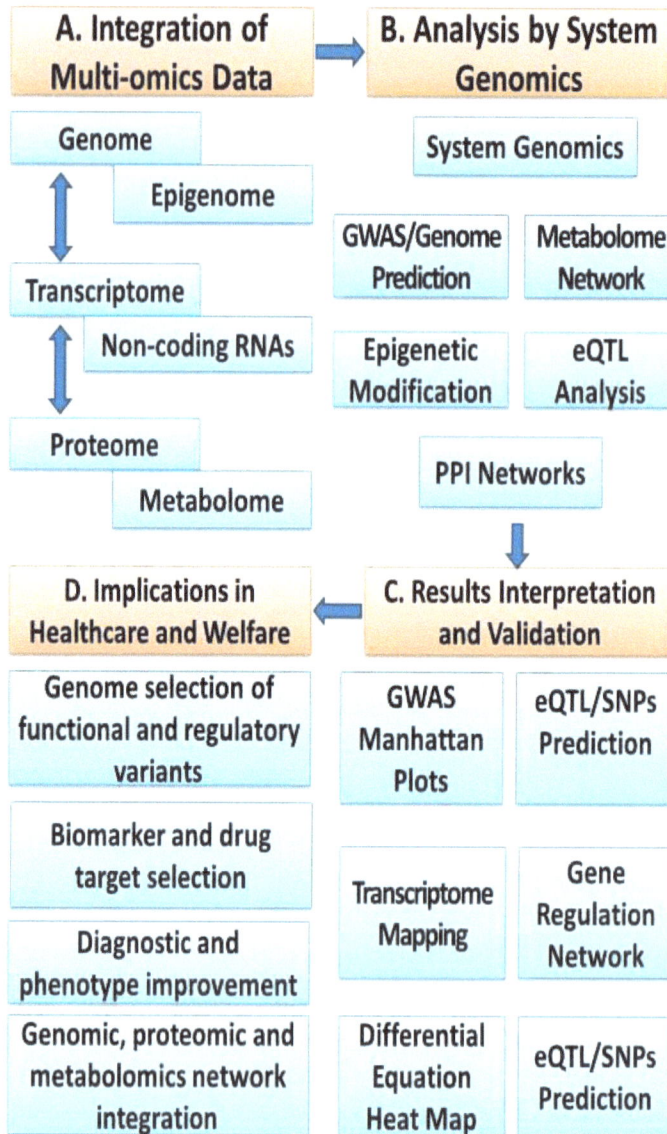

Fig. (9.2). Schematic representation of integration of multi-omics platforms/databases.

2. The approach should integrate a minimum of 2 sets of omics data which are derived from the samples that exhibit partial overlap [48].

3. The approach must be readily accessible in tool or package form to be capable of executing the process on any data set.

Several techniques and tools have been created for the multi-omics integrative data analysis and have been discussed below.

4.3. Multi-Omics Factor Analysis (MOFA)

Matrix factorization is a widespread approach, where the aim is the gathering of latent factors which discuss the interpatient variance among modalities of omics. Multi-Omics Factor Analysis is an unverified matrix factorization practice which is a simplification of the principal component evaluation to various data matrices. It is used for integration of multiomics data kinds in either the similar or partly overlapping samples [49].

4.4. MixOmics

MixOmics package [50] offers both supervised and unsupervised practices on the basis of Canonical Correlation Analysis (CCA) and Partial Least Squares (PLS) with generalizations to the multi-block data. MixOmics delivers a set of unsupervised and supervised multivariate approaches in order to perform integration of multiomics sets of data with the main emphasis on the selection of variables. This set permits the integration of multiomics datasets to cluster or classify the samples by using diverse methods for instance principal component evaluation, independent principal component evaluation, sparse partial least squares regression, partial least squares regression, canonical correlation analysis, and several supervised analyses.

4.5. Graph-based Clustering of Samples

Another powerful tool for integration of data is the clustering based on the graphs of the samples that found its application in the discovery of the subtype of disease. In the Similarity Network Fusion, the networks for single-omics subject similarity are formed, monitored by the iterative information exchange to create fused multi-omics patient network [51].

4.6. Nonnegative Matrix Factorization (NMF)

Nonnegative matrix factorization approach is generally used for evaluation of high-dimensional sets of data, and several extensions of the method are formed for improved analysis of the data of multiomics. Integrative NMF expands NMF basis for the interpretation of heterogeneous effects and the integration of multiple data [1]. Another approach depends on clustering based on permutation and was created for the identification of vigorous patient partitions. Such an approach incorporates data by understanding the difference between omics-distinct patient connectivity [52].

4.7. Multi-Omics Data Integration (miodin)

So as to address the arguments of the analysis of multiomics data, Multi-Omics Data Integration (miodin) was created. This offers a software infrastructure for building data evaluation workflows which analyzes, imports, and develops the multi-omics data. These workflows assist data from various modalities of omics, comprising proteomics, epigenomics, genomics, and transcriptomics and also from several experimental methods (mass spectrometry, sequencing, microarrays). Miodin package could be utilized for the analysis of single omics data, whereas by design, this package is proposed to update multiomics data analysis and integration [53].

4.8. Network-based Integration of Multi-omics Data (NetICS)

The network-based integration of multi-omics data approach offers an outline for integration based on the network for the data of multiomics for the prioritization of cancer genes. This foretells the genetic aberrations effect, miRNAs on both downstream protein (expression) and genes, and epigenetic changes in the interaction network [54].

4.9. moCluster

moCluster utilizes the approach of multi-table multivariate analysis in order to classify patterns across sets of multiomics data [55]. The initial step includes the classification of suppressed variables by using PCA sparse consensus. The total latent variables which are to be utilized are determined by permutation and elbow analysis. Moreover, these variables are then clustered by using established procedures for instance K-means or hierarchical and selection of the finest subtype model.

4.10. Penalized Multivariate Analysis (PMA)

The R package contains different CCA versions which assist in the evaluation of multiple sets of data integration measured by the similar sample sets. The techniques are objected at ranging CCA so as to comprise sparsity constraint, measurements of outcome as available, and the presence of more than two sets of data while forming the relation between different datasets [56].

5. CHALLENGES

Multiomics datasets integration is used to gain complete understanding of life activities and illnesses that comes with various trials. The primary heterogeneity in particular omics data, which is a big size of sets of data that leads to rigorous evaluation, and the absence of findings that assist in ordering the distinct tools make the multi-omics integration of data a challenging task [57]. One of the many multi-omics data integration challenges is that data exploitation needs imperative consideration, because it uses prior understanding and storage for designing statistical strategies to investigate the assorted data and generation of tools for data exploration which include new visualization tools and significant statistics [58].

Another substantial challenge in multi-omics data integration is the impact of BIGdata analysis. The term BIGdata describes the extent of data generated by instruments/tools [59]. This entails the development of scalable infrastructures that direct these masses of data, whereas making it accessible for proficient indexing. Another aspect that could supplement to multiomic interpretation of data is clinical knowledge. Presently, no vigorous strategy is present to incorporate non-omics data with omics data similar to clinical metadata [60]. The current advancements in this area are succeeding mostly with the strengths to minimize the challenges. More improvements in the evaluation of integration of multiomics data should aim to facilitate interoperability of various sets of data and also to make a network that assists in whole uniform evaluation of multi-omics data.

6. FUTURE ASPECTS

Clinical information is another aspect that could signify the interpretation of multi-omics data interpretation. Presently, no robust technique is available for the integration of omics and non-omics data for instance clinical metadata. The present-day advancement in this area is principally advancing with efforts in reducing the challenges. Advancements in the analysis of multiomics data integration must intend to alleviate the interoperability of several sets of data and develop an outline that can aid in unified evaluation of multi-omics data. The future work for the improvement of multiomics integration approaches could be devoted to complete metabolite and gene annotation for particular plant species, along with the development of user-friendly means using algorithms of machine learning to permit precise reconstruction of the metabolic model.

CONCLUDING REMARKS

Integrative approach by means of multiomics data is an influential approach to interpret the mechanistic aspects of material and information flow. Presently, a variety of methods and tools are available in public domain for the integration of multiomics datasets to develop meaningful understanding. As the techniques and tools mainly isolated, a uniform outline is needed which can efficiently analyze and process multi-omics data along with biologist friendly and easy interpretation and visualization.

CONSENT FOR PUBLICATION

Not Applicable.

CONFLICT OF INTEREST

The author declares no conflict of interest, financial or otherwise.

ACKNOWLEDGEMENTS

Declared none.

REFERENCES

[1]   Yang Z, Michailidis G. A non-negative matrix factorization method for detecting modules in heterogeneous omics multi-modal data. Bioinformatics 2016; 32(1): 1-8.
[http://dx.doi.org/10.1093/bioinformatics/btw552] [PMID: 26377073]

[2]   Bersanelli M, Mosca E, Remondini D, *et al.* Methods for the integration of multi-omics data: mathematical aspects. BMC Bioinformatics 2016; 17(S2) (Suppl. 2): S15.
[http://dx.doi.org/10.1186/s12859-015-0857-9] [PMID: 26821531]

[3]   Hasin Y, Seldin M, Lusis A. Multi-omics approaches to disease. Genome Biol 2017; 18(1): 83.
[http://dx.doi.org/10.1186/s13059-017-1215-1] [PMID: 28476144]

[4]   García-Sevillano MÁ, García-Barrera T, Abril N, Pueyo C, López-Barea J, Gómez-Ariza JL. Omics technologies and their applications to evaluate metal toxicity in mice M. spretus as a bioindicator. J Proteomics 2014; 104: 4-23.
[http://dx.doi.org/10.1016/j.jprot.2014.02.032] [PMID: 24631825]

[5]   Chen LC, Chen YY. Outsmarting and outmuscling cancer cells with synthetic and systems immunology. Curr Opin Biotechnol 2019; 60: 111-8.
[http://dx.doi.org/10.1016/j.copbio.2019.01.016] [PMID: 30822698]

[6]   Denman SE, Morgavi D, Mcsweeney CS. The application of omics to rumen microbiota function animal 12: 233-45.2018;
[http://dx.doi.org/10.1017/S175173111800229X]

[7]   Wanichthanarak K, Fahrmann JF, Grapov D. Genomic, proteomic, and metabolomic data integration strategies Biomarker insights. 2015; vol. 10.
[http://dx.doi.org/10.4137/BMI.S29511]

[8]   Weckwerth W, Ghatak A, Bellaire A, Chaturvedi P, Varshney RK. PANOMICS meets germplasm. Plant Biotechnol J 2020; 18(7): 1507-25.
[http://dx.doi.org/10.1111/pbi.13372] [PMID: 32163658]

[9]   Olivier M, Asmis R, Hawkins GA, Howard TD, Cox LA. The Need for Multi-Omics Biomarker Signatures in Precision Medicine. Int J Mol Sci 2019; 20(19): 4781.
[http://dx.doi.org/10.3390/ijms20194781] [PMID: 31561483]

[10]   Salgia R, Mambetsariev I, Pharaon R, *et al.* Evaluation of Omics-Based Strategies for the Management of Advanced Lung Cancer. JCO Oncol Pract 2021; 17(2): e257-65.

[http://dx.doi.org/10.1200/OP.20.00117] [PMID: 32639928]

[11]   Zhang X, Li L, Butcher J, Stintzi A, Figeys D. Advancing functional and translational microbiome research using meta-omics approaches. Microbiome 2019; 7(1): 154.
[http://dx.doi.org/10.1186/s40168-019-0767-6] [PMID: 31810497]

[12]   Chambers DC, Carew AM, Lukowski SW, Powell JE. Transcriptomics and single-cell RNA-sequencing. Respirology 2019; 24(1): 29-36.
[http://dx.doi.org/10.1111/resp.13412] [PMID: 30264869]

[13]   Moor AE, Itzkovitz S. Spatial transcriptomics: paving the way for tissue-level systems biology. Curr Opin Biotechnol 2017; 46: 126-33.
[http://dx.doi.org/10.1016/j.copbio.2017.02.004] [PMID: 28346891]

[14]   Owens NDL, De Domenico E, Gilchrist MJ. An RNA-Seq Protocol for Differential Expression Analysis. Cold Spring Harb Protoc 2019; 2019(6): pdb.prot098368.
[http://dx.doi.org/10.1101/pdb.prot098368] [PMID: 30952685]

[15]   Song Y, Xu X, Wang W, Tian T, Zhu Z, Yang C. Single cell transcriptomics: moving towards multi-omics. Analyst (Lond) 2019; 144(10): 3172-89.
[http://dx.doi.org/10.1039/C8AN01852A] [PMID: 30849139]

[16]   Han Z, Cui K, Placek K, *et al.* Diploid genome architecture revealed by multi-omic data of hybrid mice. Genome Res 2020; 30(8): 1097-106.
[http://dx.doi.org/10.1101/gr.257568.119] [PMID: 32759226]

[17]   Liu G-H, Bao Y, Qu J, *et al.* Aging Atlas: a multi-omics database for aging biology. Nucleic Acids Res 2021; 49(D1): D825-30.
[http://dx.doi.org/10.1093/nar/gkaa894] [PMID: 33119753]

[18]   Cao W, Lee H, Wu W, *et al.* Multi-faceted epigenetic dysregulation of gene expression promotes esophageal squamous cell carcinoma. Nat Commun 2020; 11(1): 3675.
[http://dx.doi.org/10.1038/s41467-020-17227-z] [PMID: 32699215]

[19]   Huthmacher C, Hoppe A, Bulik S, Holzhütter HG. Antimalarial drug targets in Plasmodium falciparum predicted by stage-specific metabolic network analysis. BMC Syst Biol 2010; 4(1): 120.
[http://dx.doi.org/10.1186/1752-0509-4-120] [PMID: 20807400]

[20]   Rienksma RA, Schaap PJ, Martins dos Santos VAP, Suarez-Diez M. Modeling host-pathogen interaction to elucidate the metabolic drug response of intracellular mycobacterium tuberculosis. Front Cell Infect Microbiol 2019; 9: 144.
[http://dx.doi.org/10.3389/fcimb.2019.00144] [PMID: 31139575]

[21]   Ideker T, Thorsson V, Ranish JA, *et al.* Integrated genomic and proteomic analyses of a systematically perturbed metabolic network. Science 2001; 292(5518): 929-34.
[http://dx.doi.org/10.1126/science.292.5518.929] [PMID: 11340206]

[22]   Kanehisa M, Goto S. KEGG: Kyoto Encyclopedia of Genes and Genomes Nucleic Acids Res 2000; 1(1).

[23]   Ruepp A, Zollner A, Maier D, *et al.* The FunCat, a functional annotation scheme for systematic classification of proteins from whole genomes. Nucleic Acids Res 2004; 32(18): 5539-45.
[http://dx.doi.org/10.1093/nar/gkh894] [PMID: 15486203]

[24]   Ashburner M, Ball CA, Blake JA, *et al.* Gene Ontology: tool for the unification of biology. Nat Genet 2000; 25(1): 25-9.
[http://dx.doi.org/10.1038/75556] [PMID: 10802651]

[25]   Kotlyar M, Rossos A E, Jurisica I. Prediction of protein-protein interactions. Current protocols in bioinformatics 2017; vol. 60(8.2): 1-8.2.
[http://dx.doi.org/10.1002/cpbi.38]

[26]   Chatr-aryamontri A, Oughtred R, Boucher L, *et al.* The BioGRID interaction database: 2017 update.

Nucleic Acids Res 2017; 45(D1): D369-79.
[http://dx.doi.org/10.1093/nar/gkw1102] [PMID: 27980099]

[27]　Salwinski L, Miller CS, Smith AJ, Pettit FK, Bowie JU, Eisenberg D. The database of interacting proteins: 2004 update. Nucleic Acids Res 2004; 32(90001): 449D-51.
[http://dx.doi.org/10.1093/nar/gkh086] [PMID: 14681454]

[28]　Orchard S, Ammari M, Aranda B, *et al.* The MIntAct project—IntAct as a common curation platform for 11 molecular interaction databases. Nucleic Acids Res 2014; 42(D1): D358-63.
[http://dx.doi.org/10.1093/nar/gkt1115] [PMID: 24234451]

[29]　Ceol A, Chatr Aryamontri A, Licata L, *et al.* MINT, the molecular interaction database: 2009 update. Nucleic Acids Res 2010; 38(Database issue) (Suppl. 1): D532-9.
[http://dx.doi.org/10.1093/nar/gkp983] [PMID: 19897547]

[30]　Dezső Z, Nikolsky Y, Nikolskaya T, *et al.* Identifying disease-specific genes based on their topological significance in protein networks. BMC Syst Biol 2009; 3(1): 36.
[http://dx.doi.org/10.1186/1752-0509-3-36] [PMID: 19309513]

[31]　Goh KI, Cusick ME, Valle D, Childs B, Vidal M, Barabási AL. The human disease network. Proc Natl Acad Sci USA 2007; 104(21): 8685-90.
[http://dx.doi.org/10.1073/pnas.0701361104] [PMID: 17502601]

[32]　Goñi J, Esteban FJ, de Mendizábal NV, *et al.* A computational analysis of protein-protein interaction networks in neurodegenerative diseases. BMC Syst Biol 2008; 2(1): 52.
[http://dx.doi.org/10.1186/1752-0509-2-52] [PMID: 18570646]

[33]　Wu S, Shao F, Sun R, Sui Y, Wang Y, Wang J. Analysis of human genes with protein–protein interaction network for detecting disease genes. Physica A 2014; 398: 217-28.
[http://dx.doi.org/10.1016/j.physa.2013.12.046]

[34]　Nguyen TP, Ho TB. Detecting disease genes based on semi-supervised learning and protein–protein interaction networks. Artif Intell Med 2012; 54(1): 63-71.
[http://dx.doi.org/10.1016/j.artmed.2011.09.003] [PMID: 22000346]

[35]　Franke L, Bakel H, Fokkens L, de Jong ED, Egmont-Petersen M, Wijmenga C. Reconstruction of a functional human gene network, with an application for prioritizing positional candidate genes. Am J Hum Genet 2006; 78(6): 1011-25.
[http://dx.doi.org/10.1086/504300] [PMID: 16685651]

[36]　Lee I, Blom UM, Wang PI, Shim JE, Marcotte EM. Prioritizing candidate disease genes by network-based boosting of genome-wide association data. Genome Res 2011; 21(7): 1109-21.
[http://dx.doi.org/10.1101/gr.118992.110] [PMID: 21536720]

[37]　Chuang HY, Lee E, Liu YT, Lee D, Ideker T. Network-based classification of breast cancer metastasis. Mol Syst Biol 2007; 3(1): 140.
[http://dx.doi.org/10.1038/msb4100180] [PMID: 17940530]

[38]　Efroni S, Schaefer CF, Buetow KH. Identification of key processes underlying cancer phenotypes using biologic pathway analysis. PLoS One 2007; 2(5): e425.
[http://dx.doi.org/10.1371/journal.pone.0000425] [PMID: 17487280]

[39]　Serra MFA, Greco D, Tagliaferri R. Data integration in genomics and systems biology 2016 IEEE Congress on Evolutionary Computation (CEC). 1272-9.Vancouver, BC, Canada 2016; pp.
[http://dx.doi.org/10.1109/CEC.2016.7743934]

[40]　Cánovas A, Reverter A, DeAtley KL, *et al.* Multi-tissue omics analyses reveal molecular regulatory networks for puberty in composite beef cattle. PLoS One 2014; 9(7): e102551.
[http://dx.doi.org/10.1371/journal.pone.0102551] [PMID: 25048735]

[41]　Westra HJ, Franke L. From genome to function by studying eQTLs. Biochim Biophys Acta Mol Basis Dis 2014; 1842(10): 1896-902.
[http://dx.doi.org/10.1016/j.bbadis.2014.04.024] [PMID: 24798236]

[42] Tsaih SW, Holl K, Jia S, *et al.* Identification of a novel gene for diabetic traits in rats, mice, and humans. Genetics 2014; 198(1): 17-29.
[http://dx.doi.org/10.1534/genetics.114.162982] [PMID: 25236446]

[43] Buchner DA, Nadeau JH. Contrasting genetic architectures in different mouse reference populations used for studying complex traits. Genome Res 2015; 25(6): 775-91.
[http://dx.doi.org/10.1101/gr.187450.114] [PMID: 25953951]

[44] Cong L, Ran FA, Cox D, *et al.* Multiplex genome engineering using CRISPR/Cas systems. Science 2013; 339(6121): 819-23.
[http://dx.doi.org/10.1126/science.1231143] [PMID: 23287718]

[45] Zhou JW, Xu QP, Yao J, Yu SM, Cao SZ. CRISPR/Cas9 genome editing technique and its application in site-directed genome modification of animals. Yi Chuan 2015; 37(10): 1011-20.
[PMID: 26496753]

[46] Whitelaw CBA, Sheets TP, Lillico SG, Telugu BP. Engineering large animal models of human disease. J Pathol 2016; 238(2): 247-56.
[http://dx.doi.org/10.1002/path.4648] [PMID: 26414877]

[47] Afgan E, Baker D, Batut B, *et al.* The Galaxy platform for accessible, reproducible and collaborative biomedical analyses: 2018 update. Nucleic Acids Res 2018; 46(W1): W537-44.
[http://dx.doi.org/10.1093/nar/gky379] [PMID: 29790989]

[48] Sangaralingam A, Dayem Ullah AZ, Marzec J, *et al.* 'Multi-omic' data analysis using O-miner. Brief Bioinform 2019; 20(1): 130-43.
[http://dx.doi.org/10.1093/bib/bbx080] [PMID: 28981577]

[49] Li Y, Wu F-X, Ngom A. A review on machine learning principles for multi-view biological data integration. Brief Bioinform 2018; 19(2): 325-40.
[PMID: 28011753]

[50] Rohart F, Gautier B, Singh A, Lê Cao KA. mixOmics: An R package for 'omics feature selection and multiple data integration. PLOS Comput Biol 2017; 13(11): e1005752.
[http://dx.doi.org/10.1371/journal.pcbi.1005752] [PMID: 29099853]

[51] Wang B, Mezlini AM, Demir F, *et al.* Similarity network fusion for aggregating data types on a genomic scale. Nat Methods 2014; 11(3): 333-7.
[http://dx.doi.org/10.1038/nmeth.2810] [PMID: 24464287]

[52] Nguyen T, Tagett R, Diaz D, Draghici S. A novel approach for data integration and disease subtyping. Genome Res 2017; 27(12): 2025-39.
[http://dx.doi.org/10.1101/gr.215129.116] [PMID: 29066617]

[53] Wei TYW, Juan CC, Hisa JY, *et al.* Protein arginine methyltransferase 5 is a potential oncoprotein that upregulates G1 cyclins/cyclin-dependent kinases and the phosphoinositide 3-kinase/AKT signaling cascade. Cancer Sci 2012; 103(9): 1640-50.
[http://dx.doi.org/10.1111/j.1349-7006.2012.02367.x] [PMID: 22726390]

[54] Dimitrakopoulos C, Hindupur SK, Häfliger L, *et al.* Network-based integration of multi-omics data for prioritizing cancer genes. Bioinformatics 2018; 34(14): 2441-8.
[http://dx.doi.org/10.1093/bioinformatics/bty148] [PMID: 29547932]

[55] Meng C, Helm D, Frejno M, Kuster B. moCluster: identifying joint patterns across multiple omics data sets. J Proteome Res 2016; 15(3): 755-65.
[http://dx.doi.org/10.1021/acs.jproteome.5b00824] [PMID: 26653205]

[56] Witten DM, Tibshirani RJ. Extensions of sparse canonical correlation analysis with applications to genomic data Statistical applications in genetics and molecular biology. 2009; vol. 8.
[http://dx.doi.org/10.2202/1544-6115.1470]

[57] Subramanian I, Verma S, Kumar S, Jere A, Anamika K. Multi-omics Data Integration, Interpretation,

and Its Application. Bioinform Biol Insights 2020; 14.
[http://dx.doi.org/10.1177/1177932219899051] [PMID: 32076369]

[58]　Gomez-Cabrero D, Abugessaisa I, Maier D, *et al.* Data integration in the era of omics: current and future challenges. BMC Syst Biol 2014; 8 (Suppl. 2): I1.
[http://dx.doi.org/10.1186/1752-0509-8-S2-I1] [PMID: 25032990]

[59]　O'Driscoll A, Daugelaite J, Sleator RD. 'Big data', Hadoop and cloud computing in genomics. J Biomed Inform 2013; 46(5): 774-81.
[http://dx.doi.org/10.1016/j.jbi.2013.07.001] [PMID: 23872175]

[60]　López de Maturana E, Alonso L, Alarcón P, *et al.* Challenges in the Integration of Omics and Non-Omics Data. Genes (Basel) 2019; 10(3): 238.
[http://dx.doi.org/10.3390/genes10030238] [PMID: 30897838]

CHAPTER 10

Single Cell Omics

Erum Dilshad[1,*], **Amna Naheed Khan**[1], **Iqra Bashir**[1], **Muhammad Maaz**[1], **Maria Shabbir**[2] and **Marriam Bakhtiar**[1]

[1] *Department of Bioinformatics and Biosciences, Faculty of Health and Life Sciences, Capital University of Science and Technology (CUST), Islamabad, Pakistan*

[2] *Healthcare Biotechnology, Attaur Rehman School of Applied Biosciences, National University of Science and Technology, Islamabad, Pakistan*

Abstract: Recent advances are nowadays providing opportunities to examine the complexities of organs and organisms at the single-cell level. The conventional cell-based analysis mainly examines the cellular processes from the bulk of cells but single-cell omics provides a more detailed insight into individual cell phenotypes, thus giving a link between the phenotype and genotype of cells. Single-cell analysis can be performed at genome, epigenome, transcriptome, proteome and metabolome levels and thus makes it possible to come across mechanisms not seen during the sequencing of bulk tissues. Researchers need to isolate single cells before the initiation of single-cell analysis. For this, various strategies like FACS, MACS, LCM, micro-manipulation and micro-fluids are used for cell isolation depending upon their physical properties and cellular biological characteristics. The analysis of single-cell data at multiple levels gives us an unusual view of multilevel transformation at the single-cell level and thus providing a better chance to discover novel biological processes. High throughput analysis of single cells at genome, transcriptome and proteome levels provides unique and important insights into cell variability and diverse processes like development, genetic expressions and severity of different symptoms in disease pathogenesis.

Keywords: Metabolomics, Omics, Proteome, Single-cell, Transcriptome.

1. INTRODUCTION

All living beings are composed of several groups of individual cells; thus, a cell can be termed a basic entity of life. The study to explore the phenotypes of different cells and the capability to observe the comportment of organs and organisms at the single-cell stage is imperative to develop and comprehend the evolving practices of these cell communities and is essential to understand the functions of diverse biological systems [1].

* **Corresponding author Erum Dilshad**: Department of Bioinformatics and Biosciences, Faculty of Health and Life Sciences, Capital University of Science and Technology (CUST), Islamabad, Pakistan; Tel: 9251111555666-324; E-mail: dr.erum@cust.edu.pk

Syeda Marriam Bakhtiar and Erum Dilshad (Eds.)

Acquiring single cells population from a heterogeneous population of tissues or cells is called single-cell omics. These populations of cells can be of various cellular states, to study either their normal development or disease mechanisms. Single-cellomics can be analyzed at genome, epigenome, transcriptome, proteome and metabolome levels with specific approaches; applications for each of the technology are mentioned in Table **10.1** [2].

Table 10.1. Single Cell-Omics Techniques with approaches and applications [2].

Life Level	Technique Level	Approaches	Applications
Single Cell	Genome	PCR, MALBAC, MDA	CNV, SNV, indel
	Epigenome	ATAC, Chlp, RRBS	Methylome, histone modifications
	Transcriptome	FISH, RT-PCR, sequencing	Cell states and types
	Proteome	Barcoding, Western blotting, staining	Cellular functions
	Metabolome	Competition assays	Genotype-Phenotype correlations

1.1. Single-cell genomics

The branch of science that deals with the all-inclusive study of genome and genome culture of a targeted sample organism is said to be genomics. The analysis of any specific cell within a tissue sample by using omics procedures is known as single-cell genomics. The single-cell genome sequencing technique is used to observe the physical features including the structural or morphological dissimilarities, aneuploidies, mutations, and genome recombination [3, 4]. The single-cell genomics technique is important for the revelation of various interactions between genetic mechanisms and cell lineage in standard and diseased tissues [5, 6]. For creating an effective treatment strategy for cancers, a precise estimation of prognosis is necessary, thus single-cell genomics has helped in allowing many new prognostic elements to be identified and confirmed. Breast cancer is the best example whereby the basis of propagated cells of a tumor in breast cancer was traced [7] and thus, now, single-cell technology is the best tool to provide a prognosis, unlike in the past [8]. The significance of SCG can be illustrated in Fig. (**10.1**).

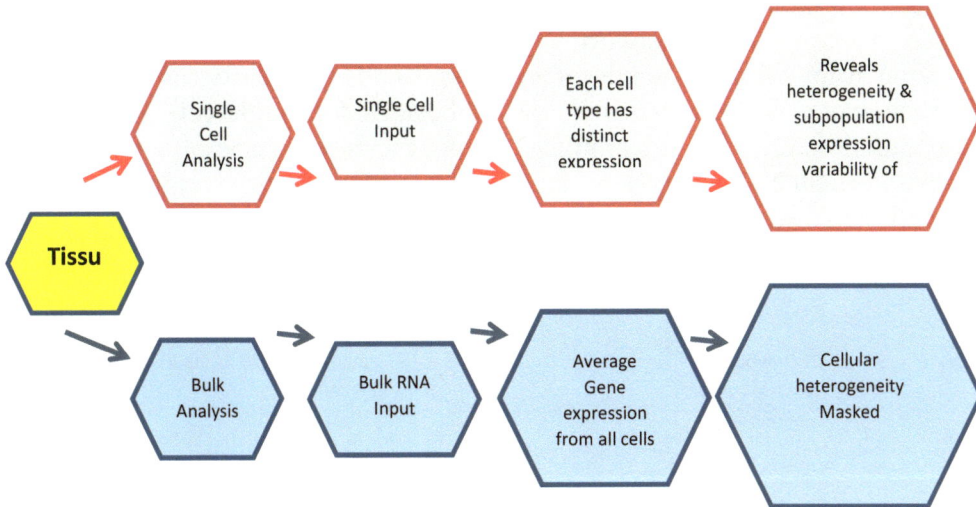

Fig. (10.1). Significance of Single Cell Genomics.

Single-cell transcriptomics

Transcriptomics is an extensive study of entire genome transcriptions for a specified sample living cell, tissue, body part, or an organism as a whole at a certain time of a developmental phase or a specified physiological situation. It is a persuasive technology used to unveil the distinct gene expressions and various RNA-associated configurations through diverse, initial embryonic development and then reprogramming. The genomics technology is also able to link a cell's genotype to its phenotype, and that is the reason for the detection of hundreds of transcripts in an array of cells and tissues [9, 10]. Single-cell transcriptomics has been functional in a range of infections including tumors, cancers, and inflammatory diseases.

The three most widely used methods for computing single-cell gene expression are single-cell quantitative PCR (qPCR), mRNA in situ hybridization, and single-cell RNA sequencing. Single-cell RNA-seq or common scRNA-seq can define the gene expression network in marked cells by combining it with over knockdown, expression, or knockout of a gene of interest [11 - 13]. Furthermore, the tools can also be used to acquire transcriptomic evidence from intra-tumoral cells and to find out the sub-populaces within a body lump by identifying alleged cancer stem cells. Besides, single-cell RNA-seq is considered a favorable technique to boost clinical diagnosis and prediction, and thus is feasible to provide a realistic plus perfect target therapy [14, 15].

It is a fact that one of the major challenges in single-cell genomics is to outline sensitive, accurate, and trustworthy tools and technologies for transcriptome sequencing from even thousands of individual cells. Similarly, as a drawback, RNA sequencing is quite expensive and laborious for single-cell analysis in a large population. Besides, the amplification phase is the cause of analysis noise and uncontrolled bias, mainly in small transcripts. The four significances of single-cell RNA sequencing are illustrated in Fig. (**10.2**), as follows [16].

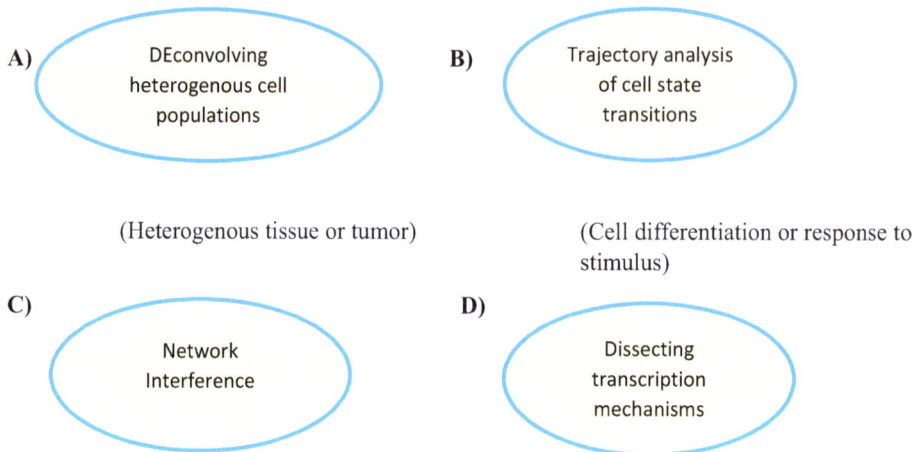

A) DEconvolving heterogenous cell populations

(Heterogenous tissue or tumor)

B) Trajectory analysis of cell state transitions

(Cell differentiation or response to stimulus)

C) Network Interference

D) Dissecting transcription mechanisms

Fig. (10.2). Significance of Single Cell Transcriptomics [16].

1.3. Single-cell Proteomics

The comprehensive characterization and study of the entire protein population and classes present at any cellular level *i.e.*, from a cell up to an organism at an explicit interval or developmental phase are called proteomics [17].

The proteomics of a cell links the genetic makeup to its phenotypic makeup by determining its response to several inner and exterior impetuses. *e.g.*, a tumor suppressor protein *i.e.*, p53 plays an imperative role in numerous cancers. Contrary to its effectiveness, many cell studies failed to reveal the potential of the true dynamic response of p53 [18]. Single-cell proteomics provides much more information about p53's response, crucial in cell signaling. Therefore, single-cell proteomics is an essential and valuable tool to understand and have an insight into genetic variations, medicines and other impetuses, particularly in the scientific trials of cancer including tumors [19]. Although, only dozens of proteins have been characterized through single-cell proteomics, yet, there is a likelihood of a more comprehensive characterization of cellular phenotypes linked to their genotypes [20, 21].

1.4. Single-cell Metabolomics

It is a precise assessment and analysis of all catalytic molecules, particles or metabolites in metabolomics under definite conditions to understand phenotypic heterogeneity. In general, metabolites are the transitional elements that are either produced in the cells or by biological processes within the cells. Metabolites are of two types *i.e.*, primary or prime metabolite or secondary-ancillary metabolites. The prime metabolite includes carbohydrates, proteins, lipids *etc.*, while the secondary metabolite includes nucleotides, oligonucleotides, amino acids, organic acid, aldehydes, ketones, fatty acids, alkaloids, steroids, drugs, *etc* [22].

Metabolomics in combination with other cellular tools like genomics, transcriptomics and proteomics provides a complete understanding of the functionality of each cell. The products of transcriptomics within a single cell are interpreted into proteins, being enzymes to catalyze transitional products of oxidation and metabolism. Thus, at the cellular level, metabolites showing a connection between genotypic and phenotypic traits provide a logical view of a single cell's performance. In this way, the phenomenon of single-cell metabolomics helps observes medication delivery concentration levels to beleaguered cells [23].

2. STRATEGIES FOR SINGLE-CELL ISOLATION

Before the initiation of single-cell analysis, it is necessary to isolate single cells. There are three important parameters used for the characterization of the performance of single-cell isolation technique [24]:

a. Efficacy means the number or quantification of cells secluded in a definite period.
b. Purity means the section of the marked cells collected after the purity phase *i.e.*, separation.
c. Recovery phase is the acquisition of only the segregated portion of the targeted cells out of the entire cellular sample having target cells.

The prevailing cell isolation techniques can be grouped into two classes, based on various principles *i.e.*, physical or biological. The physical isolation techniques are based on physical characteristics *e.g.*, extent, size, compactness, deformability and electric variations by using methodologies like membrane filtration, density gradient centrifugation, and microchip-based capture platforms. The prime benefit of a cell isolation technique based on physical properties is that it ends up without cell marking and even labelling [25].

The biological cell isolation technique is based on cellular genetic individuality, incorporating affinity methods, such as magnetic-induced cell sorting, affinity induced solid matrix, primarily based upon genetic protein expression make-up [25].

The various strategies to access the single-cell isolations are hereby mentioned in Fig. (**10.3**) as follows:

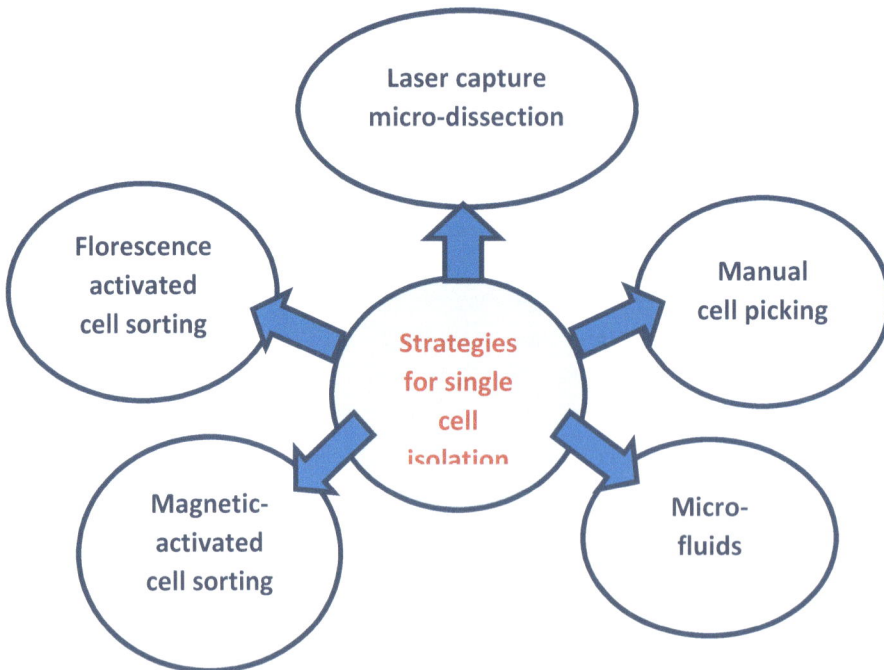

Fig. (10.3). Various Strategies to Access the Single Cell Isolations.

2.1. *Fluorescence-Activated Cell Sorting (FACS)*

Fluorescence-Activated Cell Sorting (FACS) is the most accurate, flexible and sophisticated procedure for refining, characterizing and outlining diverse brands of cells in a mixed cell population by flow cytometry based on phenotypic characteristics like granularity, fluorescence and size. FACS allows understanding of the characteristics of a single-cell population without the impact of other cells [26].

During the FACS mechanism, the targeted cells are mixed to form a suspension and then are branded with luminous probes. Various cells express unalike and exclusive molecules on the plasma membrane that fixes with specific fluorescence-conjugated single cultured antibodies. Each of the cells in the cell culture or suspension is open to a laser during the cytometry. In this way, the fluorescence detectors can classify cells based on specified distinctiveness and uniqueness. During the procedure, the instrument applies either a negative or a positive charge, as the case may be, to the bead comprising a particular cell and the static electric refraction system collects the charged droplets into proper assembly tubes for additional investigation. Although, FACS is extensively used for the segregation of extremely refined cell cultures and populations, yet, it is also clear that FACS can be used at the level of single-cell categorization [27]. A limitation of FACS is that it entails the bulk of cells in suspension, thus it miscarries to sort out single cells from a minor number of cells in suspension.

2.2. *Magnetic-activated Cell Sorting (MACS)*

Magnetic-Activated Cell Sorting (MACS), also known as immunomagnetic cell separation, is an additional but frequently used separation or segregation technique to separate diverse types of cells. It has been reported that specific cell populations can be isolated through MACS with a purity >90% purification [28]. In the MACS technique, certain enzymes, co-enzymes, antibodies and lectins are conjugated to magnetic droplets, which are then fixed to particular proteins existing on the target cells. The magnetic beads or droplets will be turned active in a magnetic external field and the resultant categorized cells will thus be polarized. When the magnetic field is turned off, the elution mechanism is utilized for the acquisition of the residual cells. The method is helpful to distinct cells on a charge basis regarding the specific antigens. The cell isolation based on the magnetic field can either be positively charged or negatively charged. In a positively charged segregation system, only magnetic coated beads are used. Afterwards, only the enticed cells are labelled, discarding the unmarked cells. On the other hand, if specific constituents are not attainable, a more promising choice is to utilize a negative segregation system that is based on a blend of antibodies for coating untreated cells. In this way, only the treated cells having been labelled are casted-off while the untreated cells having been unlabeled are kept for further application [29]. Although, between the two most common methods of cell division, MACS technology is simpler and less expensive, however, the apparent shortcomings of the MACS system lie in its initial cost of separation magnets and operating costs that include not only the value of composite droplets, in addition to column replacement. Besides, MACS is more restrictive than FACS due to immune-magnetic tools and techniques that can only differentiate between healthy and unhealthy cells. The full or restricted exposure of the molecule cannot be parted where conceivable using FACS filters [24].

2.3. *Laser Capture Micro-dissection (LCM)*

Laser Capture Micro dissection (LCM) is a cutting-edge tool for separating the unpolluted areas of a single cell in a culture or cell from solid tissue samples [30]. The technology can exploit the emerging technologies of molecular analysis, including PCR, microarrays, proteomics, *etc.*, by accurately and precisely identifying the required cells [31]. Nowadays, there are two categories of LCM technology *i.e.*, infrared Laser capture micro-dissection or briefly IRLCM technology and ultraviolet Laser capture micro-dissection or briefly UVLCM technology. The standard LCM method comprises a modified electron or optical microscope, a laser control unit, a solid position next to an infrared laser diode, a CCD camera, a monitor, and a microscope-controlled pleasure platform with vacuum cone slide control [32]. The basic laser capture micro-dissection code begins with the thought of sensory cells with a modified microscope, and then with a static laser pulse, but focused on dissolving a thin thermoplastic film on the cover of invading cells. The thermoplastic film dissolves and binds to its favorite key cells. After the removal of the thermoplastic film, the marked cells remain bound to the thermoplastic sheet, leaving all the tissues behind. Finally, the cells are then transferred to a micro-centrifuge comprising buffer elucidations for further investigation [33].

The utmost and vital benefit of Laser capture micro-dissection is its promptness even though it maintains accuracy and flexibility [34]. LCM is a reliable way to obtain pure cell communities identified by different cell types with little thought [35]. Orthodontic techniques for molecular analysis require tissue isolation that leads to contamination problems and reduces clarity and sensitivity in following cell analysis. While, LCM is a non-invasive method that does not remove connective tissue after the onset of microdissection, so the morphology of captive cells and residual tissue is well maintained with minimal tissue loss [36].

An important function of active LCM is the specific identification of isolated cells in connective tissue. Thus, it is clear that the first major limitation is the identification of interested cells with a minimal evaluation of morphological features, which requires a variety of specialists including a cytologist, pathologist, or a trained specialist in cell identification [31]. The second major limitation is that part of the tissue with small machines does not have a cover lid. Since the top slip prevents physical entrance to the apparent surface of the tissue, which is very important for any existing technique of micro-dissection, a system without a coverslip can hide mobile details at high magnification. Besides, LCM refers to several factors, including cell formation during tissue repair and ultraviolet damage to RNA or DNA from laser cutting procedures [37].

2.4. Manual Cell Picking/micro-manipulation

Among single cell division techniques, cell selection by hand is a non-invasive, efficient and effective method. Manual micro-manipulators selective LCM-like micro-manipulators are made of a modified microscope connected to micro-pipettes propelled by machine-powered engines. Each solitary cell in a culture can be detected and snapped under a modified microscope, thus allowing optimal solitude. In addition, micro-manipulation plays a key role in separating living cells compared with LCM that obtains single cells from structural tissue [24].

Micro-manipulation can be easily obtained from an electrophysiology laboratory through a patch clamp system. However, throughput is restricted and necessitates exceptionally expert specialists to accomplish it; there is an obstacle to performance when you feel complex vagaries [24].

2.5. Micro-fluidics

Micro-fluidics is regarded as a powerful technology that assists the investigation of cell surface mass as it affords precise liquid control, device miniaturization, stumpy sample consumption, little analysis expenses, and cool management of nano-litres volumes [38]. Sorting cells by microfluidic chip methodology can be assessed in four ways *i.e.*, cell-affinity based micro-fluidic chromatography, micro-fluidic cell structures disintegration, immune-magnetic droplets based on microfluidic dissociation, and dielectric dissociation methods for a wide variety of species [39].

Microfluidic devices utilize the physical and chemical characteristics at the micro-scale of various phases of matter like gases and liquids. These devices are certainly more beneficial than conventional large systems. Microfluidics runs over the principle of analysis having less sampling volumes, and limited use of chemicals and other analytical reagents thus reducing the cost of its application. This smart technology thus enables many operations to be accomplished at the same time mainly due to compacted size. The list of benefits of microfluidics is given in the following Table **10.2** [40].

Table 10.2. Advantages of Microfluidics.

Single Cell Isolation Strategy	Advantages
Microfluidics	Faster reaction time
	Enhanced analytical sensitivity
	Easier automation
	Enhanced temperature
	Portability
	Parallelization
	Integration of lab routines in one device
	Cheap

3. STRATEGIES FOR SINGLE-CELL SEQUENCING

3.1. Multiple Displacement Amplification

Multiple displacement amplification is the best procedure used in genome culture examination, being simple, and easy with high reliability. The technique is used in the amplification of minute volumes of DNA and resultantly yields good amounts of high-quality DNA. It can amplify DNA at a high response at 30°C with arbitrary primers and polymerase. The phi29 DNA polymerase can encompass primers with high reliability and efficiency, indicating the strength of strand transfer during early strand synthesis [41]. The migration process creates discarded, redesigned and enlarged DNA templates, thereby increasing the DNA to negative feedback [42].

However, the MDA also suffers from severe discrimination and a high level of allelic rejection across genetics, making the reaction more vulnerable to the production of "undesirable substances," which has led to unwanted noise and false effects.

3.2. Multiple Annealing And Looping Based Amplification Cycles

Alternatively, several growths and reduction cycles (MALBAC) have demonstrated the discovery of a reliable copy number [43], which can increase the genetic makeup of a solitary cell with an extraordinary resemblance. MALBAC is found in the pre-enlargement of the fiber which produces amplicons with corresponding endings. Therefore, full amplicons produced by the reaction seal themselves form barriers to prevent further reproduction. This also safeguards that each novel amplicon is recurring from the unique templates. Therefore, the clear benefits of MALBAC are that it can lessen magnification and selection errors as the actual descriptive magnifying elements are copied separately from the original pattern. But there is a need to increase reliability and reduce bias [44 - 46].

3.3. PCR Based scRNA Sequencing

The current single-cell RNA sequencing methodology has five steps [47]:

1. The isolation of the single-cell and RNA.

2. Conversion of RNA to complementary DNA through reverse transcription.

3. Amplification of the complementary DNA.

4. Library generation and sequencing.

5. Computational analysis of the data produced to form single-cell expression profiles.

PCR-based growth has been reported for the first time in a single cell investigation of genetic modification of cell-derived cDNAs using RNA-seq analysis and cDNA microarray [47]. Microarray retrieval is a little exposure sensitivity that is missed by many stumpy but important keywords. In comparison to microarray analysis, RNA-seq analysis increased genetic expression obtained with high accuracy and successfully increased total cDNA length. The additional benefit of PCR-based mRNA transcriptome amplification is that it sorts the sound or noise modification more noticeable amid samples and any actual RNA value that can be used. Furthermore, it can misrepresent the original variations if it is not present [48].

3.4. *In vitro* Transcription (IVT)-based Amplification

In-vitro transcription (IVT) based amplification is the principal method used to effectively increase the RNA of molecular printing investigations, which promotes simultaneous reproduction of cell analysis [49]. It needs three circles of amplification and is based on T7 RNA polymerase-mediated IVT. The key benefits of this strategy include its consistency of measurement, specified output, and reduced collection of indirect products, but have a lower effect on efficacy and time-consuming programs.

Although, single-cell RNA and DNA analysis can offer quality evidence about protein exposure, yet, they cannot provide details about protein location, concentration and translation modification. Therefore, single-cell proteomics helps us to attain the most significant details of cell signaling in cell heterogeneity. Traditional methods of protein analysis like disease immunoassays, lab gel electrophoresis, all spectrums of chromatography, and weight spectrometry require the bulk of cells to be analyzed. Therefore, the limiting factor for protein analysis at the single-cell stages is the requirement of a very small quantity of individual proteins and the deficiency of growth pathways. However, the latest techniques like microfluidics, mass spectrometry, multiparameter flow plus mass cytometry and other procedures have helped researchers to analyze cells and cell culture having greater sensitivity and clarity [24].

3.5. Mass Spectrometry

Mass spectrometry (MS) is the utmost commanding protein exploration device. However, the use of Mass spectrometry to analyze amino acids being the building blocks of proteins in solitary cells is imperfect. The reason behind this imperfectness is the absence of sensitivity to sense low amounts of protein. Recently, a flow cytometry format was developed that integrates the accuracy of mass spectrometry called weight cytometry. It would specifically allow for the measurement of more than 40 cellular parameters simultaneously in a single transfer cell to test millions of cells from a single sample [50].

3.6. Single-cell multi-Omics

The recent progress in single-cell isolation technologies provided exceptional prospects to outline mRNA, DNA, and entire proteins at a single-cell resolution. Recently, bulk multi-omics analyses have been demonstrated to help obtain all-inclusive information about cellular events. This benefit of bulk multi-omics has enabled the advancement of single-cell multi-omics analysis, which enables cell type-specific gene regulation to be examined [50 - 52].

3.7. Multi-Omics Approaches: Challenges and Opportunities

The use of multiple omics in a single cell will result in, among other things, the creation of related machine models (epi) genomic diversity and transcript/protein expression dynamics, which should also allow for a detailed examination of cellular health and disease behavior [53]. For example, some recent studies have reported scNMT-seq (single-cell nucleosome, methylation and transcription sequence) [54]. They investigated the accessibility of chromatin, DNA methylation and transcriptome simultaneously using GpCmethyltransferase to label open chromatin followed by bisulfite and RNA sequences. Methylated cytosines in the GpC context separate accessible DNA (regions that link to non-nucleosome DNA), while methylation is studied from cytosine modification events in the CpG context. By inserting an embryonic stem cell, they found novel links between both cell layers and expressed the forces that intersected between the epigenomic layers during separation. However, one limitation of scNMT-seq is the need to filter the C-C-G and G-C-G positions from raw data, which reduced the number of cytosines that can be tested compared to scBS-seq by ~ 50%. Besides, these types of omic studies also suffer from certain challenges and limitations, for example, many of which are still subjected to feeds with a low genetic predisposition. Finally, the raw data of each omic type must also be filtered separately, processed, and mapped to take into account low signal and noise levels due to locus emissions, amplification bias, and technical variations [23].

4. STRATEGIES FOR MULTI-OMICS PROFILING OF SINGLE CELLS

4.1. Combined

In the combined strategy, tests performed on similar or alike molecules can be shared to perform multi-omics of single cells. Sequencing approaches based on solitary molecules, nano-pores and real-time technology (SMRT) not only show DNA sequence but provide high sensitivity towards DNA methylation. Similarly, mass spectrometry trials of identical single cells can provide proteome and metabolome particulars. To acquire high-grade unified profiles in solo cells, further progress in experimental performance will surely be required [53].

4.2. Separate

Biomolecules of various kinds and chemical classes can be separately extracted from identical cells, then isolated, and finally analyzed. The strategy relies heavily on the property of the partition since all the tools left in the incorrect part are misplaced [53].

4.3. Split

When precise separation through chemical procedure does not occur, the lysate cell can be sorted out and processed. For example, current studies have combined the analysis of RNA and protein by lysate classification and the multiplex PCR usage to measure the transcribed RNA into a single cell, with the closest increase being followed by multiple PCR DNA antibodies repeated by another [53, 55].

4.4. Convert

The chemical transformation between the various sizes of omics brands it easier to examine them in an organized manner. Bisulfite treatment, for example, accommodates DNA methylation into DNA sequencing evidence, combined with the previous one dealing with GpCmethyltransferase which undergoes nucleosome cell formation and DNA methylation in an isolated cell [56].

4.5. Predict

It is compatible with the test techniques described above in measuring the size of omics by using computational methods. In many samples, epigenomic markers are sufficiently integrated with others to assist transcriptome and epigenome imputation, the basis for the loss of cell-type data provided from available data for other epigenomic markers [56].

The methods mentioned above provide a skeleton for scheming many detailed assessment methods. It is possible to separate a stem cell sample before DNA / RNA analysis and to incorporate a single element into the spectrometry analysis of the abundance of metabolites and proteins, allowing the first fully integrated test of multiple cells.

CONCLUDING REMARKS

Single-cell omics has brought a revolution in cellular biology. Omics technology enabled different modalities of single cells such as transcriptomes, proteomes and genomes. These brought high-resolution data about complex issues. Although all these technologies have their limitations but they provide a deep understanding of diseased tissues and phenotypes. This in turn proved to be an effective tool for the treatment of lethal diseases such as cancer.

CONSENT FOR PUBLICATION

Not applicable.

CONFLICT OF INTEREST

The author declares no conflict of interest, financial or otherwise.

ACKNOWLEDGEMENTS

Declared none.

REFERENCES

[1]   Mincarelli L, Lister A, Lipscombe J, Macaulay IC. Defining cell identity with single□cell omics. Proteomics 2018; 18(18): 1700312.
[http://dx.doi.org/10.1002/pmic.201700312] [PMID: 29644800]

[2]   Deng Y, Finck A, Fan R. Single-Cell Omics Analyses Enabled by Microchip Technologies. Annu Rev Biomed Eng 2019; 21(1): 365-93.
[http://dx.doi.org/10.1146/annurev-bioeng-060418-052538] [PMID: 30883211]

[3]   Lu S, Zong C, Fan W, *et al.* Probing meiotic recombination and aneuploidy of single sperm cells by whole-genome sequencing. Science 2012; 338(6114): 1627-30.
[http://dx.doi.org/10.1126/science.1229112] [PMID: 23258895]

[4]   Hou Y, Fan W, Yan L, *et al.* Genome analyses of single human oocytes. Cell 2013; 155(7): 1492-506.
[http://dx.doi.org/10.1016/j.cell.2013.11.040] [PMID: 24360273]

[5]   Beroukhim R, Getz G, Nghiemphu L, *et al.* Assessing the significance of chromosomal aberrations in cancer methodology and application to glioma. Proceedings of the National Academy of Sciences 2007; 104: 20007-12.
[http://dx.doi.org/10.1073/pnas.0710052104]

[6]   Ni X, Zhuo M, Su Z, *et al.* Reproducible copy number variation patterns among single circulating tumor cells of lung cancer patients. Proc Natl Acad Sci USA 2013; 110(52): 21083-8.
[http://dx.doi.org/10.1073/pnas.1320659110] [PMID: 24324171]

[7]   Demeulemeester J, Kumar P, Møller EK, *et al.* Tracing the origin of disseminated tumor cells in breast cancer using single-cell sequencing. Genome Biol 2016; 17(1): 250.
[http://dx.doi.org/10.1186/s13059-016-1109-7] [PMID: 27931250]

[8]   Liang SB, Fu LW. Application of single-cell technology in cancer research. Biotechnol Adv 2017; 35(4): 443-9.
[http://dx.doi.org/10.1016/j.biotechadv.2017.04.001] [PMID: 28390874]

[9]   Cloonan N, Forrest ARR, Kolle G, *et al.* Stem cell transcriptome profiling via massive-scale mRNA sequencing. Nat Methods 2008; 5(7): 613-9.
[http://dx.doi.org/10.1038/nmeth.1223] [PMID: 18516046]

[10]   Mortazavi A, Williams BA, McCue K, Schaeffer L, Wold B. Mapping and quantifying mammalian transcriptomes by RNA-Seq. Nat Methods 2008; 5(7): 621-8.
[http://dx.doi.org/10.1038/nmeth.1226] [PMID: 18516045]

[11]   Tang F, Barbacioru C, Wang Y, *et al.* mRNA-Seq whole-transcriptome analysis of a single cell. Nat Methods 2009; 6(5): 377-82.
[http://dx.doi.org/10.1038/nmeth.1315] [PMID: 19349980]

[12]   Kurimoto K, Saitou M. Single-cell cDNA microarray profiling of complex biological processes of differentiation. Curr Opin Genet Dev 2010; 20(5): 470-7.
[http://dx.doi.org/10.1016/j.gde.2010.06.003] [PMID: 20619631]

[13]   Kurimoto K, Yabuta Y, Ohinata Y, Shigeta M, Yamanaka K, Saitou M. Complex genome-wide transcription dynamics orchestrated by Blimp1 for the specification of the germ cell lineage in mice. Genes Dev 2008; 22(12): 1617-35.
[http://dx.doi.org/10.1101/gad.1649908] [PMID: 18559478]

[14]   Takao M, Takeda K. Enumeration, characterization, and collection of intact circulating tumor cells by cross contamination-free flow cytometry. Cytometry A 2011; 79A(2): 107-17.

[http://dx.doi.org/10.1002/cyto.a.21014] [PMID: 21246706]

[15]   Tirosh I, Izar B, Prakadan S M, *et al.* Dissecting the multicellular ecosystem of metastatic melanoma by single-cell RNA-seq. Science 2016; 352: 189-96.
       [http://dx.doi.org/10.1126/science.aad0501]

[16]   Liu S, Trapnell C. Single-cell transcriptome sequencing. Recent advances and remaining challenges 2016; 5: 182.

[17]   Barh D, Azevedo V A D, *et al.* Omics Technologies and Bio-engineering, Towards Improving Quality of Life. Academic Press 2017; 1233: 456.

[18]   Batchelor E, Loewer A, Lahav G. The ups and downs of p53: understanding protein dynamics in single cells. Nat Rev Cancer 2009; 9(5): 371-7.
       [http://dx.doi.org/10.1038/nrc2604] [PMID: 19360021]

[19]   Wu M, Singh AK. Single-cell protein analysis. Curr Opin Biotechnol 2012; 23(1): 83-8.
       [http://dx.doi.org/10.1016/j.copbio.2011.11.023] [PMID: 22189001]

[20]   Darmanis S, Gallant CJ, Marinescu VD, *et al.* Simultaneous multiplexed measurement of RNA and proteins in single cells. Cell Rep 2016; 14(2): 380-9.
       [http://dx.doi.org/10.1016/j.celrep.2015.12.021] [PMID: 26748716]

[21]   Stoeckius M, Hafemeister C, Stephenson W, *et al.* Simultaneous epitope and transcriptome measurement in single cells. Nat Methods 2017; 14(9): 865-8.
       [http://dx.doi.org/10.1038/nmeth.4380] [PMID: 28759029]

[22]   Fiehn O. Metabolomics--the link between genotypes and phenotypes. Plant Mol Biol 2002; 48(1/2): 155-71.
       [http://dx.doi.org/10.1023/A:1013713905833] [PMID: 11860207]

[23]   Kang X, Liu A, *et al.* Application of multi-omics in single cells. Annals of Biotechnology 2008; 2: 1007.

[24]   Hu P, Zhang W, Xin H, Deng G. Single Cell Isolation and Analysis. Front Cell Dev Biol 2016; 4: 116.
       [http://dx.doi.org/10.3389/fcell.2016.00116] [PMID: 27826548]

[25]   Dainiak MB, Kumar A, Galaev IY, Mattiasson B. Methods in cell separations. Adv Biochem Eng Biotechnol 2007; 106: 1-18.
       [PMID: 17660999]

[26]   Gross A, Schoendube J, Zimmermann S, Steeb M, Zengerle R, Koltay P. Technologies fors ingle-cellisolation. Int J Mol Sci 2015; 16(8): 16897-919.
       [http://dx.doi.org/10.3390/ijms160816897] [PMID: 26213926]

[27]   Schulz KR, Danna EA, Krutzik PO, Nolan GP. Single-cell phospho-protein analysis by flow cytometry. Curr Protoc Immunol 2007; Chapter 8: 17.
       [PMID: 18432997]

[28]   Miltenyi S, Müller W, Weichel W, Radbruch A. High gradient magnetic cell separation with MACS. Cytometry 1990; 11(2): 231-8.
       [http://dx.doi.org/10.1002/cyto.990110203] [PMID: 1690625]

[29]   Grützkau A, Radbruch A. Small but mighty: How the MACS®-technology based on nanosized superparamagnetic particles has helped to analyze the immune system within the last 20 years. Cytometry A 2010; 77A(7): 643-7.
       [http://dx.doi.org/10.1002/cyto.a.20918] [PMID: 20583279]

[30]   Emmert-Buck MR, Bonner RF, Smith PD, *et al.* Laser capture microdissection. Science 1996; 274(5289): 998-1001.
       [http://dx.doi.org/10.1126/science.274.5289.998] [PMID: 8875945]

[31]   Espina V, Heiby M, Pierobon M, Liotta LA. Laser capture microdissection technology. Expert Rev Mol Diagn 2007; 7(5): 647-57.

[http://dx.doi.org/10.1586/14737159.7.5.647] [PMID: 17892370]

[32]   Datta S, Malhotra L, Dickerson R, Chaffee S, Sen CK, Roy S. Laser capture microdissection: Big data from small samples. Histol Histopathol 2015; 30(11): 1255-69.
[PMID: 25892148]

[33]   Kummari E, Guo-Ross SX, Eells JB. Laser capture microdissection--a demonstration of the isolation of individual dopamine neurons and the entire ventral tegmental area. J Vis Exp 2015; 96(96): e52336.
[http://dx.doi.org/10.3791/52336] [PMID: 25742438]

[34]   Fend F, Raffeld M. Laser capture microdissection in pathology. J Clin Pathol 2000; 53(9): 666-72.
[http://dx.doi.org/10.1136/jcp.53.9.666] [PMID: 11041055]

[35]   Bonner RF, Emmert-Buck M, Cole K, *et al.* Laser capture microdissection: molecular analysis of tissue. Science 1997; 278(5342): 1481-1483, 1483.
[http://dx.doi.org/10.1126/science.278.5342.1481] [PMID: 9411767]

[36]   Esposito G. Complementary Techniques. Adv Exp Med Biol 2007; 593: 54-65.
[http://dx.doi.org/10.1007/978-0-387-39978-2_6] [PMID: 17265716]

[37]   Allard WJ, Matera J, Miller MC, *et al.* Tumor cells circulate in the peripheral blood of all major carcinomas but not in healthy subjects or patients with nonmalignant diseases. Clin Cancer Res 2004; 10(20): 6897-904.
[http://dx.doi.org/10.1158/1078-0432.CCR-04-0378] [PMID: 15501967]

[38]   Whitesides GM. The origins and the future of microfluidics. Nature 2006; 442(7101): 368-73.
[http://dx.doi.org/10.1038/nature05058] [PMID: 16871203]

[39]   Nagrath S, Sequist LV, Maheswaran S, *et al.* Isolation of rare circulating tumour cells in cancer patients by microchip technology. Nature 2007; 450(7173): 1235-9.
[http://dx.doi.org/10.1038/nature06385] [PMID: 18097410]

[40]   Dean FB, Hosono S, Fang L, *et al.* Comprehensive human genome amplification using multiple displacement amplification. Proc Natl Acad Sci USA 2002; 99(8): 5261-6.
[http://dx.doi.org/10.1073/pnas.082089499] [PMID: 11959976]

[41]   Xu X, Hou Y, Yin X, *et al.* Single-cell exome sequencing reveals single-nucleotide mutation characteristics of a kidney tumor. Cell 2012; 148(5): 886-95.
[http://dx.doi.org/10.1016/j.cell.2012.02.025] [PMID: 22385958]

[42]   Zong C, Lu S, Chapman AR, Xie XS. Genome-wide detection of single-nucleotide and copy-number variations of a single human cell. Science 2012; 338(6114): 1622-6.
[http://dx.doi.org/10.1126/science.1229164] [PMID: 23258894]

[43]   Marcy Y, Ishoey T, Lasken RS, *et al.* Nanoliter reactors improve multiple displacement amplification of genomes from single cells. PLoS Genet 2007; 3(9): e155.
[http://dx.doi.org/10.1371/journal.pgen.0030155] [PMID: 17892324]

[44]   Wu AR, Neff NF, Kalisky T, *et al.* Quantitative assessment of single-cell RNA-sequencing methods. Nat Methods 2014; 11(1): 41-6.
[http://dx.doi.org/10.1038/nmeth.2694] [PMID: 24141493]

[45]   Stoakes Shelley Farrar. Single-Cell Genomics. News-Medical 2019.

[46]   Brady G, Niscove N. [361 Construction of cDNA libraries from single cells. Methods Enzymol 1993; 225: 611-23.
[http://dx.doi.org/10.1016/0076-6879(93)25039-5] [PMID: 8231874]

[47]   Pan X. Single cell analysis: from technology to biology and medicine. Single Cell Biol 2014; 3(1): 106.
[PMID: 25177539]

[48]   Liu N, Liu L, Pan X. Single-cell analysis of the transcriptome and its application in the characterization of stem cells and early embryos. Cell Mol Life Sci 2014; 71(14): 2707-15.

[http://dx.doi.org/10.1007/s00018-014-1601-8] [PMID: 24652479]

[49]   Mellors JS, Jorabchi K, Smith LM, Ramsey JM. Integrated microfluidic device for automated single cell analysis using electrophoretic separation and electrospray ionization mass spectrometry. Anal Chem 2010; 82(3): 967-73.
[http://dx.doi.org/10.1021/ac902218y] [PMID: 20058879]

[50]   Macaulay IC, Ponting CP, Voet T. Single-cell multiomics: multiple measurements from single cells. Trends Genet 2017; 33(2): 155-68.
[http://dx.doi.org/10.1016/j.tig.2016.12.003] [PMID: 28089370]

[51]   Geiger R, Rieckmann JC, Wolf T, *et al.* L-arginine modulates T cell metabolism and enhances survival and anti-tumor activity. Cell 2016; 167(3): 829-842.e13.
[http://dx.doi.org/10.1016/j.cell.2016.09.031] [PMID: 27745970]

[52]   Bock C, Farlik M, Sheffield NC. Multi-omics of single cells: strategies and applications. Trends Biotechnol 2016; 34(8): 605-8.
[http://dx.doi.org/10.1016/j.tibtech.2016.04.004] [PMID: 27212022]

[53]   Clark SJ, Argelaguet R, Kapourani CA, *et al.* scNMT-seq enables joint profiling of chromatin accessibility DNA methylation and transcription in single cells. Nat Commun 2018; 9(1): 781.
[http://dx.doi.org/10.1038/s41467-018-03149-4] [PMID: 29472610]

[54]   Darmanis S, Gallant CJ, Marinescu VD, *et al.* Simultaneous multiplexed mea-surement of RNA and proteins in single cells. Cell Rep 2016; 14(2): 380-9.
[http://dx.doi.org/10.1016/j.celrep.2015.12.021] [PMID: 26748716]

[55]   Small EC, Xi L, Wang JP, Widom J, Licht JD. Single-cell nucleosome mapping reveals the molecular basis of gene expression heterogeneity. Proc Natl Acad Sci USA 2014; 111(24): E2462-71.
[http://dx.doi.org/10.1073/pnas.1400517111] [PMID: 24889621]

[56]   Ernst J, Kellis M. Large-scale imputation of epigenomic datasets for systematic annotation of diverse human tissues. Nat Biotechnol 2015; 33(4): 364-76.
[http://dx.doi.org/10.1038/nbt.3157] [PMID: 25690853]

CHAPTER 11

Pharmacogenomics

Shumaila Azam[1], **Sahar Fazal**[1,*], **Attiya Kanwal**[2], **Muhammad Saad Khan**[5], **Narjis Khatoon**[1], **Muneeba Ishtiaq**[1], **RabbiahManzoor Malik**[1, 3], **Sana Elahi**[1] and **Fakhra Nazir**[1, 4]

[1] *Department of Bioinformatics and Biosciences, Capital University of Science and Technology, (CUST), Islamabad, Pakistan*

[2] *International Islamic University Islamabad (IIUI), Islamabad, Pakistan*

[3] *Wah Medical College, WahCantt, Pakistan*

[4] *Centre for Bioresource Research, Islamabad, Pakistan*

[5] *Department of Biosciences, COMSATS University Islamabad, Sahiwal, Pakistan*

Abstract: The ongoing development in new genotyping methods necessitates an understanding of their potential benefits and limits in terms of pharmacogenomics utility. We give an overview of technologies that can be used in pharmacogenomics research and clinical practice in this chapter. The Human Genome Project's completion has paved the way for the development of clinical instruments for patient evaluation. Pharmacogenomics may enable the identification of patients who are most likely to benefit from a specific drug, as well as those for whom the expense and risk are greater than the advantages. Both drug therapy's safety and efficacy may improve. In the future, genotyping may be used to tailor drug treatment for large groups of individuals, lowering drug treatment costs and improving therapeutic efficacy and overall health.

Keywords: Clinical Pharmacogenetics Implementation Consortium (CPIC), Dutch Pharmacogenetics Working Group (DPWG, Pharmacogenomics (PGx), PharmGKB, US Food and Drug Administration (FDA).

1. INTRODUCTION

Scientists have been attempting to recognize the causes of ailments at the genetic level since Mendel's discovery of genes in 1865 and the Human Genome Project (HGP) in 2003 [1]. Following the completion of the HGP, new projects have continued to use the genetic sequencing data obtained from that project [1]. We now have more knowledge than ever before about how our genes influence development, growth, health, and even drug metabolism [2]. In 2003, The

---

* **Corresponding author Sahar Fazal**: Department of Bioinformatics and Biosciences, Capital University of Science and Technology, Islamabad, Pakistan; E-mail: sahar@cust.edu.pk

Syeda Marriam Bakhtiar and Erum Dilshad (Eds.)

National Human Genome Research Institute instigated the project "Encyclopedia of DNA Elements" [3] the aim of which is to locate all coding elements/sequences in the human genome [3]. In many inherited diseases, next-generation sequencing has established a potent method in disease-related variants identification, whereas to detect variants in previously identified genes associated with disease, selective sequencing is found to be useful [4, 5].

The Cancer Genome Atlas [6] has helped us better understand the molecular markers associated with many types of cancer. The TCGA has also proven valuable in detecting molecular similarities between different cancer patients and types of cancer, as well as in documenting the heterogeneity of all cancers [6]. In addition, a rising number of organizations and universities are creating pharmacogenetics testing clinical facilities and support infrastructures [7, 8]. The Pharmacogenomics Research Network (PGRN) is made up of three major center-grant programs with the goal of improving precision medicine by identifying and understanding genetic variants that influence therapeutic effects and cause adverse medication effects in patients [9]. Two of the three PGRN projects aim to make pharmacogenomics and precision medicine services more accessible [9]. To obtain information, The PharmGKB base (https://www.pharmgkb.org/) and a PGRN hub (http://www.pgrn.org/) have been developed to coordinate the activities of the new PGRN [9]. The scientific community's access to genomic data is the major hurdle to full adoption of pharmacogenomics [10]. ClinVar [11] is a free resource of papers and supporting information on the connections between human genetic variations and phenotypes. This database offers information on how human genetic diversity affects patients' health [11]. ClinVar works with the Clinical Genome Resource (ClinGen; https://www.clinical genome.org/) to determine the clinical importance of genes and their variations in precision medicine and research [12]. The NOMAD registry is a database of healthy people's genetic information that allows researchers to discuss and exchange their discoveries. Thanks to breakthroughs in genomics, scientists can now generate therapeutic therapies and diagnostic tests at a faster rate than ever before [13, 14].

Due to the ability to sequence, DNA and RNA at a faster rate and at a low cost, clinicians can efficiently detect and identify rare disorders [4, 5, 14]. Rare disease patients may have to wait a long period for an accurate diagnosis [15, 16]. Rather than putting patients in the dark with delayed therapy for their sickness, genetic testing gives them peace of mind and hope [17, 18]. The National Institutes of Health will launch "All of Us," a new programme in the spring of 2018 that will collect data from at least one million people in the United States in order to speed up research and improve health. This programme will have a substantial impact on the future delivery of precision medicine [19]. Data provided through genetic testing is exceedingly difficult to understand [21]. The biggest challenge, according to the scientific community [21], is to understand the effects after acquiring the DNA sequence and finding a genetic mutation. Genetics' ultimate goal is to discover a link between genetic variation and a specific illness or metabolic pathway [22]. On the other hand, the pool of new variants is enormous, with the possibility of having no established link to a specific condition [22]. As a result, genetics must transform genomic data into information that doctors can utilize to make decisions [22]. Physicians indicated they did not know how to apply pharmacogenetic testing in clinical practice in a recent study [23, 24]. Researchers and scientists in this sector must provide information, guidance, and education to physicians who lack confidence when ordering pharmacogenetic testing in order to bridge the gap between science and healthcare [20].

Before prescribing a treatment based on a single biomarker, a physician must have a thorough understanding of the patient (integrated medicine) [20]. In response to the growing need for pharmacogenomics information and guidance, the FDA has released a list of pharmacogenomic biomarkers in drug labelling on its website [25]. Biomarkers identified on the FDA website include differences in the germline or somatic genes (polymorphisms, mutations), genetic etiological functional impairments, variations in gene expression, and chromosomal abnormalities [26]. Some drug labels state what a clinician can do based on biomarkers, which may or may not require pharmacogenetic testing [26]. Specific variants in the genetic code are linked to variances in medication reactivity, the chance of an individual having certain drug side effects, and variations in the rate and degree of drug metabolism. We are at a vital juncture in medical science and pharmacy practice. Pharmacogenomics (PGx) is the study of the connection between the human genome and the science of pharmacology [27]. Most pharmacy schools' curricula have just lately introduced genetics and PGx courses. Previous generations of pharmacists may not have been exposed to the genetic concepts that drive PGx.

The goal of this chapter is to go through fundamental principles in genetics and genetic variation in order to lay the groundwork for comprehending crucial and well-illustrated gene-drug interactions. Wherever possible, we employ drugs with genetic testing guidelines on the labeling or professional clinical practice recommendations from the US Food and Drug Administration (FDA). There will also be several genuine, online PGx references offered. The moment has come for pharmacists and scientists to embrace these developments in drug therapy and prepare to translate gene-drug therapy. The Human Genome Project's findings spawned pharmacogenomics. The Human Genome Project (HGP) began in 1990 as a global effort to identify and comprehend the structure of every human gene. The HGP is without a doubt our lifetime's greatest scientific achievement, having far-reaching ramifications for medical science and pharmacy practice. The major goal of the project was to break the human genetic code by merging the expertise of experts from universities and research centers across the United States, the United Kingdom, France, Germany, Japan, and China. This international collaboration shows the public benefit that may be achieved when scholars work together to pursue a common aim. The sequencing or mapping of the 2.91 billion base pairs within the molecule deoxyribonucleic acid (DNA) laying out the genetic blueprint was accomplished years ahead of schedule in April 2003 [28]. The human genome is the full code, and it is found in the nucleus of practically every human cell. The investigation into how variations in this code affect human health is only the beginning. The HGP has cleared the door for completely personalized medicine, in which disease causes and treatments are linked to markers or patterns in a person's DNA sequence. Pharmacists are the best doctors for translating gene-drug interactions into clinical practice and adopting PGx-driven drug therapy. Pharmacists may be expected to personalize medicine selection and dosing, as well as to inform patients and clinicians about the risks associated with PGx, by explaining the core vocabulary and concepts of PGx and giving educational materials to help you stay up to date with these rising trends in medical science and Medicare. This analysis attempts to open a window into the future of drug therapy.

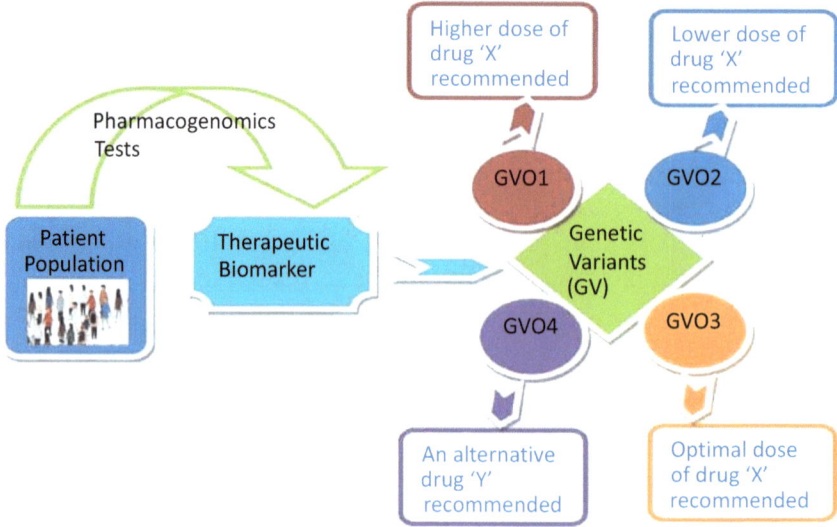

Fig. (11.1). Graphical abstract of how pharmacogenomics leads to better drug therapy.

1.1. Application of Pharmacogenomics

Pharmacogenomics has the potential to revolutionize medicine by replacing broad techniques of screening and treatment with a more individualized approach that takes into account both clinical considerations and the patient's biology. As previously stated, genetic variation can have a significant impact on the type of a medicine's effect on an individual (whether it works or causes an adverse event), as well as the amount of drug required to achieve the intended effect. Pharmacogenomics will have an impact on how pharmaceuticals are taken, dosed, and monitored for side effects, as a result of this. Clinical annotation of a patient's whole genome sequence revealed the patient's possible tolerance to clopidogrel, a positive reactivity to lipid-lowering medications, and a lower initial dose threshold for warfarin on a person-by-person basis [29].

In addition to standard clinical techniques, doctors will use pharmacogenomics to determine which medicines are more or less likely to work, which patients will require more or less care to obtain a therapeutic response, and which drugs should be avoided due to bad effects. To attain these objectives, research laboratory findings must be translated into clinical practice, and the pharmacogenomics process must be integrated into the existing medical system. While there are examples of how pharmacogenomics could affect drug prescribing, adverse effect prediction, and more, the actual use of pharmacogenomics is still in its early stages. The day when all clinicians routinely use genetics to drug dose is becoming closer as pharmacogenomics knowledge grows and the infrastructure for its use grows. Overcoming regulatory impediments, developing methods to continuously update known data, equipping clinicians with expertise, and integrating genomics into medicine are all challenges that must be overcome. Scientists have been working to find solutions to these issues, and pharmacogenomics is likely to be one of the first major clinical uses of personalized genetic medicine. The FDA regulates medications and their labeling in the United States. Contact between scientists and the FDA is also required for pharmacogenomics information to be included on medicine labels. The type of investigation, sample size, repeatability, and degree of the effect will all be considered in the evaluation [30]. One advantage of pharmacogenomics is that the links between genetics and pharmacological effects are more obvious and immediate than in other translational bioinformatics ideas, such as disease risk assessment, where scientists must contend with "lost heritability" and combinations of modest risks. As a result, pharmacogenomic principles do not require the same level of scrutiny as other treatments that require a randomized clinical study to verify efficacy. Rather than delivering a novel treatment, the vast majority of pharmacogenomics research just raises clinicians' awareness of previously approved medications. Doctors already examine their patients' clinical histories when making prescription selections (*e.g.*, weight, gender, presumed organ function, drug reactions, and compliance). There is no opposition to including the genetic information variable as long as it does not detract from the present standard of care [31]. Once a biomarker has been proven to be important, this will be the time to make other decisions, such as whether biomarker testing should be mandatory or just advised. Along with the biomarker's predictive value, socioeconomic variables would need to be considered. The use of pharmacogenomics data may be totally up to the clinician's discretion unless the FDA has formalized its involvement in their application. Once a pharmacogenetic biomarker has been approved, it can be used in clinical trials. Biomarkers characterizing the patient population that should get the drug will be printed under "indication,", biomarkers related to drug mechanism could be printed under "clinical pharmacology," and biomarkers related to protection might be printed under "adverse effects" on the drug's label. When it comes to updating new knowledge, the FDA and doctors may have to be cautious as the number of pharmacogenetics organizations have increased [30]. New drug-gene interactions are also being investigated using pharmacogenetic studies. The volume of recent responses significantly exceeds anyone's ability to assess them. As a result, bioinformatics will be critical in bringing data to the patient. For extracting structured literature material and upgrading knowledge systems like PharmGKB, text mining is useful. Finally, the data would be gathered into a central database, making the analysis accessible to everyone. A robust, FDA-modified database or evidence-based licensed drug-gene interactions that doctors may use in their practice will be required for global adoption. For example, PharmGKB is frequently utilized as a scientific tool for evaluating drug-gene interactions. These kinds of programs serve as a model for the systems that will be in place once sequenced genomes are widely available for medical purposes. Finally, personal genomics must become thoroughly embedded in modern medicine in order for pharmacogenomics to become extensively employed. It is critical to inform doctors and patients about the benefits of genomic medicine, dispel any misconceptions, and prevent ethical issues. Furthermore, genetic testing laboratories that meet the Clinical Laboratory Improvement Amendments (CLIA) regulatory standards of the US government should be established to offer patients with genomic data that is regarded as appropriate for clinical application. Finally, health firms would consent to pay for genetic testing. The cost-related debates will soon be moot, as the cost of sequencing continues to fall drastically [31]. Finally, insurance companies would agree to pay for genetic testing. The cost-related arguments will soon be a thing of the past, since the cost of sequencing continues to plummet [31]. Despite the fact that pharmacogenetics is a fast-growing area, getting research findings from the bench to the bedside remains a barrier. As a result of ongoing research and development in this field, these problems will be overcome, ushering in a new era of tailored drug therapy.

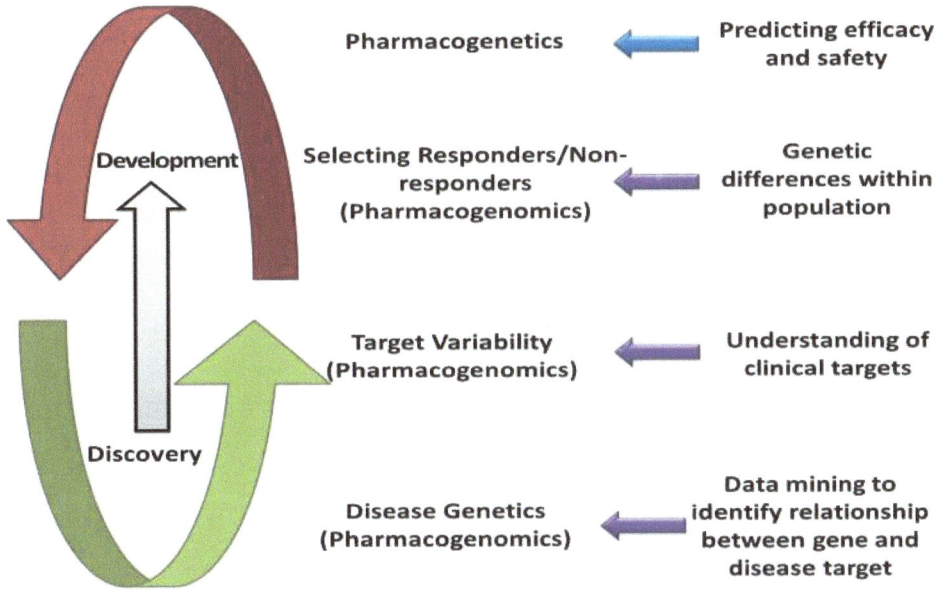

Fig. (11.2). Application of pharmacogenomics/genetics for clinical use [31].

1.2. Translating Pharmacogenomics

Many challenges to turning PGx test results into clinical action have evolved since the first pharmacogenetics implementation programs were launched. As a result, many lessons were learnt, and options for resolving some of these difficulties began to appear. A variety of strategies could be used to aid the conversion of information received from pharmacogenetics genotypes into prescription medicines. Apart from the numerous platforms for extracting genotypes, one of the initial difficulties was how to turn the results of a genetic test into diagnostic action. The Clinical Pharmacogenetics Implementation Consortium (CPIC) [34] and the Dutch Pharmacogenetics Working Group (DPWG) [32, 33] recognized the need for more defined guidance. Both organizations' suggestions provide clinicians with dosing protocols or alternative treatment techniques [36, 37] for specific carefully selected gene-drug pairings that have a considerable, evidence-based effect on the impact of pharmacotherapy [38], as well as determining which pharmacogenetics are eligible for research. The similarities between these recommendations for the same gene drug were apparent, and inconsistencies were typically explained by the use of alternative dosing approaches [35]. All of the discrepancies between the guidelines are being investigated further in order to improve them through collaborative efforts. As recommendations expand and grow, and new material becomes accessible, it's critical to build strategies for keeping information up to date [39]. This can make establishing a method that regularly changes the recommendations a technological issue.

1.3. Challenges in Pharmacogenomics

A growing understanding of the association between genetic variations and drug response heterogeneity has developed and exposed numerous key problems [41] that must be addressed in order to join and deepen the clinical practice.

1.4. Design and Interpretation of Pharmacogenetics and Pharmacogenomics Studies

The discovery of a link between a clinical trait, such as medication reaction, and a genetic variant or a set of genetic variants is becoming more common in the medical literature. Many of these relationships, however, have not been confirmed in clinical trials [41, 42], with false-positive interactions being one typical cause. Another issue could be subtle differences in patient research classifications, such as ethnicity or the idea of endpoints. Pharmacogenetics testing, like other diagnostic procedures, would be done only when its predictive value is established.

1.5. Regulatory Issues in Genetic Testing

Frameworks for controlling genotyping experiments, the degree to which pharmacogenetics research can be integrated into the development of new drugs before or after large-scale clinical trials, and whether and how pharmacogenetics knowledge should be integrated into labeling requirements that notify physicians and patients are all regulatory concerns. The US Food and Medication Administration has begun an effort to collect pharmacogenetics information that could assist resolve many of these concerns during drug development [43, 44]; certain drug labels have already been changed to provide pharmacogenetics detail, as previously indicated.

1.6. Development of New Genomic Technologies

Providing the clinician with accurate genetic data for decision-making involves a very quick turnover or an atmosphere in which drug treatment can be fairly undertaken after the genetic test are accessible (for example, in chronic disorders, such as hypertension). Technology is advancing quite quickly in this field. Within 5 to 10 years, a third example, in which the entire genome of a particular person is sequenced and accessible for decision-making, seems possible. This would cost less than several thousand dollars in whole-genome sequencing, adequate knowledge management systems, and alternative insights to genomic quantitative tests.

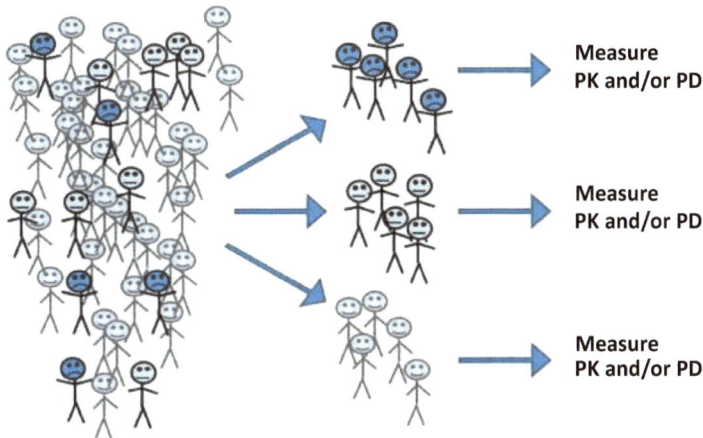

Fig. (11.3). Study Designs in Clinical Pharmacogenetics and Pharmacogenomics Research.

1.7. Ethical Issues

The discovery of genetic variants correlated with enhanced pharmacokinetics posed concerns as to whether it was possible to demonize groups and individuals privileged with such genetic variants (for example, by refusing insurance) [44, 45].

1.8. Education

The genetic code is a resource, and enforcing its promise in reality will necessitate a great deal of knowledge [44]. Even for prevalent and well-defined genetic variations with replicable and significant implications for disease or prescribed drugs, medical identification has been gradual. This could indicate a lack of comprehension or clarity in studies that shows an additional clinical benefit before administering opioids to comprehend genetic features. Increased educational initiatives for the medical and lay communities will be necessary to recognize the benefits and downsides of new clinical evidence focusing on genomes.

1.9. Cost

One reason for the sluggish uptake of pharmacogenetic testing is because there is effectively less proof. This is a dynamic dilemma that includes not only the cost of genotyping, but also other expenditures, such as the cost of caring for a medication therapy patient who is prone to terrible and unavoidable consequences. However, it is critical to determine a genotype just once in a lifetime, and the cost of the tests currently available is frequently less than the cost of the medications.

2. ANTICIPATED BENEFITS OF PHARMACOGENOMICS

2.1. More Powerful Medicines

Pharmaceutical companies would be able to create treatments based on proteins, enzymes, and RNA molecules linked to genes and disorders. This might aid drug research by allowing pharmaceutical companies to create medications that are more specific to specific ailments. Not only would this selectivity boost therapeutic results, but it will also reduce damage to nearby healthy cells.

2.2. Better, Safer Drugs the First Time

Doctors would be able to evaluate the genetic profile of a patient and recommend the best possible drug treatment from the start, instead of the traditional trial-an--error approach of coordinating individuals with the right medications. Not only will this take the trial and error out of choosing the correct prescription, but as the risk of adverse reactions is reduced, it will also speed up response time and improve protection. Pharmacogenomics has the potential to reduce the 100,000 deaths and 2 million hospitalizations that occur each year in the United States as a result of severe medication reactions [45].

2.3. More Accurate Methods of Determining Appropriate Drug Dosages

Dosages based on a person's genetics—how well the body absorbs the drug and how long it takes to ingest it—will replace current weight and age-based techniques. This would boost the treatment's value while lowering the risk of toxicity.

2.4. Advanced Screening for Disease

Fully understanding one's genetic code would enable an individual at an early age to make appropriate behavioral and environmental conditions to prevent or reduce the seriousness of a genetic disorder. Similarly, comprehensive knowledge of specific chronic diseases would enable proper scrutiny, and therapies to optimize their therapy can be implemented at the most appropriate stage.

2.5. Better Vaccines

Antibiotics made of genetic material, including DNA or RNA, offer all the advantages without all the complications of current vaccines. They will trigger the immune response, but diseases will not be triggered. They will be cheap, durable, simple to store, and capable to be built at once to hold many variants of a pathogen.

2.6. Improvements in the Drug Discovery and Approval Process

Pharmaceutical companies may be able to explore new medications more quickly if they use gene targeting. Previously unsuccessful medicine candidates can be resurrected when they are linked with the niche population they represent. When testing is targeted at certain genetic population groupings, the drug approval procedure should be streamlined, resulting in increased success rates. By selecting only those individuals capable of reacting to a treatment, the expense and risk of clinical trials can be minimized.

2.7. Decrease in the Overall Cost of Health Care

Decreases in the variety of serious drug reactions, the number of unsuccessful drug tests, the time it takes for a drug to be authorized, the period of time patients are on treatment, the number of drugs patients need to take in order to obtain successful therapy, the impact of the epidemic on the body (through early diagnosis), and an improvement in the variety of potential drug targets would encourage a slight reduction in the cost of healthcare.

3. PHARMACOGENOMICS TODAY

The pharmacogenomics area is also in its infancy. The use is primarily very limited, but in clinical trials, new methods are under review. Pharmacogenomics will enable tailor-made drug production to address a variety of health problems in the future, particularly coronary heart disease, Alzheimer's, leukemia, HIV/AIDS, and asthma.

4. FUTURE OF PHARMACOGENOMICS

CONCLUSION

According to studies, a substantial majority of medical practitioners believe in or consider pharmacogenomics to be applicable in clinical research. More resources should be committed to education or training initiatives in order to make physicians feel more at ease evaluating the results and boost their overall performance in the profession. Existing implementation activities are now making more educational possibilities available. Furthermore, consortia such as the CPIC have made recommendations for making genetic discoveries easier to assimilate and comprehend, and when these are accompanied by automatic decision-making assistance systems for practitioners, preliminary training for healthcare professionals should be appropriate. Significant pharmacogenetic variations have been discovered by clinical researchers, which can be exploited to alter the way drugs are administered for implementation. Between several hurdles, more clarification of the variants interviewed is required for the systematic application of preemptive PGx. By setting explicit criteria for variations that need to be validated for allele classification as well as offering simple directions for applying the translation tables, it is possible to acquire a single approach for the reliable translation of variants into metabolizing phenotypes. PharmVar, for example, is a database that focuses on nomenclature uniformity. Economic and efficiency analyses have demonstrated the enormous benefits of genotype-guided therapy, and more research into the use of PGx is currently underway. All of these current activities have helped to solve many PGx implementation issues, making the pharmacogenomics pledge a reality.

Biobanks might be viewed as underutilized resources for both finding uncommon variations and conducting validation studies. They can also be utilized to look into PGx implementation issues and solutions in general. The present comprehensive and longitudinal data on biobank participants can be used to convert genetic data from pharmacogenes into advice for safer and more cost-effective drug therapy. Furthermore, allowing biobank participants to provide input on the related PGx elements enables for more research to be conducted to assess the benefit of preemptive PGx testing, underlining the potential significance of biobanks in PGx adoption. As research advances, more evidence of gene-drug interactions will emerge, and current implementation hurdles will be overcome. Patients' PGx data will be widely available in the near future, allowing for improved treatment success and lower societal expenses. Though different solutions have disadvantages, we should not let the ideal become the enemy of the good and avoid implementing what has already been shown to improve clinical outcomes and reduce adverse effects in a cost-effective manner.

CONSENT FOR PUBLICATION

Not applicable.

CONFLICT OF INTEREST

The author declares no conflict of interest, financial or otherwise.

ACKNOWLEDGEMENTS

Declared none.

REFERENCES

[1]   Ansari JA, Ali S, Ansari MA. A Brief Focus on Hepatoprotective Leads from Herbal Origin. Int J Pharmacol 2011; 7(2): 212-6.
        [http://dx.doi.org/10.3923/ijp.2011.212.216]

[2]   Gross T, Daniel J. Overview of pharmacogenomic testing in clinical practice. Ment Health Clin 2018; 8(5): 235-41.
        [http://dx.doi.org/10.9740/mhc.2018.09.235]

[3]   Kalow W. Pharmacogenetics and pharmacogenomics: origin, status, and the hope for personalized medicine. Pharmacogenomics J 2006; 6(3): 162-5.
        [http://dx.doi.org/10.1038/sj.tpj.6500361]

[4]   Helgadottir A, Manolescu A, Thorleifsson G, *et al.* The gene encoding 5-lipoxygenase activating protein confers risk of myocardial infarction and stroke. Nat Genet 2004; 36(3): 233-9.
        [http://dx.doi.org/10.1038/ng1311]

[5]   Hakonarson H, Thorvaldsson S, Helgadottir A, *et al.* Effects of a 5-Lipoxygenase–Activating Protein Inhibitor on Biomarkers Associated With Risk of Myocardial Infarction. JAMA 2005; 293(18): 2245.
        [http://dx.doi.org/10.1001/jama.293.18.2245]

[6]   Klein RJ, Zeiss C, Chew EY, *et al.* Complement Factor H Polymorphism in Age-Related Macular Degeneration. Science 2005; 308(5720): 385-9.
        [http://dx.doi.org/10.1126/science.1109557]

[7]   Edwards AO, Ritter R III, Abel KJ, Manning A, Panhuysen C, Farrer LA. Complement Factor H Polymorphism and Age-Related Macular Degeneration. Science 2005; 308(5720): 421-4.
        [http://dx.doi.org/10.1126/science.1110189]

[8]   Haines JL, Hauser MA, Schmidt S, *et al.* Complement Factor H Variant Increases the Risk of Age-Related Macular Degeneration. Science 2005; 308(5720): 419-21.
        [http://dx.doi.org/10.1126/science.1110359]

[9]   Guessous I, Gwinn M, Khoury MJ. Genome-wide association studies in pharmacogenomics: untapped potential for translation. Genome Med 2009; 1(4): 46.
        [http://dx.doi.org/10.1186/gm46]

[10]   Crawford DC, Nickerson DA. Definition and Clinical Importance of Haplotypes. Annu Rev Med 2005; 56(1): 303-20.
        [http://dx.doi.org/10.1146/annurev.med.56.082103.104540]

[11]   Johnson JA. Pharmacogenetics: potential for individualized drug therapy through genetics. Trends Genet 2003; 19(11): 660-6.
        [http://dx.doi.org/10.1016/j.tig.2003.09.008]

[12]   Gershon ES, Alliey-Rodriguez N, Grennan K. Ethical and public policy challenges for

pharmacogenomics. Dialogues Clin Neurosci 2014; 16(4): 567-74.
[http://dx.doi.org/10.31887/DCNS.2014.16.4/egershon]

[13] Ingelman-Sundberg M, Rodriguez-Antona C. Pharmacogenetics of drug-metabolizing enzymes: implications for a safer and more effective drug therapy. Philos Trans R Soc Lond B Biol Sci 2005; 360(1460): 1563-70.
[http://dx.doi.org/10.1098/rstb.2005.1685]

[14] Ikediobi ON, Shin J, Nussbaum RL, Phillips KA. Addressing the Challenges of the Clinical Application of Pharmacogenetic Testing. Clin Pharmacol Ther 2009; 86(1): 28-31.
[http://dx.doi.org/10.1038/clpt.2009.30]

[15] Hopkins MM, Ibarreta D, Gaisser S, *et al.* Putting pharmacogenetics into practice. Nat Biotechnol 2006; 24(4): 403-10.
[http://dx.doi.org/10.1038/nbt0406-403]

[16] Woelderink A, Ibarreta D, Hopkins MM, Rodriguez-Cerezo E. The current clinical practice of pharmacogenetic testing in Europe: TPMT and HER2 as case studies. Pharmacogenomics J 2006; 6(1): 3-7.
[http://dx.doi.org/10.1038/sj.tpj.6500341]

[17] Weinshilboum R, Wang L. Pharmacogenomics: bench to bedside. Nat Rev Drug Discov 2004; 3(9): 739-48.
[http://dx.doi.org/10.1038/nrd1497]

[18] Kam H, Jeong H. Pharmacogenomic Biomarkers and Their Applications in Psychiatry. Genes (Basel) 2020; 11(12): 1445.
[http://dx.doi.org/10.3390/genes11121445]

[19] Limou S, Winkler CA, Wester CW. "HIV pharmacogenetics and pharmacogenomics: From bench to bedside," in Genomic and Precision Medicine. Elsevier 2019; pp. 185-222.
[http://dx.doi.org/10.1016/B978-0-12-801496-7.00013-7]

[20] Slatko BE, Gardner AF, Ausubel FM. Overview of Next-Generation Sequencing Technologies. Curr Protoc Mol Biol 2018; 122(1).
[http://dx.doi.org/10.1002/cpmb.59]

[21] Levy SE, Myers RM. Advancements in Next-Generation Sequencing. Annu Rev Genomics Hum Genet 2016; 17(1): 95-115.
[http://dx.doi.org/10.1146/annurev-genom-083115-022413]

[22] Yang W, Wu G, Broeckel U, *et al.* Comparison of genome sequencing and clinical genotyping for pharmacogenes. Clin Pharmacol Ther 2016; 100(4): 380-8.
[http://dx.doi.org/10.1002/cpt.411]

[23] Londin ER, Clark P, Sponziello M, Kricka LJ, Fortina P, Park JY. Performance of exome sequencing for pharmacogenomics. Per Med 2015; 12(2): 109-15.
[http://dx.doi.org/10.2217/pme.14.77]

[24] Russell LE, Zhou Y, Almousa AA, Sodhi JK, Nwabufo CK, Lauschke VM. Pharmacogenomics in the era of next generation sequencing – from byte to bedside. Drug Metab Rev 2021; 53(2): 253-78.
[http://dx.doi.org/10.1080/03602532.2021.1909613]

[25] Rasmussen-Torvik LJ, Almoguera B, Doheny KF, *et al.* Concordance between Research Sequencing and Clinical Pharmacogenetic Genotyping in the eMERGE-PGx Study. J Mol Diagn 2017; 19(4): 561-6.
[http://dx.doi.org/10.1016/j.jmoldx.2017.04.002]

[26] Ng D, Hong CS, Singh LN, Johnston JJ, Mullikin JC, Biesecker LG. Assessing the capability of massively parallel sequencing for opportunistic pharmacogenetic screening. Genet Med 2017; 19(3): 357-61.
[http://dx.doi.org/10.1038/gim.2016.105]

[27]   Cohn I, Paton TA, Marshall CR, *et al.* Genome sequencing as a platform for pharmacogenetic genotyping: a pediatric cohort study. NPJ Genom Med 2017; 2(1): 19.
[http://dx.doi.org/10.1038/s41525-017-0021-8]

[28]   Gordon AS, Fulton RS, Qin X, Mardis ER, Nickerson DA, Scherer S. PGRNseq. Pharmacogenet Genomics 2016; 26(4): 161-8.
[http://dx.doi.org/10.1097/FPC.0000000000000202]

[29]   Chua EW, Cree SL, Ton KNT, *et al.* Cross-Comparison of Exome Analysis, Next-Generation Sequencing of Amplicons, and the iPLEX® ADME PGx Panel for Pharmacogenomic Profiling. Front Pharmacol 2016; 7.
[http://dx.doi.org/10.3389/fphar.2016.00001]

[30]   Ingelman-Sundberg M, Sim SC. Intronic polymorphisms of cytochromes P450. Hum Genomics 2010; 4(6): 402.
[http://dx.doi.org/10.1186/1479-7364-4-6-402]

[31]   Bush WS, Crosslin DR, Owusu-Obeng A, *et al.* Genetic variation among 82 pharmacogenes: The PGRNseq data from the eMERGE network. Clin Pharmacol Ther 2016; 100(2): 160-9.
[http://dx.doi.org/10.1002/cpt.350]

[32]   Wang L, Weinshilboum R. Thiopurine S-methyltransferase pharmacogenetics: insights, challenges and future directions. Oncogene 2006; 25(11): 1629-38.
[http://dx.doi.org/10.1038/sj.onc.1209372]

[33]   Bielinski SJ, Olson JE, Pathak J, *et al.* Preemptive Genotyping for Personalized Medicine: Design of the Right Drug, Right Dose, Right Time—Using Genomic Data to Individualize Treatment Protocol. Mayo Clin Proc 2014; 89(1): 25-33.
[http://dx.doi.org/10.1016/j.mayocp.2013.10.021]

[34]   Peterson JF, Field JR, Shi Y, *et al.* Attitudes of clinicians following large-scale pharmacogenomics implementation. Pharmacogenomics J 2016; 16(4): 393-8.
[http://dx.doi.org/10.1038/tpj.2015.57]

[35]   van der Wouden CH, Cambon-Thomsen A, Cecchin E, *et al.* Implementing Pharmacogenomics in Europe: Design and Implementation Strategy of the Ubiquitous Pharmacogenomics Consortium. Clin Pharmacol Ther 2017; 101(3): 341-58.
[http://dx.doi.org/10.1002/cpt.602]

[36]   Mills MC, Rahal C. A scientometric review of genome-wide association studies. Commun Biol 2019; 2(1): 9.
[http://dx.doi.org/10.1038/s42003-018-0261-x]

[37]   Sherman RM, Forman J, Antonescu V, *et al.* Assembly of a pan-genome from deep sequencing of 910 humans of African descent. Nat Genet 2019; 51(1): 30-5.
[http://dx.doi.org/10.1038/s41588-018-0273-y]

[38]   Green RC, Berg JS, Grody WW, *et al.* ACMG recommendations for reporting of incidental findings in clinical exome and genome sequencing. Genet Med 2013; 15(7): 565-74.
[http://dx.doi.org/10.1038/gim.2013.73]

[39]   van El CG, Cornel MC, Borry P, *et al.* Whole-genome sequencing in health care. Eur J Hum Genet 2013; 21(6): 580-4.
[http://dx.doi.org/10.1038/ejhg.2013.46]

[40]   Horn R, Parker M. Health professionals' and researchers' perspectives on prenatal whole genome and exome sequencing: 'We can't shut the door now, the genie's out, we need to refine it'. PLoS One 2018; 13(9): e0204158.
[http://dx.doi.org/10.1371/journal.pone.0204158]

[41]   Thorogood A, Cook-Deegan R, Knoppers BM. Public variant databases: liability? Genet Med 2017; 19(7): 838-41.

[http://dx.doi.org/10.1038/gim.2016.189]

[42]   Burke W, Matheny Antommaria AH, Bennett R, *et al.* Recommendations for returning genomic incidental findings? We need to talk! Genet Med 2013; 15(11): 854-9.
[http://dx.doi.org/10.1038/gim.2013.113]

[43]   Daly AK. Genome-wide association studies in pharmacogenomics. Nat Rev Genet 2010; 11(4): 241-6.
[http://dx.doi.org/10.1038/nrg2751]

[44]   Phillips EJ, Mallal SA. Pharmacogenetics of drug hypersensitivity. Pharmacogenomics 2010; 11(7): 973-87.
[http://dx.doi.org/10.2217/pgs.10.77]

[45]   Pirmohamed M. Pharmacogenetics: past, present and future. Drug Discov Today 2011; 16(19-20): 852-61.
[http://dx.doi.org/10.1016/j.drudis.2011.08.006]

[46]   Yang JJ, Plenge RM. Genomic Technology Applied to Pharmacological Traits. JAMA 2011; 306(6).
[http://dx.doi.org/10.1001/jama.2011.1125]

CHAPTER 12

Biomaterials in Gene Therapy for Soft and Hard Tissues

Sarmad Mehmood[1], Sajjad Haider[2], Muhammad Naeem[3], Raees Khan[4], Muhammad Faheem[3], Bushra Bano[4], Syeda Marriam Bakhtiar[5], Atif Ali Khan Khalil[3], Fazli Subhan[3], Syed Babar Jamal[3,*] and Adnan Haider[3,*]

[1] *Department of Pathology, CMH Institute of Medical Sciences, Bahawalpur, Pakistan*

[2] *Department of Chemical Engineering, King Saud University, Riyadh, Saudi Arabia*

[3] *Department of Biological Sciences, National University of Medical Sciences, Rawalpindi, Pakistan*

[4] *Institute of Basic Medical Sciences, Khyber Medical University, Peshawar, Pakistan*

[5] *Department of Bioinformatics and Bioscience, Capital University of Science and Technology, Islamabad, Pakistan*

Abstract: Bone healing and formation are under the control of growth factors. Among these factors, bone morphogenetic proteins (BMPs) have a vital role in bone and cartilage maintenance and formation. BMP itself belongs to the superfamily of transforming growth factor β (TGFβ). Although, the use of recombinant BMPs has no significant association with the treatment of bone fractures, arthroplasty, pseudoarthrosis or other bone-related diseases. Recent advancements in genetic engineering have led to the foundation of gene therapy. Gene therapy uses genes to be incorporated in the living cells to replace defective genes or manipulate gene expression for therapeutic purposes. Gene therapy is emerging for the treatment of diseases with approval in Europe where it is in the marketing surveillance phase (Phase IV Clinical trial). This technique has also been tested for the incorporation of osteogenic genes in stem cells for repairing spinal fusion and recovering defects in bones in preclinical models. Therefore, gene therapy has the potential for the treatment of different diseases and has the advantage over the use of recombinant proteins. In this chapter, we have discussed gene therapy, its mechanism, delivery system and its use in tissue engineering (soft and bone tissue) for clinical application.

Keywords: Gene Delivery, Gene Therapy, Scaffolds, Polymeric Composites.

* **Corresponding authors Adnan Haider and Syed Babar Jamal:** Department of Biological Science, National University of Medical Sciences, Rawalpindi, Pakistan; E-mail: adnan.haider@numspak.edu.pk and Department of Biological Science, National University of Medical Sciences, Rawalpindi, Pakistan; E-mail: babar.jamal@numspak.edu.pk

1. INTRODUCTION

Many clinical conditions have characteristic features of bone growth under the stimulus of osteogenic cytokines and proteins [1]. In the last decade, *in vivo* investigations have shown that growth factors can stimulate bone healing and bone formation [2]. Osteogenic cytokines are studied recently for understanding the osteoinductive ability of demineralized bone matrix [3], along with bone morphogenetic proteins (BMP) interactions with muscle bone [4]. BMPs are members of the transforming growth factor (TGF) superfamily and play an important role in bone and cartilage maintenance and development. Recent studies have revealed that the BMP pathway has also been associated to adult skeletal muscle mass control. Therefore, BMPs come forward as an essential player involved in the regulation of both homeostasis and muscle formation. BMP-2 and BMP-7 have already been approved for the treatment of spinal fusion and non-union fractures [5]. Recombinant BMPs presented higher healing rates and lesser infections with reduction in failure risk [6], also exhibiting a higher fusion rate contrary to autograft [7]. On the other hand, protein delivery has shown potential in the field of bone tissue engineering. Application of the recombinant proteins are often challenged regarding delivery as this protein based therapy is not feasible in terms of shorter half-life of protein along with poor retention in the defected site [8]. Moreover, expensive and high doses are required for protein delivery contrary to conventional bone repairing methods [9]. Apart from that, the use of recombinant BMPs, bone loss, and delayed bone healing are all linked to revision joint arthroplasty, tumor excision, spine and trauma. Keeping the aforementioned hurdles, it is pivotal for the researchers working in the field to look for the alternate method through which bone repair and formation can be stimulated.

Recent advancement in gene therapy has gained much popularity and attraction as the first gene therapy based product (Glybera®, uniQure, Amsterdam, The Netherlands) was approved in Europe and proved successful in post marketing surveillance phase (Phase IV Clinical trial) [10]. Glybera®, a gene delivery system created by Amsterdam-based uniQure, has been approved for patients with a rare lipid processing impairment known as lipoprotein lipase deficiency (LPLD), which affects only 1 to 2 people in a million [11]. Gene therapy has shown to have a promising potential in overcoming hurdles which occur in conventional protein-based delivery system. Different animal studies have highlighted the potential of gene therapy to be capable of delivering osteogenic drug molecules to precise anatomical levels for a longer period of time [12]. In preclinical models, genetic engineering of stem cells with the addition of osteogenic genes showed promising outcomes in repairing spinal fusion, advanced fractures, and the recovery of defective bones [13].

Gene delivery exploits protein synthesis by using natural cellular machinery which is a central dogma of life. Furthermore, endogenously synthesized proteins may have greater efficacy as compared to recombinant and exogenous counterparts [14]. Nucleic acid delivery to the site provides osteogenic growth factors with an increase in retaining time at the site [15]. In this book chapter, we have discussed in detail about the mechanism and current strategies opted for bone tissue engineering including both viral and non-viral delivery techniques providing future prospective on the potential use of tissue engineering *via* gene therapy in clinical use.

2. MECHANISM OF GENE THERAPY

In gene therapy, gene is transferred to suitable cells which ultimately penetrates the nucleus. Vectors are required for carrying genes and protecting them from negative charges of the genes and nucleases. Gene delivery is broadly classified into viral and non-viral categories depending upon the type of vector used, with every type having its own benefits and limitation, for example, viral vectors exhibited higher transfection efficiency along with toxicity and immunogenicity making patients vulnerable to the side effects. However, non-viral vectors have shown lesser transfection efficiency with non-immunogenic and safe results.

2.1. Delivery of Gene for Gene Therapy

2.1.1. Gene Release

In the gene therapy process, an abnormal copy of gene, which is responsible for a particular disease, is replaced by the normal copy of the gene. Releasing of genes into stem cells is the major hurdle in gene therapy. Vectors, which are efficient, specific, able to be purified in higher concentrations and non-immunogenic are used for releasing genes or a number of genes depending upon the requirement into stem cells. Vectors must not trigger inflammatory responses and should rectify deficiencies, inhibit harmful activities and increase normal processing of cells. Furthermore, it should be safe for both persons being administered with the gene and the person administering the gene of interest harboring vector. Conclusively, the vector should be able to express transgene for patient's entire life in general [16].

2.1.2. Hematopoietic Stem Cells and Gene Therapy

Because of their ability of self-renovation and longevity, hematopoietic stem cells have proved ideal for gene therapy. Using gene therapy technology, induced pluripotent stem cells (iPS) are generated by combining stem cells and gene therapy vectors. For making additional phenotypes from this derived cell, differentiated induced pluripotent stem cells (iPS) are used. Liver transplants are recommended for patients suffering from chronic liver infection and disease caused by hepatitis virus (*e.g.* , hepatitis B and C), who may opt for mature hepatocytes (hepatic transplantation) transplantation or those derived from iPS [17]. Similarly, Short hairpin RNA directed against the virus could reduce the risk of reinfection by the hepatitis virus and immunise the transplanted cells, allowing them to repopulate the liver and restore normal liver function [17].

2.1.3. Gene Therapy via T Cells of a Chimeric Antigen (CAR-T)

Immunotherapy including reprogramming of the patient's immune cells (T lymphocytes) to recognize and target tumor T cells is known as chimeric antigen recipient T (CAR-T) cell treatment. Recently the therapy is modified by fusion of single chain fragment variable (scFv) to a transmembrane domain and an intracellular signaling unit called chain CD3 zeta [18]. Combination of a signaling domain with a well-characterized monoclonal antibody is used to increase recognition of tumor specific epitope and activating T cells without the involvement of other molecules in the histocompatibility complex. CAR was improved by integrating co-stimulating molecules essential for signal transduction. CD28 is often used for CAR generation. This recipient functions as a second activist, enhancing proliferation of T cells and helping in increasing the cytokines expression [19]. Recently, the incorporation of a co-stimulatory domain is reported to have enhanced the CAR function. CD134 or CD137 acts as co-stimulatory molecules are used for this purpose. The most recent CAR includes scFv the initial chain of CD3-ζ, as well as the stimulatory chains of CD28, CD134 and CD137 [20]. The third-generation CAR exhibited improvement in activating T cell of the Akt route (protein kinase B), regulating cell cycle, showing greater persistence of T cells when compared to the second generation of CAR [21].The CAR recognized non-tumor cells as well which present target epitope, it's the worst effect of CAR-T therapy. Tumor antigens are also expressed in cells which are normal. For example, the CD19 antigen is present in both malignant and normal B cells, and CAR is not designed to distinguish between them [22]. Cytokine release syndrome (CRS) is caused by toxicity due to CAR-T therapy. Immune system activation resulted by CAR-T infusion can trigger an increase in inflammatory cytokines levels [23]. The recent modifications have been made in the design of vectors and CAR-T trials provide balance and safety for increasing efficacy in clinical application. There has been a significant improvement in results of CAR trials when compared generation wise. The findings obtained for CAR-T toxicity would play a role towards the betterment of future trials.

2.1.4. CRISPR-Cas9

In 1980s, genome of *Escherichia coli* was identified with a variable sequence inserted by a repeated sequence with unknown functions. In 2005, it was assumed that those variable sequences are of extra-chromosomal origin, who have a role in immune memory against plasmids and phages originating the CRISPR system which was not known until then (Clustered Regularly Interspaced Short Palindromic Repeats) and Cas (Associated Proteins), that was considered from 2012 as a major biotechnological method for gene editing [24]. This is supposed to be originated from immune-adaptive system of procaryontes, the mechanism recognizes foreign invading genetic material, cleaves it into smaller fragments followed by an integration in its own DNA. The following sequence is triggered by reinfection with the same agent: transcription of the CRISPR locus, RNAm processing, and creation of tiny fragments of RNA (crRNAs) that form complexes with the Cas proteins, assisting in the recognition of alien nucleic acids and finally discarding/destroying them [24]. CRISPR uses a natural mechanism to allow editing of a targeted DNA sequence in an organism's genome *via* using three molecules: nuclease (Cas9), which cleaves double-strand DNA; an RNA guide, which directs the complex to the target region; and the target DNA [25]. Cas-9 is involved in the identification of this complex as well as mediates in cleavage of the DNA double strand and donor DNA separation. Integration of foreign (exogenous) DNA takes place resulting in allele substitution. The recent advances in this technology enabled genetic editing using CRISPR of human somatic cells under translational trials. Recently betterment in specificity, safety, effectiveness and optimization of this therapy is reported [26]. Researchers from the University of Utah and California reported correction of the sickle cell causing mutations in the hemoglobin gene. CD34+ cells were isolated and edited *via* CRISPR-Cas9 from patients suffering from sickle cell anemia. After 16 weeks, results exhibited reduced level of expression of mutated and increased expression of the wild type [27]. This is highly suitable for monogenic genetic pathologies, which are rare but still account for 10 thousand diseases already reported [28].

2.1.5. Ethical Issues

The genetically modified germlines are the topic of interest these days with the involvement of bioethics for understanding risks in the procedures and their moral implications. Many people advocate for the use of gene therapy in somatic cells especially in case of Duchenne muscular dystrophy and cystic fibrosis. In 2015, Chinese researchers reported the modification of embroyonic cells using CRISPR-Cas9 which gained international attention with the implication of bioethics laws for this case. Another Chinese group used CRISPR-Cas9 for inducing resistance to HIV by inserting the CCR5 gene mutation. An examination of the genetic code revealed success in 1:6 which clearly shows the requirement of betterment in the procedure by further trials in animal models [29].These recent reported advancements started a new debate on gene editing therapies. Japanese ethical committee reports that these experiments were carried out under ethical laws with the permission of egg donors. The first ever experiment on human embryo was approved in the United Kingdom (UK). American research groups showed conservative thoughts not supporting these types of experiments [29].

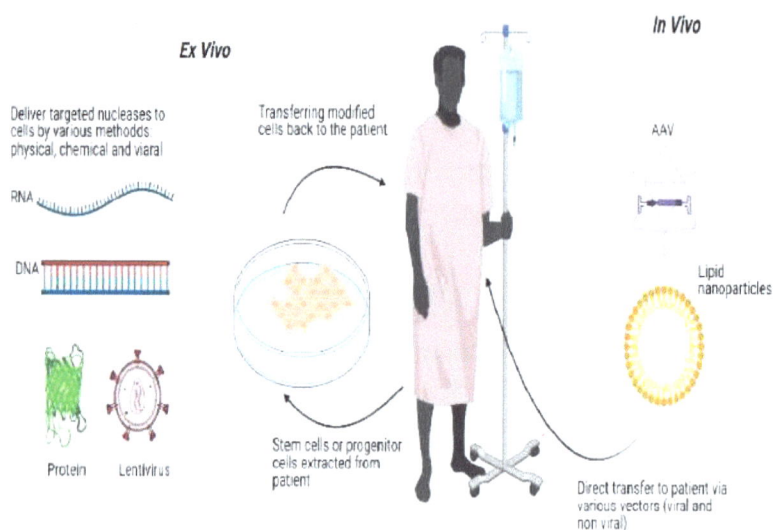

Fig. (12.1). Mechanisms of gene therapy. Various *Ex vivo* and *In vivo* mechanisms of gene therapy has been described, demonstrating how this technique could be used as a potential therapy.

3. TYPES OF GENE DELIVERY CARRIERS

Researchers have synthesized and designed non-viral vectors that can mimic transfection similar to viral vectors with a safe and non-immunogenic outcome. There are various viral and non-viral vectors associated with bone tissue repair and regenerative medicine. Both the aforementioned vectors have exhibited tremendous potential of delivering genes at various targeted sites. However, each vector has its own merits and demerits. Ideal vectors must have low toxicity, high transfection efficacy, no immunogenicity and consistent gene expression.

3.1. Viral Vectors

It is already understood that gene delivery can be performed with the help of viral and non-viral vectors. Both vectors have their benefits and the selection of vectors primarily depends on the target cells and the desired expression. Viral delivery is assumed to be the most advantageous method of gene delivery which depends upon viral envelope proteins for transferring the gene of interest into the cytoplasm and further to the nucleus resulting in the expression of the gene of interest. Viral vectors are reported to have a highly evolved and sophisticated mechanism for transferring DNA into target cells [30]. The viral vectors can either integrate into the host genome, resulting in stable gene expression, or stay in the cell as an episomal vector, which is lost during cell division. The virulent gene of the virus due to which virus has pathogenicity is replaced by our gene of interest [31]. As a result of this modification, viral vector loses pathogenicity and induces osteogenesis. Various viral vectors are studied based on their natural property to enter into cells and integration enabled by the removal of virulence and disease-causing property. This approach has been used to create a large number of viruses, which have been used in over 1200 human gene therapy experiments [32]. Most common of them are retrovirus, adenovirus, adeno-associated viruses (AAVs) and lentivirus [33]. Adenoviruses are considered useful for gene delivery as they can invade a broad range of cells and can be purified in high titers. The adeno-viruses delivery genes presented a higher gene expression for osteogenesis (bone formation) [20]. For tissue repair, these vectors are considered to have various advantages such as non-integrating, easy preparation, and higher transduction efficiency. Betz *et al.* presented an ideal expression pattern for healing of bone fractures [34], which showed expression results in 2-3 weeks for *in vivo* administration of first-generation adenoviral vectors, following a sudden fall of expression with almost no expression at 6 weeks [35]. Retroviral and lentiviral vectors exhibit the similar mode of integration as of adenovirus, but they have a long and sustained gene expression with low immunogenicity as was shown in the case of treatment of large segmental defects after trauma using the BMP-2 osteogenic gene for bone tissue repair [36]. These vectors may show an unregulated overexpression of gene resulting in a hurdle for gene delivery processes. Inducible expression systems have been developed for overcoming unregulated overexpression. An inducible promoter is inactivated or activated by external chemical agents like tetracycline which help in regulating the expression of osteogenic gene [37]. Adeno-associated viruses (AAVs) are considered safer than retro, adeno and lentiviral vectors. AAVs are preferred for delivery because of their overall safety, high titer, milder immune response and their ability to invade various cells. AAV shows milder immune response when compared to adenovirus, making AAV an ideal option for researchers working on *in vivo* delivery of genes. Furthermore, AAVs do not integrate into the host cell genome which makes them a better option than lentivirus and retrovirus having random integration disrupting gene function. Moreover, the AAV's ability to avoid integrating into the genome of the host cell allows it to reduce the impact of insertional mutagenesis. Apart from that, the AAV vector genome does not possess viral coding sequences, vector in itself is not associated with any inflammatory response or toxicity (with the exception of neutralizing antibodies, which may restrict re-administration) [38]. AAV studies have shown promising results for bone tissue engineering [39]. In the last decade, AAV has appeared to be the favorite/favored viral vector for gene therapy. In 2012, Glybera®, an AAV vector used for the treatment of LPLD, got approval as the first ever gene therapy product in western world [40]. However, in terms of cost and purity, the production of these vectors is a challenge. Apart from that, gene delivery vectors are a promising avenue for gene enhanced bone tissue engineering [41].

3.1.1. Polymeric Vectors

Polymers are formed from monomers. There are mainly two types of polymers i.e Natural and Synthetic polymers. In biomedical devices and more specifically in tissue regeneration, both polymers (natural and synthetic) have been frequently used mostly for drug carrying/delivering purposes due to their biocompatible and biodegradable properties. Here we have gone through both natural and synthetic polymers in depth, as well as their prospective applications in gene therapy.

3.1.2. Natural Polymeric Vectors

Because of their biocompatibility, biodegradability, low/non-toxicity, and ability to be modified, natural polymer-based vectors are used in gene therapy. These properties makes polymeric vectors pivotal in gene therapy [42]. Among the natural polymers, chitosan, obtained by deacytylation of chitin has been opted as a carrier for gene delivery due to the aforementioned properties [43]. The chitosan and the gene form complexes and cause the delivery of genes into the cells although their transfection efficiency is low and without specificity. Therefore, modified chitosan is used for increasing transfection efficiency for getting the required cell specificity. The modification of chitosan is carried out *via* chemicals such as urocanic acid [44], mannose [45] polyethylenimine (PEI) [38], folic acid [46], galactose [47], lactobionic acid [48], dextran [49], and spermine (SPE) [50]. According to reports, chemical modification of chitosan is reported to be the most suitable option for delivering gene exhibiting synergistic effects [51]. Alginate, an anionic linear copolymer of beta-D-mannuronic acid and alpha-L-glucuronic acid residues, is used in genes delivery [52], due to the its gelation with bivalent cations such as $Ca2^+$, biocompatible, non-toxicity [53]. Therefore, in alginate hydrogel polyplexes in the form of nanoparticles could be used [54]. The sustained and gradual release of BMP-2 for osteogenic *in vitro* and osteogenesis differentiation *in vivo* has been demonstrated using alginate-mediated transfection with plasmid DNA [55]. Furthermore, due to its biodegradable and biocompatible qualities, gelatin generated by denaturing collagen was employed as a vector. Crosslinking of gelatin is done by treating it with glutaraldehyde which helps in regulating gene release from gelatin [56].

3.1.3. Synthetic Polymeric Vectors

Synthetic polymers are known for their improved flexibility, safety and the easy of their fabrication. These polymers get electrostatically attached with genes and condense the gene to form nanoparticles; this results in the protection of genes and helps in penetrating the cells due to their small size. Such complexes are known as polyplexes [57]. Among synthetic polymers, Polyethylenimine (PEI) is a synthetic polymer that has been utilized as a standard for gene delivery because of its proton sponge effect, which causes burst gene release from the endosome [58]. Despite the fact that PEI's high molecular weight (25 kDa) is associated with cytotoxicity [59], and nanoparticle aggregation under ionic conditions [60], these issues were resolved by using low molecular weight (LMW) degradable PEIs as well as cross-linked PEIs for intracellular degradation such as enzymatic degradation, hydrolysis at low endosomal pH, simple hydrolysis and cytosol specific reductive degradation *via* glutathione [61]. Due to rapid in-situ degradation/fragmentation into LMW water soluble fragments, which are eventually removed by the cells, these PEIs showed low toxicity and higher transfection efficiency [62]. PEI has also been found to be effective in a number of tissues, including the kidney [63], the central nervous system [51], tumors [64], and the lungs [65].

From degradable PEIs, polysorbitol-based osmotically active transporter (PSOAT) synthesized from low molecular weight PEI and sorbitol dimethacrylate (SDM) synthesized *via* Michael addition reaction (mechanism), demonstrated accelerated transfection capability with an intriguing cellular internalization mechanism. The proton sponge effect by PEI and hyperosmotic activity by polysorbitol showed a synergistic effect triggered by better transfection capacity of PSOAT [66]. Furthermore, when SDM was replaced with sorbitol diacrylate, the cytotoxicity of hydrophobic methyl moieties in SDM was reduced, and polysorbitol mediated transporter survival was higher on contrary to PSOAT, as well as increased gene transfection because of the caveolae endocytic pathway [67]. Similarly, polyxylitol [68] and polymannitol [69] based hyperosmotic transporters were prepared for transporting carriers for gene delivery purpose.

Dendrimers are becoming a topic of great interest for researchers for delivering gene either wholly or with chemical modification with other polymers or by the modification of surface of dendrimer [70]. Dendrimers are structured dendritic polymers made up of repeated branched units commonly called dendrimers. Numerous types of dendrimers [70] have been studied for genes delivery. Among those dendrimers, poly (prophylenimine) and poly (amidoamine) (PAMAM) are mostly studied for gene delivery. The degraded PAMAM dendrimer-based material Super Fect as a gene transfection reagent is available having good potential. Even though less literature is available due to lesser transfection efficacy and cytotoxicity [71]. Chemical modification of dendrimers is done to increase the transfection efficiency and to minimize toxicity. Hence, the structure function relationship of these modified dendrimers is required to be studied in detail in order to elucidate their potential efficacy in gene delivery process. Cyclodextrin (CD) has shown promise to be considered a candidate for gene delivery mainly because of the presence of the active site (functional group) which can be tailored depending on the target site to which the gene is to be delivered [82]. Because of their ability to make inclusion complexes with guests that fit in their hydrophobic cavity, CD is widely used. Chemical medication is considered to be a powerful tool for improving CD application in gene therapy, and it is reported that some cationic and neutral derivatives of CD enhanced adenoviral-mediated gene expression. It has also been reported that cationic CD derivatives interact with the adenoviral surface bearing a negative charge. The interactions inhibit nonspecific interactions and facilitate their entry into epithelial cells of the intestine. The CD derivatives improve bioavailability and viral dispersion causing adenoviral vectors' absorption in the cells even after prolonged storage [72]. Polymer materials containing CD-containing were studied for pharmaceutical and biomedical purposes. The CD-containing polymeric materials were used for the first time for gene delivery purpose by Gonzalz *et al.* [73] and the CD-based polymer technology was the first polymer gene carrier to be chosen for clinical studies of siRNA delivery.

3.2. Non-Viral Vectors

Non-viral vectors are lipid-based carriers and inorganic nanoparticles [74]. Plasmid DNA is a double-stranded circular molecule, small and easily produced in bacteria, possessing promoters and copy DNAs (cDNAs) are mostly used for non-viral gene delivery [75]. The pDNA was used at the start for gene delivery and now it has been established that all types of DNAs which have a negative charge can be used for gene delivery. The principle behind this is the electrostatic interaction between positively charged components forming polyplexes and negatively charged nucleic acid. In order to enter the nucleus, these polyplexes must first penetrate the cellular and nuclear membranes, as well as remove DNA from transfection complexes [57, 76].

4. BIOMATERIALS FOR GENE THERAPY

Biomaterials are an important factor for tissue regeneration for wound healing and in creating and maintaining a space for tissue growth and supporting cell migration and adhesion resulting in integration with the host [77]. The regenerative capacity of these materials can be increased by the local delivery of growth factors and cytokines that can result in the induction of tissue formation. Gene delivery is a unique strategy for obtaining a sustained protein production within the wound as the intrinsic cells have the transgene which can also be called as transduced or transfected for viral and nonviral vectors, respectively, which would ultimately function as a bioreactor for the protein of interest. For gene therapy vectors, the physical properties do not depend on the sequence so various combinations of sequences can be delivered without the modification of the delivery vector. Vectors may be plasmids, which are a circular strand of DNA, relatively stable and can be delivered directly from the material consisting of nucleic acids packaged into the nonviral and viral systems that have increased efficacy related to plasmids [78]. Fabricated biomaterial scaffolds can be loaded with these vectors and used for releasing payload in a regulated manner maintaining a higher concentration vector which ultimately increases the probability of cellular internalization.

Hurdles to gene delivery include the transport of vectors to the cell surface, trafficking and internalization to the nucleus for initiation of transgene expression. Biomedical scaffolds delivering vectors are basically targeting mass transport limitations; however, the scaffold design may affect other processes like internalization pathways [79]. Cells which are present in or near the material express the transgene and this expression can trigger regeneration. The design of the scaffold is of utmost importance depending upon porosity, degradation rate and architecture which influence the rate of cell growth and identity of infiltrating cells, which affect the expression of the transgene. Several important issues need to be addressed here for vector, material and implant site including (i) the duration and extent of transgene expression, (ii) the identity of cells expressing the transgene and infiltrating cells, (iii) the number of cells adjacent to the implant expressing transgene, (iv) the impact of vector and material and their response to the foreign body and (v) suitable factors for the expression of a transgene and for maximum tissue formation. Studies involving and mixing gene therapy and tissue engineering technology are making good progress in therapeutic applications. Microporous scaffolds and hydrogels were studied as a passage for the delivery of viral and non-viral vectors which show mechanisms of a biomaterial gene transfer improving the delivery of transgene and increasing the efficacy of this technology [80]. The *in vivo* expression of a transgene for the identification of cells expressing the transgene was characterized for naked plasmid and lentiviral delivery from microporous scaffolds. This mediation is also studied for varied affinities for binding the vectors, presenting design parameter as crucial for the development of scaffolds for regenerative medicine applications. Release strategies have been found for maintaining increased plasmid concentration and enhancing gene transfer. The duration of the transgene expression and plasmid release kinetics has also been studied. Microspheres made up of copolymers of glycolide and lactide were used for the fabrication with the modification of catioionic polymer polydomamine (PD). In their study, they used polydomamine (PD) for enhancing incorporation and obtaining slow and sustained release from the fabricated scaffolds [81].

They entrapped plasmid in the porous scaffold, the pores in the scaffolds, allows cell infiltration. The scaffold's central layer can be changed to control DNA release (*e.g.* , addition of cationic polymer). There was no significant difference in the duration of transgene expression between PD modified and unmodified scaffolds after *in vivo* implantation. The regulated scaffold with dried plasmid on the exterior surface showed a rapid release. Altering the design of the plasmid from a cytomegalovirus to ubiquitin C promoter, increased the expression duration significantly. The study showed that the vector design and the initial release dose affect the extent and transgene expression duration for several weeks [81, 82].

Gene transfer can also be promoted by modifying the interaction of biomaterial with the vector. Alteration of the interaction between the vector and the material was studied by exploiting binding between phosphatidylserine (PS); which is a constituent of the plasma membrane and lentivirus [80]. PS was used with microspheres which were made up of the copolymers of glycolide (PLG) and lactide *via* emulsion method. In this study, lentivirus, but not adenovirus, associated with PS-PLG microspheres with specific binding to PS relative to PLG alone resulted in good yield of immobilized lentivirus from transduced cells with an increased amount of expression in transgene contrary to the virus alone. Microspheres were incorporated into porous tissue engineering scaffolds exhibiting localized and long term expression *in vivo* with extended retention of lentivirus [80]. Lentivirus delivery into a spinal cord model showed maximum expression at the implant site with a gradient expression caudally and rostrally. There are numerous applications utilizing these specific binding properties of lentiviral vectors in model systems investigating tissue development and regenerative medicine. Lentiviruses are usually integrating viruses but controlled integrating variants are also designed. Integration may or may not be required depending upon the requirement for expression. However, integration is being controlled with the addition of genes that halt the transgene expression once the drug is administered to the patient [78].

Hydrogels are found to be particularly beneficial for localized gene delivery providing tissue growth [83], and as a new method for inducing the expression of integrated genes, however it may result in the insufficient duration of expression for regeneration [77]. Hydrogel is a matrix of hydrophilic polymer made up of over 90% water, showing physical properties similar to native tissues which can be easily altered *via* crosslinking [84]. Natural hydrogels like collagen have an innate ability for supporting cell adhesion, however, synthetic hydrogels based on poly (ethylene glycol) (PEG) should be modified for supporting cell migration. Peptide sequences are added during crosslinking allowing degradation and cell adhesion and subsequently achieving functionality [85]. Proteolytic degradation of the peptide crosslinkers by cell-secreted enzymes results in cell migration. Studies showed that transgene expression is related with cell migration through the hydrogel [79]; however, matrix is degraded by migrating cells resulting in the loss of substantial quantities of DNA [82].

5. GENE THERAPY IS SOFT AND HARD TISSUE (EXAMPLES)

5.1. Muscle Tissue

Muscle has been reported to be a potent target for gene delivery. Studies have shown minimal turnover of muscle cells for achieving increased and prolonged transient expression and expression from integrated DNA. Muscle tissue can be a good option for providing therapeutic levels of clotting factors for many months [86]. New approaches have investigated the efficacy of genetically induced neovascularization on muscle flaps survival. When delivered to muscle flaps, genes encoding platelet-derived growth factor-AA and vascular endothelial growth factor are known to stimulate neovascularization and have a protective effect on muscle flaps [87].

5.2. Nerve Tissue

The goal of nerve tissue regeneration is to achieve a precise and rapid healing that innervates distal structures without inducing neuroma or severe scarring. In grafted nerves, where healing can be selectively promoted across the junctions between the graft and native nerve, guided healing is pivotal. Nerve cells present in the brain and spinal cord have been studied for viral vector mediated gene transfer. HSV and adenoviral vectors are usually used for gene transferring to nerve tissues. HSV, being neurotropic is suitable for this purpose. Recently peripheral nerves have been developed for gene transfer using LacZ-containing plasmid DNA, delivered to nerve anastomosis through DNA-soaked sutures in rabbit model, reported successful transfer of the transgene at the junction of anastomosis, providing an evidence for using gene therapy technique for the recovery of nerve function [88].

5.3. Bone Tissues

Bone is prone to injury and is one of the frequently repaired organs of the human body [89]. Functional treatment of bone loss associated with cancer, trauma, or fracture nonunion is considered a significant challenge in plastic and orthopaedic surgery. Tissue engineering is considered these days as an efficacious and alternative treatment for bone repair and several studies have been reported using bioresorbable scaffolds having pores and fibrous in nature for bone regeneration [90]. The genetically modified osteoblasts are then combined with polymeric matrices, *e.g.* growth stimulating factors or bone-morphogenic protein (BMP-2) [91].Similar results were reported the overexpression of BMP-2 for genetically modified mesenchymal stem cells [92]. Eriksson *et al.*, studied the micro-seeding method for bone transfection *via* BMP-2 [93]. In the mouse model, the bone under study was exposed and periosteum was raised which allowed its microseeding under the surface prior to getting back to the place. Significantly higher expression levels were found of the BMP-2 gene [94].

5.4. Non-Viral Gene Therapy for Bone Engineering

Catioionic polymers, peptides, calcium phosphate and other inorganic nanomaterials are studied *in vivo* for their properties of gene transfer into the target cell [95]. Among all of these chemical moieties, cationic polymers and cationic liposomes are the most used carriers for nucleic acid and gene delivery these days [96]. Opposite charges present on surface are useful in forming complexes (polyplexes or lipoplexes) with the molecules of negatively charged nucleic acids. These systems have a drawback such as low transfection efficiency over viral vectors specifically when transfected cells like MSCs are the target. Although, recently lipid development has shown promising results in transfection studies [97]. Nonetheless, being non-biodegradable both cationic polymers and lipids are toxic for the cells and contamination risk of the whole body is high. It can be concluded that the synthesis of non-viral gene therapy which is less toxic and presents higher efficiency is the most difficult task for researchers working in the field of gene therapy [98]. Recent research has revealed that the transfection of adipose tissue derived MSCs with the G4 PAMAM/BMP-2 plasmid dendriplex successfully induces differentiation of the cells into the osteogenic phenotype, even at the modest transfection levels [99]. The use of an alginate hydrogel to deliver BMP-2 cDNA has also exhibited promising results. *In vivo* ectopic osteogenesis is reported to be achieved when BMP-2 (biologically active) is released from the BMSC present in the gel over 5 weeks period [100]. Other hydrogels such as hyaluronic acid or fibrin can also be used for transporting osteogenic genes accelerating fracture healing and inducing bone formation [101].

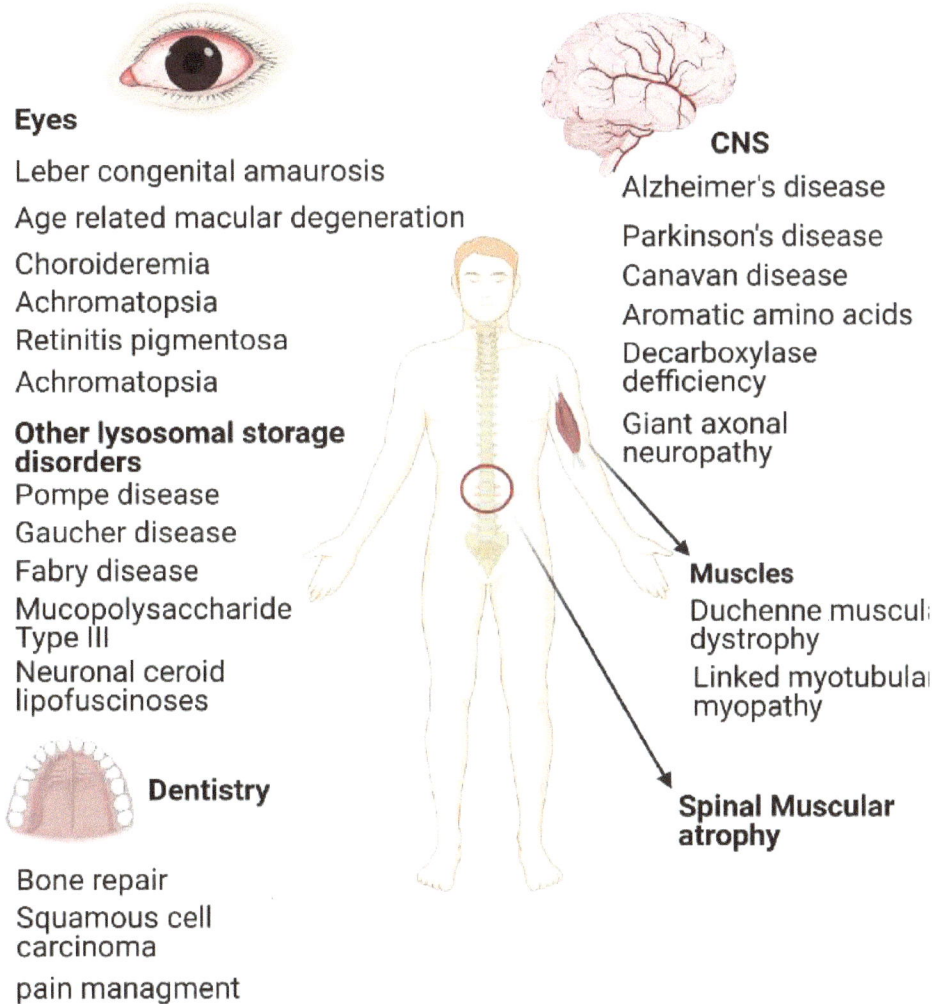

Eyes

Leber congenital amaurosis

Age related macular degeneration

Choroideremia
Achromatopsia
Retinitis pigmentosa
Achromatopsia

Other lysosomal storage disorders
Pompe disease
Gaucher disease
Fabry disease
Mucopolysaccharide Type III
Neuronal ceroid lipofuscinoses

Dentistry

Bone repair
Squamous cell carcinoma
pain managment

CNS
Alzheimer's disease
Parkinson's disease
Canavan disease
Aromatic amino acids
Decarboxylase defficiency
Giant axonal neuropathy

Muscles
Duchenne muscula dystrophy
Linked myotubula myopathy

Spinal Muscular atrophy

Fig. (12.2). Applications of gene therapy. Some of the potential applications of gene therapy in various pathologcal conditions have been described. These include various medical conditions of the eyes, muscles, central nervous system, spinal muscular atrophy, various lysosomal storage disorders and dentistry [106].

Sonoporation is also known as a method for transducing cells [102], microbubbles are moved under the effect of ultrasound for transfecting cells. In ectopic and orthotopic animals, a novel nonviral osteoinductive *in vivo* gene therapy approach was investigated [103]. Co-expression plasmids of BMP-2 and BMP7 were examined for 5 days with and without sonoporation. In ectopic model, bioluminescence imaging and luciferase plasmid reported transduction efficiency. Transduction efficiency was marked with increased luminescence in sonoporated animals when compared with the passive gene delivery [103]. BMP-2/BMP-7 or BMP-9 reported increased bone formation when sonoporated as compared to passive gene delivery [104]. Similar results were obtained in orthotopic application on a rat femur non-union model by opting sonoporation technique as sonoporated animals exhibited increased union rate [103, 105].

6. FUTURE PROSPECTS

Development of imminent novel therapies for the treatment of wounds, diseases and disorders is utmost of importance. Gene therapy is the most promising approach for reversing fundamental abnormalities. However, major clinical studies have shown promising results in the translation of gene therapy for clinical trials. Further clinical trials with an emphasis on details will improve gene therapies. Transduction efficiency is a major hurdle in gene therapy. For increasing transduction efficiency, the selection of vector, optimization of the dose of drug and development of more efficient gene therapy method for immunogenic effect is required. Another major hurdle is the selection criteria for patients and endpoints which play an extremely pivotal role in the success of gene therapy. In most of the clinical trials, patients who have an advanced degree of disease are recruited not giving successful results. There is an utmost need for recognizing valid endpoints for future trials. Finally, current clinical trials of gene therapy have proved to be safe. This is definitely encouraging for conducting more clinical trials and testing their therapeutic effects for developing new and improved gene delivery systems.

CONCLUDING REMARKS

In the recent times, gene therapy has emerged as a powerful tool for disease treatment. Although, there are limitations for gene delivery system but many different systems have emerged to overcome this hurdle. Recently, biomaterials have also been taken into account for gene delivery system. Gene therapy has been performed into different soft and hard tissues like muscles, nerves and bones. Addressing the ethical concerns associated with gene therapy, it is believed that gene therapy would have a strong impact on the treatment of diseases in the future.

CONSENT FOR PUBLICATION

Not applicable.

CONFLICT OF INTEREST

The author declares no conflict of interest, financial or otherwise.

ACKNOWLEDGEMENTS

Declared none.

REFERENCES

[1]   AI-Aql ZS, Alagl AS, Graves DT, Gerstenfeld LC, Einhorn TA. Molecular mechanisms controlling bone formation during fracture healing and distraction osteogenesis. J Dent Res 2008; 87(2): 107-18.
        [http://dx.doi.org/10.1177/154405910808700215] [PMID: 18218835]

[2]   Lind M. Growth factors: Possible new clinical tools: A review. Acta Orthop Scand 1996; 67(4): 407-17.
        [http://dx.doi.org/10.3109/17453679609002342] [PMID: 8792750]

[3]   Urist MR. Bone: Formation by Autoinduction. Science 1965; 150(3698): 893-9.
        [http://dx.doi.org/10.1126/science.150.3698.893] [PMID: 5319761]

[4]   Sartori R, Sandri M. BMPs and the muscle–bone connection. Bone 2015; 80: 37-42.
        [http://dx.doi.org/10.1016/j.bone.2015.05.023] [PMID: 26036170]

[5]   Friedlaender G E, *et al.* Osteogenic protein-1 (bone morphogenetic protein-7) in the treatment of tibial nonunions: a prospective, randomized clinical trial comparing rhOP-1 with fresh bone autograft. The Journal of bone and joint surgery American 2001; 83(2): S151.
        [http://dx.doi.org/10.2106/00004623-200100002-00010]

[6]   Govender S, Csimma C, Genant HK, *et al.* BMP-2 Evaluation in Surgery for Tibial Trauma (BESTT) Study Group. Recombinant human bone morphogenetic protein-2 for treatment of open tibial fractures: a prospective, controlled, randomized study of four hundred and fifty patients. J Bone Joint Surg Am 2002; 84(12): 2123-34.
        [http://dx.doi.org/10.2106/00004623-200212000-00001] [PMID: 12473698]

[7]   Boden SD, Zdeblick TA, Sandhu HS, Heim SE. The use of rhBMP-2 in interbody fusion cages. Definitive evidence of osteoinduction in humans: a preliminary report. Spine 2000; 25(3): 376-81.
        [http://dx.doi.org/10.1097/00007632-200002010-00020] [PMID: 10703113]

[8]   Talwar R, Di Silvio L, Hughes FJ, King GN. Effects of carrier release kinetics on bone morphogenetic protein-2-induced periodontal regeneration *in vivo.* J Clin Periodontol 2001; 28(4): 340-7.
        [http://dx.doi.org/10.1034/j.1600-051x.2001.028004340.x] [PMID: 11314890]

[9]   Uludag H, Gao T, Porter TJ, Friess W, Wozney JM. Delivery systems for BMPs: factors contributing to protein retention at an application site. J Bone Joint Surg Am 2001; 83(Pt 2) (Suppl. 1): S1-, 128-S1-135.
        [http://dx.doi.org/10.2106/00004623-200100002-00007] [PMID: 11314790]

[10]   Ylä-Herttuala S. Endgame: glybera finally recommended for approval as the first gene therapy drug in the European union. Mol Ther 2012; 20(10): 1831-2.
        [http://dx.doi.org/10.1038/mt.2012.194] [PMID: 23023051]

[11]   Melchiorri D, Pani L, Gasparini P, *et al.* Regulatory evaluation of Glybera in Europe — two committees, one mission. Nat Rev Drug Discov 2013; 12(9): 719-9.
        [http://dx.doi.org/10.1038/nrd3835-c1] [PMID: 23954897]

[12]   Solheim E. Growth factors in bone. Int Orthop 1998; 22(6): 410-6.
        [http://dx.doi.org/10.1007/s002640050290] [PMID: 10093814]

[13]   Barba M, *et al.* Spinal fusion in the next generation: gene and cell therapy approaches. Scientific
        World Journal 2014; 28: 406159.

[14]   Evans CH, Robbins PD. Possible orthopaedic applications of gene therapy. J Bone Joint Surg Am
        1995; 77(7): 1103-14.
        [http://dx.doi.org/10.2106/00004623-199507000-00021] [PMID: 7608237]

[15]   Shea LD, Smiley E, Bonadio J, Mooney DJ. DNA delivery from polymer matrices for tissue
        engineering. Nat Biotechnol 1999; 17(6): 551-4.
        [http://dx.doi.org/10.1038/9853] [PMID: 10385318]

[16]   Misra S. Human gene therapy: a brief overview of the genetic revolution. J Assoc Physicians India
        2013; 61(2): 127-33.
        [PMID: 24471251]

[17]   Kay MA. State-of-the-art gene-based therapies: the road ahead. Nat Rev Genet 2011; 12(5): 316-28.
        [http://dx.doi.org/10.1038/nrg2971] [PMID: 21468099]

[18]   Gross G, Waks T, Eshhar Z. Expression of immunoglobulin-T-cell receptor chimeric molecules as
        functional receptors with antibody-type specificity. Proc Natl Acad Sci USA 1989; 86(24): 10024-8.
        [http://dx.doi.org/10.1073/pnas.86.24.10024] [PMID: 2513569]

[19]   Chambers CA, Allison JP. Co-stimulation in T cell responses. Curr Opin Immunol 1997; 9(3): 396-
        404.
        [http://dx.doi.org/10.1016/S0952-7915(97)80087-8] [PMID: 9203422]

[20]   Betz OB, Betz VM, Nazarian A, *et al.* Direct percutaneous gene delivery to enhance healing of
        segmental bone defects. J Bone Joint Surg Am 2006; 88(2): 355-65.
        [http://dx.doi.org/10.2106/00004623-200602000-00015] [PMID: 16452748]

[21]   Zhong XS, Matsushita M, Plotkin J, Riviere I, Sadelain M. Chimeric antigen receptors combining 4-
        1BB and CD28 signaling domains augment PI3kinase/AKT/Bcl-XL activation and CD8+ T cell-
        mediated tumor eradication. Mol Ther 2010; 18(2): 413-20.
        [http://dx.doi.org/10.1038/mt.2009.210] [PMID: 19773745]

[22]   Maude SL, Frey N, Shaw PA, *et al.* Chimeric antigen receptor T cells for sustained remissions in
        leukemia. N Engl J Med 2014; 371(16): 1507-17.
        [http://dx.doi.org/10.1056/NEJMoa1407222] [PMID: 25317870]

[23]   Wilkins O, Keeler AM, Flotte TR. CAR T-cell therapy: progress and prospects. Hum Gene Ther
        Methods 2017; 28(2): 61-6.
        [http://dx.doi.org/10.1089/hgtb.2016.153] [PMID: 28330372]

[24]   Marraffini LA, Sontheimer EJ. CRISPR interference: RNA-directed adaptive immunity in bacteria and
        archaea. Nat Rev Genet 2010; 11(3): 181-90.
        [http://dx.doi.org/10.1038/nrg2749] [PMID: 20125085]

[25]   Cong L, Ran FA, Cox D, *et al.* Multiplex genome engineering using CRISPR/Cas systems. Science
        2013; 339(6121): 819-23.
        [http://dx.doi.org/10.1126/science.1231143] [PMID: 23287718]

[26]   Gori JL, Hsu PD, Maeder ML, Shen S, Welstead GG, Bumcrot D. Delivery and specificity of
        CRISPR/Cas9 genome editing technologies for human gene therapy. Hum Gene Ther 2015; 26(7):
        443-51.
        [http://dx.doi.org/10.1089/hum.2015.074] [PMID: 26068008]

[27]   DeWitt MA, *et al.* Selection-free genome editing of the sickle mutation in human adult hematopoietic
        stem/progenitor cells. Sci Transl Med 2016; 8(360): 360ra134.
        [http://dx.doi.org/10.1126/scitranslmed.aaf9336]

[28]   Tebas P, Stein D, Tang WW, *et al.* Gene editing of CCR5 in autologous CD4 T cells of persons infected with HIV. N Engl J Med 2014; 370(10): 901-10.
[http://dx.doi.org/10.1056/NEJMoa1300662] [PMID: 24597865]

[29]   Callaway E. Second Chinese team reports gene editing in human embryos. Nature 2016.
[http://dx.doi.org/10.1038/nature.2016.19718]

[30]   Wegman F, Öner FC, Dhert WJA, Alblas J. Non-viral gene therapy for bone tissue engineering. Biotechnol Genet Eng Rev 2013; 29(2): 206-20.
[http://dx.doi.org/10.1080/02648725.2013.801227] [PMID: 24568281]

[31]   Verma IM, *et al.* Gene therapy: promises, problems and prospects. Genes and resistance to disease. Springer 2000; pp. 147-57.
[http://dx.doi.org/10.1007/978-3-642-56947-0_13]

[32]   Ginn SL, Alexander IE, Edelstein ML, Abedi MR, Wixon J. Gene therapy clinical trials worldwide to 2012 - an update. J Gene Med 2013; 15(2): 65-77.
[http://dx.doi.org/10.1002/jgm.2698] [PMID: 23355455]

[33]   Oligino TJ, Yao Q, Ghivizzani SC, Robbins P. Vector systems for gene transfer to joints. Clin Orthop Relat Res 2000; 379(379) (Suppl.): S17-30.
[http://dx.doi.org/10.1097/00003086-200010001-00004] [PMID: 11039748]

[34]   Betz VM, Betz OB, Harris MB, Vrahas MS, Evans CH. Bone tissue engineering and repair by gene therapy. Front Biosci 2008; 13(13): 833-41.
[http://dx.doi.org/10.2741/2724] [PMID: 17981592]

[35]   Cao H, Koehler DR, Hu J. Adenoviral vectors for gene replacement therapy. Viral Immunol 2004; 17(3): 327-33.
[http://dx.doi.org/10.1089/vim.2004.17.327] [PMID: 15357899]

[36]   Sugiyama O, Sung An D, Kung SPK, *et al.* Lentivirus-mediated gene transfer induces long-term transgene expression of BMP-2 *in vitro* and new bone formation *in vivo*. Mol Ther 2005; 11(3): 390-8.
[http://dx.doi.org/10.1016/j.ymthe.2004.10.019] [PMID: 15727935]

[37]   Peng H, Usas A, Gearhart B, Young B, Olshanski A, Huard J. Development of a self-inactivating tet-on retroviral vector expressing bone morphogenetic protein 4 to achieve regulated bone formation. Mol Ther 2004; 9(6): 885-94.
[http://dx.doi.org/10.1016/j.ymthe.2004.02.023] [PMID: 15194055]

[38]   Kay MA, Glorioso JC, Naldini L. Viral vectors for gene therapy: the art of turning infectious agents into vehicles of therapeutics. Nat Med 2001; 7(1): 33-40.
[http://dx.doi.org/10.1038/83324] [PMID: 11135613]

[39]   Gafni Y, Pelled G, Zilberman Y, *et al.* Gene therapy platform for bone regeneration using an exogenously regulated, AAV-2-based gene expression system. Mol Ther 2004; 9(4): 587-95.
[http://dx.doi.org/10.1016/j.ymthe.2003.12.009] [PMID: 15093189]

[40]   Salmon F, Grosios K, Petry H. Safety profile of recombinant adeno-associated viral vectors: focus on alipogene tiparvovec (Glybera ®). Expert Rev Clin Pharmacol 2014; 7(1): 53-65.
[http://dx.doi.org/10.1586/17512433.2014.852065] [PMID: 24308784]

[41]   Morrison C. $1-million price tag set for Glybera gene therapy. Nature Publishing Group 2015.

[42]   Dang J, Leong K. Natural polymers for gene delivery and tissue engineering. Adv Drug Deliv Rev 2006; 58(4): 487-99.
[http://dx.doi.org/10.1016/j.addr.2006.03.001] [PMID: 16762443]

[43]   Ravi Kumar MNV. A review of chitin and chitosan applications. React Funct Polym 2000; 46(1): 1-27.
[http://dx.doi.org/10.1016/S1381-5148(00)00038-9]

[44]   Kim TH, Ihm JE, Choi YJ, Nah JW, Cho CS. Efficient gene delivery by urocanic acid-modified

chitosan. J Control Release 2003; 93(3): 389-402.
[http://dx.doi.org/10.1016/j.jconrel.2003.08.017] [PMID: 14644588]

[45] Jiang HL, Kim YK, Arote R, *et al.* Mannosylated chitosan-graft-polyethylenimine as a gene carrier for Raw 264.7 cell targeting. Int J Pharm 2009; 375(1-2): 133-9.
[http://dx.doi.org/10.1016/j.ijpharm.2009.03.033] [PMID: 19481699]

[46] Jiang HL, Xu CX, Kim YK, *et al.* The suppression of lung tumorigenesis by aerosol-delivered folate–chitosan-graft-polyethylenimine/Akt1 shRNA complexes through the Akt signaling pathway. Biomaterials 2009; 30(29): 5844-52.
[http://dx.doi.org/10.1016/j.biomaterials.2009.07.017] [PMID: 19640582]

[47] Jiang HL, Kwon JT, Kim EM, *et al.* Galactosylated poly(ethylene glycol)-chitosan-graft-polyethylenimine as a gene carrier for hepatocyte-targeting. J Control Release 2008; 131(2): 150-7.
[http://dx.doi.org/10.1016/j.jconrel.2008.07.029] [PMID: 18706946]

[48] Kim TH, Park IK, Nah JW, Choi YJ, Cho CS. Galactosylated chitosan/DNA nanoparticles prepared using water-soluble chitosan as a gene carrier. Biomaterials 2004; 25(17): 3783-92.
[http://dx.doi.org/10.1016/j.biomaterials.2003.10.063] [PMID: 15020154]

[49] Park YK, Park YH, Shin BA, *et al.* Galactosylated chitosan–graft–dextran as hepatocyte-targeting DNA carrier. J Control Release 2000; 69(1): 97-108.
[http://dx.doi.org/10.1016/S0168-3659(00)00298-4] [PMID: 11018549]

[50] Jiang HL, Lim HT, Kim YK, *et al.* Chitosan-graft-spermine as a gene carrier *in vitro* and *in vivo*. Eur J Pharm Biopharm 2011; 77(1): 36-42.
[http://dx.doi.org/10.1016/j.ejpb.2010.09.014] [PMID: 20932903]

[51] Abdallah B, Hassan A, Benoist C, Goula D, Behr JP, Demeneix BA. A powerful nonviral vector for *in vivo* gene transfer into the adult mammalian brain: polyethylenimine. Hum Gene Ther 1996; 7(16): 1947-54.
[http://dx.doi.org/10.1089/hum.1996.7.16-1947] [PMID: 8930654]

[52] Jiang G, Min SH, Oh EJ, Hahn SK. DNA/PEI/Alginate polyplex as an efficient *in vivo* gene delivery system. Biotechnol Bioprocess Eng; BBE 2007; 12(6): 684-9.
[http://dx.doi.org/10.1007/BF02931086]

[53] Kong HJ, Kim ES, Huang YC, Mooney DJ. Design of biodegradable hydrogel for the local and sustained delivery of angiogenic plasmid DNA. Pharm Res 2008; 25(5): 1230-8.
[http://dx.doi.org/10.1007/s11095-007-9526-7] [PMID: 18183476]

[54] Krebs MD, Salter E, Chen E, Sutter KA, Alsberg E. Calcium phosphate-DNA nanoparticle gene delivery from alginate hydrogels induces *in vivo* osteogenesis. J Biomed Mater Res A 2010; 92(3): 1131-8.
[PMID: 19322877]

[55] Wegman F, Geuze RE, van der Helm YJ, Cumhur Öner F, Dhert WJA, Alblas J. Gene delivery of bone morphogenetic protein-2 plasmid DNA promotes bone formation in a large animal model. J Tissue Eng Regen Med 2014; 8(10): 763-70.
[http://dx.doi.org/10.1002/term.1571] [PMID: 22888035]

[56] Chew SA, Kretlow JD, Spicer PP, *et al.* Delivery of plasmid DNA encoding bone morphogenetic protein-2 with a biodegradable branched polycationic polymer in a critical-size rat cranial defect model. Tissue Eng Part A 2011; 17(5-6): 751-63.
[http://dx.doi.org/10.1089/ten.tea.2010.0496] [PMID: 20964581]

[57] Pack DW, Hoffman AS, Pun S, Stayton PS. Design and development of polymers for gene delivery. Nat Rev Drug Discov 2005; 4(7): 581-93.
[http://dx.doi.org/10.1038/nrd1775] [PMID: 16052241]

[58] Boussif O, Lezoualc'h F, Zanta MA, *et al.* A versatile vector for gene and oligonucleotide transfer into cells in culture and *in vivo*: polyethylenimine. Proc Natl Acad Sci USA 1995; 92(16): 7297-301.

[http://dx.doi.org/10.1073/pnas.92.16.7297] [PMID: 7638184]

[59]   Jere D, Jiang HL, Arote R, *et al.* Degradable polyethylenimines as DNA and small interfering RNA carriers. Expert Opin Drug Deliv 2009; 6(8): 827-34.
[http://dx.doi.org/10.1517/17425240903029183] [PMID: 19558333]

[60]   Chollet P, Favrot M C, Hurbin A, Coll J L. Side-effects of a systemic injection of linear polyethylenimine–DNA complexes. The Journal of Gene Medicine: A cross-disciplinary journal for research on the science of gene transfer and its clinical applications 2002; 4(1): 84-91.
[http://dx.doi.org/10.1002/jgm.237]

[61]   Jiang HL, Kim TH, Kim YK, Park IY, Cho MH, Cho CS. Efficient gene delivery using chitosan–polyethylenimine hybrid systems. Biomed Mater 2008; 3(2): 025013.
[http://dx.doi.org/10.1088/1748-6041/3/2/025013] [PMID: 18477817]

[62]   Kim TH, Jiang H-L, Jere D, *et al.* Chemical modification of chitosan as a gene carrier *in vitro* and *in vivo.* Prog Polym Sci 2007; 32(7): 726-53.
[http://dx.doi.org/10.1016/j.progpolymsci.2007.05.001]

[63]   Boletta A, Benigni A, Lutz J, Remuzzi G, Soria MR, Monaco L. Nonviral gene delivery to the rat kidney with polyethylenimine. Hum Gene Ther 1997; 8(10): 1243-51.
[http://dx.doi.org/10.1089/hum.1997.8.10-1243] [PMID: 9215741]

[64]   Coll JL, Chollet P, Brambilla E, Desplanques D, Behr JP, Favrot M. *In vivo* delivery to tumors of DNA complexed with linear polyethylenimine. Hum Gene Ther 1999; 10(10): 1659-66.
[http://dx.doi.org/10.1089/10430349950017662] [PMID: 10428211]

[65]   Goula D, Benoist C, Mantero S, Merlo G, Levi G, Demeneix BA. Polyethylenimine-based intravenous delivery of transgenes to mouse lung. Gene Ther 1998; 5(9): 1291-5.
[http://dx.doi.org/10.1038/sj.gt.3300717] [PMID: 9930332]

[66]   Islam MA, Shin JY, Firdous J, *et al.* The role of osmotic polysorbitol-based transporter in RNAi silencing *via* caveolae-mediated endocytosis and COX-2 expression. Biomaterials 2012; 33(34): 8868-80.
[http://dx.doi.org/10.1016/j.biomaterials.2012.08.049] [PMID: 22975426]

[67]   Islam MA, Yun CH, Choi YJ, *et al.* Accelerated gene transfer through a polysorbitol-based transporter mechanism. Biomaterials 2011; 32(36): 9908-24.
[http://dx.doi.org/10.1016/j.biomaterials.2011.09.013] [PMID: 21959011]

[68]   Garg P, Pandey S, Seonwoo H, *et al.* Hyperosmotic polydixylitol for crossing the blood brain barrier and efficient nucleic acid delivery. Chem Commun (Camb) 2015; 51(17): 3645-8.
[http://dx.doi.org/10.1039/C4CC09871D] [PMID: 25645149]

[69]   Park TE, Singh B, Li H, *et al.* Enhanced BBB permeability of osmotically active poly(mannitol-c--PEI) modified with rabies virus glycoprotein *via* selective stimulation of caveolar endocytosis for RNAi therapeutics in Alzheimer's disease. Biomaterials 2015; 38: 61-71.
[http://dx.doi.org/10.1016/j.biomaterials.2014.10.068] [PMID: 25457984]

[70]   Yang J, Zhang Q, Chang H, Cheng Y. Surface-engineered dendrimers in gene delivery. Chem Rev 2015; 115(11): 5274-300.
[http://dx.doi.org/10.1021/cr500542t] [PMID: 25944558]

[71]   Akhtar S, Chandrasekhar B, Attur S, Yousif MHM, Benter IF. On the nanotoxicity of PAMAM dendrimers: Superfect® stimulates the EGFR–ERK1/2 signal transduction pathway *via* an oxidative stress-dependent mechanism in HEK 293 cells. Int J Pharm 2013; 448(1): 239-46.
[http://dx.doi.org/10.1016/j.ijpharm.2013.03.039] [PMID: 23538097]

[72]   Croyle MA, Cheng X, Wilson JM. Development of formulations that enhance physical stability of viral vectors for gene therapy. Gene Ther 2001; 8(17): 1281-90.
[http://dx.doi.org/10.1038/sj.gt.3301527] [PMID: 11571564]

[73]   Gonzalez H, Hwang SJ, Davis ME. New class of polymers for the delivery of macromolecular

therapeutics. Bioconjug Chem 1999; 10(6): 1068-74.
[http://dx.doi.org/10.1021/bc990072j] [PMID: 10563777]

[74]   Mintzer MA, Simanek EE. Nonviral vectors for gene delivery. Chem Rev 2009; 109(2): 259-302.
[http://dx.doi.org/10.1021/cr800409e] [PMID: 19053809]

[75]   Gill DR, Pringle IA, Hyde SC. Progress and Prospects: The design and production of plasmid vectors.
Gene Ther 2009; 16(2): 165-71.
[http://dx.doi.org/10.1038/gt.2008.183] [PMID: 19129858]

[76]   Kim YD, Pofali P, Park TE, *et al.* Gene therapy for bone tissue engineering. Tissue Eng Regen Med
2016; 13(2): 111-25.
[http://dx.doi.org/10.1007/s13770-016-9063-8] [PMID: 30603391]

[77]   De Laporte L, Shea LD. Matrices and scaffolds for DNA delivery in tissue engineering. Adv Drug
Deliv Rev 2007; 59(4-5): 292-307.
[http://dx.doi.org/10.1016/j.addr.2007.03.017] [PMID: 17512630]

[78]   Waehler R, Russell SJ, Curiel DT. Engineering targeted viral vectors for gene therapy. Nat Rev Genet
2007; 8(8): 573-87.
[http://dx.doi.org/10.1038/nrg2141] [PMID: 17607305]

[79]   Shepard JA, Huang A, Shikanov A, Shea LD. Balancing cell migration with matrix degradation
enhances gene delivery to cells cultured three-dimensionally within hydrogels. J Control Release
2010; 146(1): 128-35.
[http://dx.doi.org/10.1016/j.jconrel.2010.04.032] [PMID: 20450944]

[80]   Shin S, Tuinstra HM, Salvay DM, Shea LD. Phosphatidylserine immobilization of lentivirus for
localized gene transfer. Biomaterials 2010; 31(15): 4353-9.
[http://dx.doi.org/10.1016/j.biomaterials.2010.02.013] [PMID: 20206382]

[81]   Avilés MO, Lin CH, Zelivyanskaya M, *et al.* The contribution of plasmid design and release to *in vivo*
gene expression following delivery from cationic polymer modified scaffolds. Biomaterials 2010;
31(6): 1140-7.
[http://dx.doi.org/10.1016/j.biomaterials.2009.10.035] [PMID: 19892398]

[82]   Gower RM, Shea LD. Biomaterial scaffolds for controlled, localized gene delivery of regenerative
factors. Adv Wound Care (New Rochelle) 2013; 2(3): 100-6.
[http://dx.doi.org/10.1089/wound.2011.0325] [PMID: 24527333]

[83]   Shikanov A, Smith RM, Xu M, Woodruff TK, Shea LD. Hydrogel network design using
multifunctional macromers to coordinate tissue maturation in ovarian follicle culture. Biomaterials
2011; 32(10): 2524-31.
[http://dx.doi.org/10.1016/j.biomaterials.2010.12.027] [PMID: 21247629]

[84]   Andreopoulos FM, Beckman EJ, Russell AJ. Light-induced tailoring of PEG-hydrogel properties.
Biomaterials 1998; 19(15): 1343-52.
[http://dx.doi.org/10.1016/S0142-9612(97)00219-6] [PMID: 9758034]

[85]   Drury JL, Mooney DJ. Hydrogels for tissue engineering: scaffold design variables and applications.
Biomaterials 2003; 24(24): 4337-51.
[http://dx.doi.org/10.1016/S0142-9612(03)00340-5] [PMID: 12922147]

[86]   Prud'homme GJ, Lawson BR, Chang Y, Theofilopoulos AN. Immunotherapeutic gene transfer into
muscle. Trends Immunol 2001; 22(3): 149-55.
[http://dx.doi.org/10.1016/S1471-4906(00)01822-6] [PMID: 11286730]

[87]   Machens HG, Morgan JR, Berthiaume F, Stefanovich P, Reimer R, Berger AC. Genetically modified
fibroblasts induce angiogenesis in the rat epigastric island flap. Langenbecks Arch Surg 1998; 383(5):
345-50.
[http://dx.doi.org/10.1007/s004230050146] [PMID: 9860229]

[88]   Zhang S, Zhang J, Zhang Y, Liu L. Direct gene transfer into rabbit peripheral nerve *in vivo*. Journal of

Tongji Medical University= Tong ji yi ke da xue xue bao 2001; 21(1): 52-5.

[89]   Langer R, Vacanti J. Tissue engineering. Science 260: 920-926. Tissue Engineering: The Union Of Biology And Engineering 1993; 98.

[90]   Thomson RC, Yaszemski MJ, Powers JM, Mikos AG. Fabrication of biodegradable polymer scaffolds to engineer trabecular bone. J Biomater Sci Polym Ed 1996; 7(1): 23-38.
       [http://dx.doi.org/10.1163/156856295X00805] [PMID: 7662615]

[91]   Laurencin C, Attawia MA, Lu LQ, *et al.* Poly(lactide-co-glycolide)/hydroxyapatite delivery of BMP-2-producing cells: a regional gene therapy approach to bone regeneration. Biomaterials 2001; 22(11): 1271-7.
       [http://dx.doi.org/10.1016/S0142-9612(00)00279-9] [PMID: 11336299]

[92]   Turgeman G, Pittman DD, Müller R, *et al.* Engineered human mesenchymal stem cells: a novel platform for skeletal cell mediated gene therapy. J Gene Med 2001; 3(3): 240-51.
       [http://dx.doi.org/10.1002/1521-2254(200105/06)3:3<240::AID-JGM181>3.0.CO;2-A]   [PMID: 11437329]

[93]   Eriksson E, Yao F, Svensjö T, *et al. In vivo* gene transfer to skin and wound by microseeding. J Surg Res 1998; 78(2): 85-91.
       [http://dx.doi.org/10.1006/jsre.1998.5325] [PMID: 9733623]

[94]   Hoeller D, Petrie N, Yao F, Eriksson E. Gene therapy in soft tissue reconstruction. Cells Tissues Organs 2002; 172(2): 118-25.
       [http://dx.doi.org/10.1159/000065610] [PMID: 12426488]

[95]   Jun Loh X, Lee TC. Gene delivery by functional inorganic nanocarriers. Recent Pat DNA Gene Seq 2012; 6(2): 108-14.
       [http://dx.doi.org/10.2174/187221512801327361] [PMID: 22670611]

[96]   Won YW, Lim KS, Kim YH. Intracellular organelle-targeted non-viral gene delivery systems. J Control Release 2011; 152(1): 99-109.
       [http://dx.doi.org/10.1016/j.jconrel.2011.01.013] [PMID: 21255626]

[97]   Sarker SR, Aoshima Y, Hokama R, Inoue T, Sou K, Takeoka S. Arginine-based cationic liposomes for efficient *in vitro* plasmid DNA delivery with low cytotoxicity. Int J Nanomedicine 2013; 8: 1361-75.
       [PMID: 23630419]

[98]   Shan Y, Luo T, Peng C, *et al.* Gene delivery using dendrimer-entrapped gold nanoparticles as nonviral vectors. Biomaterials 2012; 33(10): 3025-35.
       [http://dx.doi.org/10.1016/j.biomaterials.2011.12.045] [PMID: 22248990]

[99]   Santos JL, Oramas E, Pêgo AP, Granja PL, Tomás H. Osteogenic differentiation of mesenchymal stem cells using PAMAM dendrimers as gene delivery vectors. J Control Release 2009; 134(2): 141-8.
       [http://dx.doi.org/10.1016/j.jconrel.2008.11.007] [PMID: 19070635]

[100] Wegman F, Bijenhof A, Schuijff L, Öner FC, Dhert WJA, Alblas J. Osteogenic differentiation as a result of BMP-2 plasmid DNA based gene therapy *in vitro* and *in vivo*. Eur Cell Mater 2011; 21: 230-42.
       [http://dx.doi.org/10.22203/eCM.v021a18] [PMID: 21409753]

[101] Kaipel M, Schützenberger S, Hofmann AT, *et al.* Evaluation of fibrin-based gene-activated matrices for BMP2/7 plasmid codelivery in a rat nonunion model. Int Orthop 2014; 38(12): 2607-13.
       [http://dx.doi.org/10.1007/s00264-014-2499-3] [PMID: 25192687]

[102] Mehier-Humbert S, Bettinger T, Yan F, Guy RH. Ultrasound-mediated gene delivery: Kinetics of plasmid internalization and gene expression. J Control Release 2005; 104(1): 203-11.
       [http://dx.doi.org/10.1016/j.jconrel.2005.01.011] [PMID: 15866346]

[103] Feichtinger GA, Hofmann AT, Slezak P, *et al.* Sonoporation increases therapeutic efficacy of inducible and constitutive BMP2/7 *in vivo* gene delivery. Hum Gene Ther Methods 2014; 25(1): 57-71.

[http://dx.doi.org/10.1089/hgtb.2013.113] [PMID: 24164605]

[104] Osawa K, Okubo Y, Nakao K, Koyama N, Bessho K. Osteoinduction by microbubble-enhanced transcutaneous sonoporation of human bone morphogenetic protein-2 The Journal of Gene Medicine: A cross☐disciplinary journal for research on the science of gene transfer and its clinical applications 2009; 11(7): 633-41.
[http://dx.doi.org/10.1002/jgm.1331]

[105] Balmayor ER, van Griensven M. Gene therapy for bone engineering. Front Bioeng Biotechnol 2015; 3: 9.
[http://dx.doi.org/10.3389/fbioe.2015.00009] [PMID: 25699253]

[106] Gonçalves GAR, Paiva RMA. Gene therapy: advances, challenges and perspectives. Einstein (Sao Paulo) 2017; 15(3): 369-75.
[http://dx.doi.org/10.1590/s1679-45082017rb4024] [PMID: 29091160]

CHAPTER 13

Induced Pluripotent Stem Cells

Ambrin Fatima[1,*], Uzma Abdullah[2] and Zafar Ali[3]

[1] *Department of Biological and Biomedical Sciences, The Aga Khan University, Karachi, Pakistan*

[2] *University Institute of Biochemistry and Biotechnology, PMAS-Arid Agriculture University, Rawalpindi, Pakistan*

[3] *Centre for Biotechnology and Microbiology, University of Swat, Swat, Pakistan*

Abstract: A limiting factor for the identification of disease mechanisms and development of new therapies has been the access to a model system/s that can faithfully recapitulate key features of the disease and more precise clinical translations of new treatments. Stem cells in this regard are very promising, but the ethical issues related to totipotent embryonic stem cells and functional constraints to unipotent somatic stem cells have led to focus on induced pluripotent stem cells to avoid both functional and ethical constraints. The introduction of human Induced Pluripotent Stem Cell (iPSC) technology provides a model system to replicate diseases in humans. In this technology, human somatic cells can be "reprogrammed" by the transgene expression of four transcription factors into stem cells called iPSC. In this chapter, it will be discussed how iPSCs can be used for disease modelling, drug discovery and regenerative medicine.

Keywords: Disease modelling, Embryonic Stem Cells, Induced Pluripotent Stem Cells.

1. HUMAN EMBRYONIC STEM CELLS

A stem cell is defined by two key characteristics namely; self-renewability (unlimited potential to make copies of itself) and differentiability (give rise to almost any human cell type). Human embryonic stem cells (hESCs) are pluripotent stem cells derived from the inner cell mass of embryos (blastocyst stage 4–5 days post fertilization, at the stage of 50-150 cells) [1]. hESCs are mostly obtained from donors after they are deemed unsuitable for implantation and appropriate consent has been obtained. For the isolation of hESCs, the inner cell mass is separated from the trophectoderm and initially plated onto a layer of feeder cells (non-dividing cells that provide growth factors, adhesion molecules, and extracellular matrix) to form an hESC cell line [1, 2].

[*] **Corresponding author Ambrin Fatima**: Department of Biological and Biomedical Sciences, The Aga Khan University, Karachi, Pakistan; E-mail: ambrin.fatima@aku.edu

Syeda Marriam Bakhtiar and Erum Dilshad (Eds.)
All rights reserved-© 2022 Bentham Science Publishers

The first hESC line was developed by James Thomson in 1998, from the cells derived from surplus embryos after *in vitro* fertilization [3]. The hESCs are pluripotent, and under optimal laboratory conditions can be differentiated *in-vitro* into any cell type of the body. The pluripotency and unlimited capacity for self-renewal of hESCs have created a huge interest both in disease modelling and as possible tools for regenerative medicine (Fig. **13.1**). However, this excitement has been attenuated due to ethical and political considerations as well as few scientific limitations that have reduced the scientific progress in the field of hESCs.

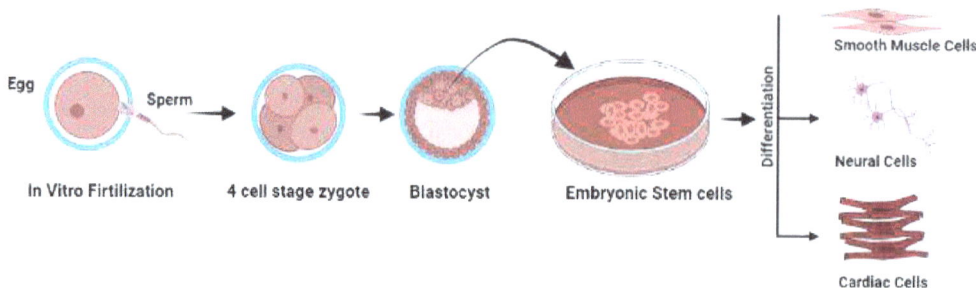

Fig. (13.1). General scheme of development of embryonic stem cell lines and their pluripotency.

New doors were opened with the development of methods for reprogramming somatic cells with properties akin to ESCs. These are called induced pluripotent stem cells (iPSCs). This technology has changed the prospects of the field of stem cell and regenerative medicine.

1.1. Human Induced Pluripotent Stem Cells: Origins and Properties

The modern work on iPSCs is built on the pioneering work of Sir John Gurdon [4] [5], a British developmental biologist, who showed programing of somatic nucleus to a pluripotent state through the process of somatic cell nuclear transfer. In 2006, two Japanese researchers Shinya Yamanaka and Kazutoshi Takahashi extended Goudon's work and attempted to generate mouse stem cells in the laboratory conditions. They achieved this by employing forced and transgenic expression of transcription factors (*i.e. Oct 3/4*, *Sox2*, *c-Myc* and *Klf4*) in murine dermal fibroblasts [6]. It was the first proof of concept and received with huge enthusiasm. The same process of generating human iPSCs (hiPSCs) was repeated in 2007, this time human fibroblasts were used for generating hiPSCs [7].

This time, through virus mediated over-expression of a human ortholog by using Yamanaka factors (OCT4, SOX2, KLF4 and c-MYC) (Fig. **13.2**), they were able to induce pluripotency in cultured dermal fibroblasts. The generated pluripotent stem cells which were highly analogous to human embryonic stem cells in terms of transcriptional activity, epigenetic patterns and morphology [7 - 9]. Therefore, these cells were termed as induced pluripotent stem cells (iPSC). In 2012, Shinya Yamanaka and John Gurdon received the Nobel Prize in physiology or medicine for their work of reprograming somatic cells into stems cells that are capable of differentiating into any cell of the body.

The iPSCs technology offers a substitute of accessible tissue types and thus enormous possibilities in research and therapeutics. However, it also has certain inherent challenges, such as all cells do not complete this forced reprogramming journey, some remain in a partially reprogrammed state. Moreover, the stressful reprogramming process, involving the increased expression of oncogenes like KLF-4 and c-MYC, can introduce gene chromosomal anomalies. Therefore, reprogrammed iPSCs are subsequently screened for morphology, pluripotency, chromosomal stability, genetic aberrations and differentiation potential [9].

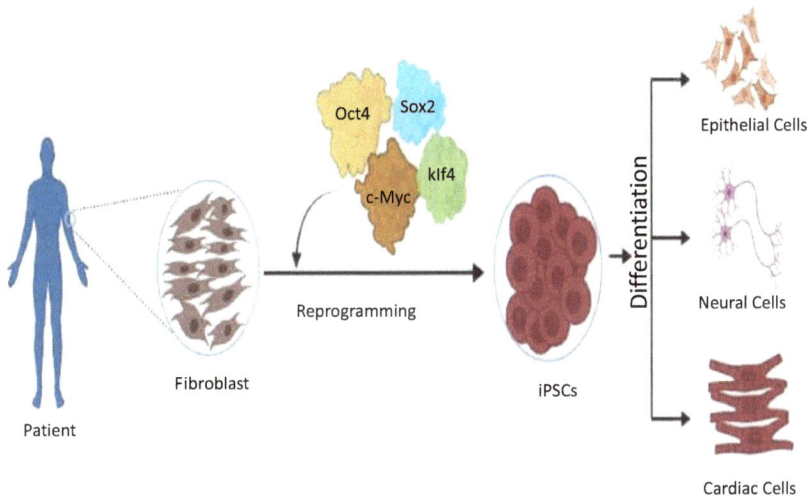

Fig. (13.2). A schematic representation of the human iPSC generation from patient fibroblast by introduction of cocktail of reprogramming factors, such as (OCT4, SOX2, KLF4, and C-MYC) and pluripotency of generated iPSCs.

1.2. Applications of Induced Pluripotent Stem Cells

Surpassing initial expectations, 15 years since discovery, iPSCs have revolutionized biology and proved an invaluable tool for disease modelling, developmental biology, regenerative medicine and drug discovery and has proven its universality for cellular reprogramming in different somatic cells.

1.3. Disease modelling

The recapitulation of human disease in animals to study pathophysiology and therapeutics testing has traditionally relied heavily on model animals such as mice and Zebrafish. Due to a relatively short generation time and large number of offsprings, evolutionary conversion of mammalian genomes has made these an indispensable tool to explore the underlying disease mechanisms. However, despite the high degree of conversion, human's divergence from model organisms can be placed in millions of years apart (96 and 450 million years for rodents and Zebrafish respectively) [10]. Consequently, it is not surprising to see differences in the phenotypes and response between human and model organisms [11, 12] that limit the scope and reliability of the findings.

Therefore, a bottleneck for the analysis of disease mechanisms in several genetic disease especially neurological disorders has been the access to biological materials as well as appropriate model systems that can faithfully recapitulate pathophysiology of human diseases. Cancer cell lines derived from humans (Hela, HeK293) have also been used *in-vitro* for decades to study human diseases. These cell lines acquired chromosomal and other genetic anomalies due to high passage number over the time and thus no longer are true representative of disease underpinnings [13].

The human iPSCs provide unprecedented opportunities of modelling human diseases *in-vivo* and circumvent the limitations of other disease models described above. Reprogramming patient somatic cells into iPSCs retains the genetic signature of patients and subsequent differentiation on iPSCs in disease specific cell types allows scientists to model patient's altered pathophysiology in a petri dish thus called disease in a dish (Fig. **13.3**).

Reprogramming cells from a patient into a pluripotent form followed by differentiation into disease specific cell types can generate an unlimited source of human tissues carrying the genetic variations that caused or facilitated disease development [14]. Human iPSCs have been generated for modelling of a wide range of genetic disorders both monogenic, complex disorders [15, 16] as well as acquired disorders (*e.g.* myeloproliferative neoplasms and myelodysplastic syndromes) [17, 18]. Furthermore, the possibility of genomic editing through CRISPR/Cas9 further broadens its scope and enables to induce or rescue mechanisms in isogenic (having the same or closely similar genotypes) iPSCs. It has thus dramatically improved our capability of determining the molecular and cellular perturbations underlying the disease. Employing such multi-disciplinary approaches have unravelled novel players in the pathogenesis of several previously poorly managed disorders such as, Rett's syndrome, Fragile X syndrome, Down syndrome, Dravet syndrome, ataxia, autism spectrum disorder, schizophrenia, ALS, Alzheimer's disease, cardiovascular disorders [19 - 21].

Modelling genetic disorders requires selection of an appropriate differentiation method to generate cell types representative of the developmental stage or onset for the phenotype being investigated. A couple of differentiation protocols and their rationale have been illustrated below.

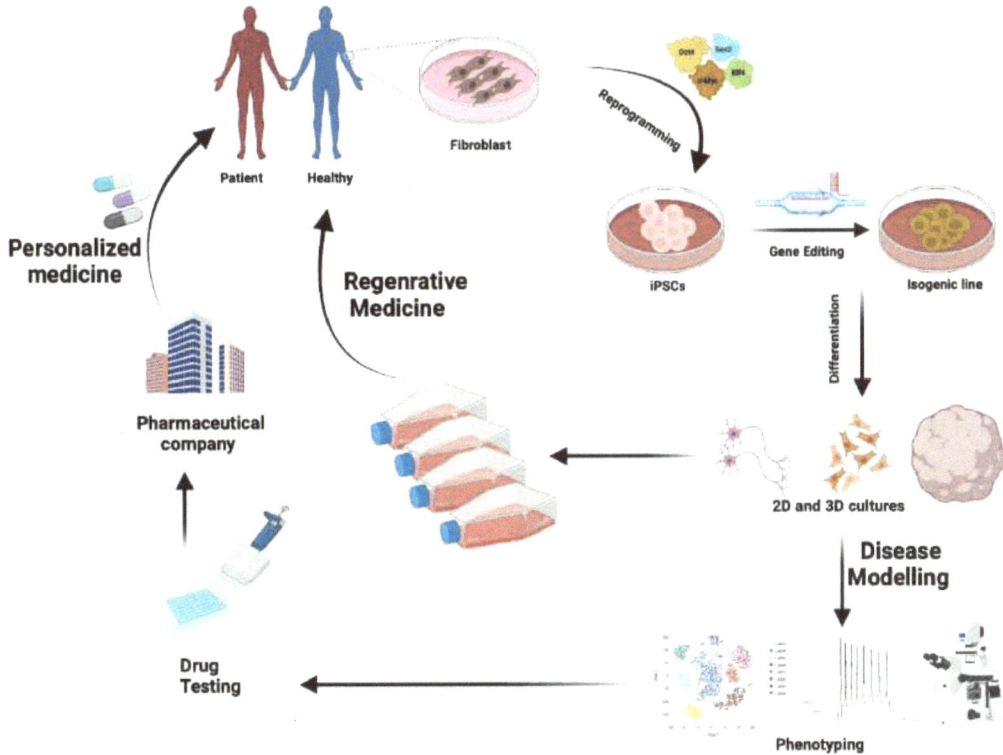

Fig. (13.3). Applications of iPSCs in disease modelling, drug discovery/ personalized medicine and regenerative medicine.

1.4. Embryoid Bodies: An *in vitro* Model of Embryogenesis

Pluripotent stem cells, when differentiate spontaneously, form self-organizing aggregates called embryoid bodies (EBs). These are constituted by descendants of the three embryonic germ layers [22]. Under the local activation of the Wnt pathway, these EBs establish anteroposterior polarity and form a primitive streak-like region. The cells in this region undergo EMT and form mesoendodermal precursors. Conversely, neuroectodermal differentiation is derived by inhibition of the Wnt signalling along the anterior axis [23]. Therefore, EBs recapitulate early gastrulation events making them a powerful tool to study early embryonic developmental programs *in vitro*. In combination with molecular tools for genetic editing, labelling and cell sorting, EBs offer an accessible model to test gene function during development and differentiation [24].

1.5. 2D Models

Initially, most of the disease modelling studies through iPSC used a conventional 2D monolayer culture platform. In a 2D model, iPSCs are plated directly on a polystyrene or glass (coated with substrates that mimic ECM composition) and subsequently differentiated into cell type of interest. Because iPSCs can be differentiated into disease-relevant cells and can faithfully replicate pathomechanism of the patients. 2D iPSC models have been widely employed in dissecting the functional underpinnings of monogenic as well as polygenic diseases of different organs [21, 25, 26].

Conventional 2D iPSCs cultures provide reproducible and relatively cost-effective tools to model human disorders and developmental processes. Despite the incontestable importance of 2D models, they however do not mimic the more complex organization and heterotypic setting in which the cells generally reside *in vivo*. For example, in the human heart, only about 30% of the total cells represent cardiomyocytes, the remaining 70% consist of non-myocytes, such as endothelial cells, vascular smooth muscle cells, fibroblasts, leukocytes, and various extracellular matrix components [27]. Thus, essential queries regarding the actual complex 3D status remain unresolved, specifically those related to non-cell autonomous pathogenesis and structurally related disease phenotype [28]. These limitations led to efforts to create more complex 3D models.

1.6. 3D Models (Examples)

Organoids are 3D cultures maintained *in vitro* that can be derived directly from the primary tissue or differentiated from embryonic or induced human pluripotent stem cells (hPS cells). Because of the greater diversity of cell composition, the lack of cellular interactions with artificial plastic substrates, and the undirected formation of complex 3D structures seen in the developing brain, organoids resembling neural tissue have the potential to create more realistic cellular environments for modelling the cell biology of the nervous system. The development of human brain organoids is relatively straight forward and starts from differentiating human pluripotent stem cells into embryoid bodies that are subsequently directed towards neuroectodermal lineage. The developmental precursors, once developed in cell aggregates, proceed spontaneously towards brain tissue patterning and develop brain organoid.

Other organoids, however, are more complex to develop. For example, for liver primordia, hepatocyte precursors (hepatoblasts) only cannot differentiate into diverse lineages of endothelial, mesenchymal cells. However, mixture of these with hepatoblasts would assemble *in vitro* and acquire the architecture that mimics a developing human liver primordium.

The protocols get more complex when developing other organoids, for example for endoderm-derived organs (such as intestine, stomach or lungs), stepwise protocol mimicking the fetal development is required. It involves modulating different signaling mechanisms though the combination of morphogens and/or inhibitors in precise timings and concentrations, that thus lead to desired epithelial tissue in a required architecture. Media formulations and culture matrix and are also optimized to aid the cells in achieving terminal differentiation into desired cell types [29, 30].

1.7. Drug Testing and Personalized Medicine

Drug discovery is an arduous and expensive process. On average, more than $1.8 billion and almost a decade are required from the discovery to the commercial launch of a new drug [31]. Previous attempts of drug discovery relied heavily on mice and other model organisms that differ from human in genetics, anatomy, and physiology thus do not faithfully recapitulate the disease physiology leading to overall low success rate of drugs during clinical development [32]. An alternate option to overcome the challenges of animal models has been the use of primary cells from humans, however, the limited access, genetic background, ethical concerns and their limited expansion capacity make them unsuitable for high-throughput drug screening [33].

The opportunity to generate disease-specific iPSCs derived diverse cell types offers a suitable model for high-throughput drug screenings in clinically relevant human cell types thus helping to better understand pharmacogenomics and hence accelerate drug discovery [34].

One of the first iPSCs based drug screening was carried out in neuronal cultures derived from patients with Rett syndrome [35] (followed by more studies using iPSCs derived cell lineages [16, 36].

These studies demonstrate the exceptional potential of iPSC technology in personalized medicine to predict patient outcomes they may allow the use of tailored drugs according to patients' genetic and epigenetic background [37].

1.8. Stem Cell Therapy and Regenerative Medicine

Conventionally, cell therapy was restricted to blood stem cells and bone marrow until the recent advancement in pluripotent stem cell technology to have the ability to produce clinically relevant cell types which is a fast-developing field in regenerative medicine. A big plus of using iPSCs derived cells over conventional therapies is the possibility of patient derived autologous cells therapies. One of the major advantages of iPSCs base autologous cell therapies is that these are tolerated by immune system and overcome the side effects from immunosuppression and immune rejection caused by allogeneic transplantation. The discovery of iPSC-based technology offers a promising cell source for autologous cell transplantation for various degenerative diseases without side effects from immunosuppression and allograft rejection.

One of the bottlenecks in the use of iPSCs is the high cost associated with generation and validation of these cells. Generation and validation of a research grade iPSC line requires 6-9 months and $10,000–$25,000 respectively. The cost elevates to approximately US $800,00 for generation and validation of a clinical grade iPSC line [9, 33]. Therefore, many researcher are working on the identification and banking of high-quality iPSCs donor lines (called super doner) those can be close immunological match to a huge proportion of the population. These donor lines with matched major human leukocyte antigen (HLA) markers reduce the cost and thus maximize the utility and efficiency of an iPSCs line. In Japan, it has been proposed that 50 HLA homozygous super donor lines could match over 90% of the Japanese population [38]. Similarly, the generation of iPSCs line from150 HLA homozygous donors could match approximately 93% of the UK population [39].

Despite obvious potential of these HLA-matched iPSC lines, none (even for perfectly matched major HLAs) has yet made the way to human trials due the possibility that minor antigens could cause rejection. Even the autologous iPSC-derived transplants have raised concerns due to the observation of immunogenic teratoma formation in the transplantation of mouse iPSCs into syngeneic rodents [40]. The recent development of the CRISPR/Cas9 system has enhanced the feasibility of HLA-edited iPSCs.

Further rodent trials, including a mouse model reconstituting human immune system, produced contradictory findings. Some of these found autologous transplants to be immune tolerant, while others found a substantial immune response for some types of iPSC-derived cells. Thus, it is speculated that an autologous immune response may be caused by an aberrant antigen expression induced by differentiation *in vitro* and might be cell-type specific. The aberrant antigen expression has been observed in iPSC-derived smooth muscle cells but not in iPSC-derived retinal pigment cells. Therefore, even for autologous transplantation, preclinical studies could benefit from the potential immune response analysis [41, 42]. In the future, the generation of CRISPR edited universal iPSCs and cell specific preclinical trials can rapidly advance the clinical application of regenerative medicine-based therapies and can contribute greatly to medical care.

Besides these immunological aspects, iPSCs derived cells carry an inherent challenge of precise delivery of the cell product to the region of interest. Cells must be precisely integrated both physically and electrically to provide meaningful improvements and avoid potentially detrimental side effects.

1.9. CHALLENGES TO IPSC-BASED DISEASE MODELLING AND DRUG DISCOVERY/CONCLUSION

The technology of iPSC offers countless new possibilities but several challenges must be overcome before many of these could be materialized, especially in the field of drug screening and pathway discovery. For example, a fundamental concern is the faithfulness of recapitulation of phenotypes *in vitro* and accuracy of them to predict disease behavior in vivo. Despite considerable success in recapitulating certain clinical features of familial dysautonomia, Spinal Muscular Atrophy (SMA) and Rett syndrome in iPSC-derived neural cells, it is lagging behind in other disorders such as Parkinson's disease [33]. This limitation is attributed to three main factors; the disease onset in patients, the cell- autonomous nature of the disorder and the complexity of the causative genetic mutation. For example, the above-mentioned disorders are manifested early in life, may have a strong cell-autonomous component and are caused by single genes mutations, whereas Parkinson's disease generally occurs later in life and is complex in nature caused by both environmental and genetic factors. However, it is still a point of active research which of these three factors most strongly influence our ability to recapitulate a phenotype *in vitro* [43].

CONSENT FOR PUBLICATION

Not applicable.

CONFLICT OF INTEREST

The author declares no conflict of interest, financial or otherwise.

ACKNOWLEDGEMENTS

Declared none.

REFERENCES

[1]   Evans MJ, Kaufman MH. Establishment in culture of pluripotential cells from mouse embryos. Nature 1981; 292(5819): 154-6.
        [http://dx.doi.org/10.1038/292154a0] [PMID: 7242681]

[2]   Martin GR. Isolation of a pluripotent cell line from early mouse embryos cultured in medium conditioned by teratocarcinoma stem cells. Proc Natl Acad Sci USA 1981; 78(12): 7634-8.
        [http://dx.doi.org/10.1073/pnas.78.12.7634]

[3]   Thomson JA, Itskovitz-Eldor J, Shapiro SS, *et al*. Embryonic stem cell lines derived from human blastocysts. Science 1998; 282(5391): 1145-7.
        [http://dx.doi.org/10.1126/science.282.5391.1145] [PMID: 9804556]

[4]   Gurdon J B. The Developmental Capacity of Nuclei taken from Intestinal Epithelium Cells of Feeding Tadpoles. J Embryol Exp Morphol 1962; 10: 622-40.
        [http://dx.doi.org/10.1242/dev.10.4.622]

[5]   Gurdon JB, Laskey RA, Reeves OR. The developmental capacity of nuclei transplanted from keratinized skin cells of adult frogs. Development 1975; 34(1): 93-112.
        [http://dx.doi.org/10.1242/dev.34.1.93] [PMID: 1102625]

[6]   Takahashi K, Yamanaka S. Induction of pluripotent stem cells from mouse embryonic and adult fibroblast cultures by defined factors. Cell 2006; 126(4): 663-76.
        [http://dx.doi.org/10.1016/j.cell.2006.07.024] [PMID: 16904174]

[7]   Takahashi K, Tanabe K, Ohnuki M, *et al*. Induction of pluripotent stem cells from adult human fibroblasts by defined factors. Cell 2007; 131(5): 861-72.
        [http://dx.doi.org/10.1016/j.cell.2007.11.019] [PMID: 18035408]

[8]   Maherali N, Sridharan R, Xie W, *et al*. Directly reprogrammed fibroblasts show global epigenetic remodeling and widespread tissue contribution. Cell Stem Cell 2007; 1(1): 55-70.
        [http://dx.doi.org/10.1016/j.stem.2007.05.014] [PMID: 18371336]

[9]   Stadtfeld M, Hochedlinger K. Induced pluripotency: history, mechanisms, and applications. Genes Dev 2010; 24(20): 2239-63.
        [http://dx.doi.org/10.1101/gad.1963910] [PMID: 20952534]

[10]   Kumar S, Hedges SB. A molecular timescale for vertebrate evolution. Nature 1998; 392(6679): 917-20.
        [http://dx.doi.org/10.1038/31927] [PMID: 9582070]

[11]   Bracken MB. Why animal studies are often poor predictors of human reactions to exposure. J R Soc Med 2009; 102(3): 120-2.
        [http://dx.doi.org/10.1258/jrsm.2008.08k033] [PMID: 19297654]

[12]   Perlman RL. Mouse models of human disease: An evolutionary perspective. Evol Med Public Health 2016; 2016(1): eow014.
        [http://dx.doi.org/10.1093/emph/eow014] [PMID: 27121451]

[13]   Wilding JL, Bodmer WF. Cancer cell lines for drug discovery and development. Cancer Res 2014; 74(9): 2377-84.
        [http://dx.doi.org/10.1158/0008-5472.CAN-13-2971] [PMID: 24717177]

[14]   Soldner F, Jaenisch R. Medicine. iPSC disease modeling. Science 2012; 338(6111): 1155-6.
        [http://dx.doi.org/10.1126/science.1227682] [PMID: 23197518]

[15]   Spitalieri P, Talarico VR, Murdocca M, Novelli G, Sangiuolo F. Human induced pluripotent stem cells

for monogenic disease modelling and therapy. World J Stem Cells 2016; 8(4): 118-35.
[http://dx.doi.org/10.4252/wjsc.v8.i4.118] [PMID: 27114745]

[16]   Avior Y, Sagi I, Benvenisty N. Pluripotent stem cells in disease modelling and drug discovery. Nat Rev Mol Cell Biol 2016; 17(3): 170-82.
[http://dx.doi.org/10.1038/nrm.2015.27] [PMID: 26818440]

[17]   Arai S, Miyauchi M, Kurokawa M. Modeling of hematologic malignancies by iPS technology. Exp Hematol 2015; 43(8): 654-60.
[http://dx.doi.org/10.1016/j.exphem.2015.06.006] [PMID: 26135030]

[18]   Kotini AG, Chang CJ, Chow A, *et al.* Stage-Specific Human Induced Pluripotent Stem Cells Map the Progression of Myeloid Transformation to Transplantable Leukemia. Cell Stem Cell 2017; 20(3): 315-328.e7.
[http://dx.doi.org/10.1016/j.stem.2017.01.009] [PMID: 28215825]

[19]   Boland MJ, Nazor KL, Tran HT, *et al.* Molecular analyses of neurogenic defects in a human pluripotent stem cell model of fragile X syndrome. Brain 2017; 140(3): aww357.
[http://dx.doi.org/10.1093/brain/aww357] [PMID: 28137726]

[20]   Xie N, Gong H, Suhl JA, Chopra P, Wang T, Warren ST. Reactivation of FMR1 by CRISPR/Cas9-mediated deletion of the expanded CGG-repeat of the fragile X chromosome. PLoS One 2016; 11(10): e0165499.
[http://dx.doi.org/10.1371/journal.pone.0165499] [PMID: 27768763]

[21]   Yagi T, Ito D, Okada Y, *et al.* Modeling familial Alzheimer's disease with induced pluripotent stem cells. Hum Mol Genet 2011; 20(23): 4530-9.
[http://dx.doi.org/10.1093/hmg/ddr394] [PMID: 21900357]

[22]   Itskovitz-Eldor J, Schuldiner M, Karsenti D, *et al.* Differentiation of human embryonic stem cells into embryoid bodies compromising the three embryonic germ layers. Mol Med 2000; 6(2): 88-95.
[http://dx.doi.org/10.1007/BF03401776] [PMID: 10859025]

[23]   ten Berge D, Koole W, Fuerer C, Fish M, Eroglu E, Nusse R. Wnt signaling mediates self-organization and axis formation in embryoid bodies. Cell Stem Cell 2008; 3(5): 508-18.
[http://dx.doi.org/10.1016/j.stem.2008.09.013] [PMID: 18983966]

[24]   Brickman JM, Serup P. Properties of embryoid bodies. Wiley Interdiscip Rev Dev Biol 2017; 6(2): 1-11.
[http://dx.doi.org/10.1002/wdev.259] [PMID: 27911036]

[25]   Matsa E, Ahrens JH, Wu JC. Human induced pluripotent stem cells as a platform for personalized and precision cardiovascular medicine. Physiol Rev 2016; 96(3): 1093-126.
[http://dx.doi.org/10.1152/physrev.00036.2015] [PMID: 27335446]

[26]   Firth AL, *et al.* HHS Public Access 2015; 12(9): 1385-90.
[http://dx.doi.org/10.1016/j.celrep.2015.07.062.Functional]

[27]   Pinto AR, Ilinykh A, Ivey MJ, *et al.* Revisiting Cardiac Cellular Composition. Circ Res 2016; 118(3): 400-9.
[http://dx.doi.org/10.1161/CIRCRESAHA.115.307778] [PMID: 26635390]

[28]   Liu C, Oikonomopoulos A, Sayed N, Wu JC. Modeling human diseases with induced pluripotent stem cells: from 2D to 3D and beyond. Development 2018; 145(5): dev156166.
[http://dx.doi.org/10.1242/dev.156166] [PMID: 29519889]

[29]   Passier R, Orlova V, Mummery C. Complex Tissue and Disease Modeling using hiPSCs. Cell Stem Cell 2016; 18(3): 309-21.
[http://dx.doi.org/10.1016/j.stem.2016.02.011] [PMID: 26942851]

[30]   Kim J, Koo BK, Knoblich JA. Human organoids: model systems for human biology and medicine. Nat Rev Mol Cell Biol 2020; 21(10): 571-84.
[http://dx.doi.org/10.1038/s41580-020-0259-3] [PMID: 32636524]

[31] Mohs RC, Greig NH. Drug discovery and development: Role of basic biological research. Alzheimers Dement (N Y) 2017; 3(4): 651-7.
[http://dx.doi.org/10.1016/j.trci.2017.10.005] [PMID: 29255791]

[32] Philippakis AA, Azzariti DR, Beltran S, *et al.* The Matchmaker Exchange: a platform for rare disease gene discovery. Hum Mutat 2015; 36(10): 915-21.
[http://dx.doi.org/10.1002/humu.22858] [PMID: 26295439]

[33] Doss MX, Sachinidis A. Current Challenges of iPSC-Based Disease Modeling and Therapeutic Implications. Cells 2019; 8(5): 403.
[http://dx.doi.org/10.3390/cells8050403] [PMID: 31052294]

[34] Ebert AD, Liang P, Wu JC. Induced pluripotent stem cells as a disease modeling and drug screening platform. J Cardiovasc Pharmacol 2012; 60(4): 408-16.
[http://dx.doi.org/10.1097/FJC.0b013e318247f642] [PMID: 22240913]

[35] Marchetto MCN, Carromeu C, Acab A, *et al.* A model for neural development and treatment of Rett syndrome using human induced pluripotent stem cells. Cell 2010; 143(4): 527-39.
[http://dx.doi.org/10.1016/j.cell.2010.10.016] [PMID: 21074045]

[36] Chang CJ, Kotini AG, Olszewska M, *et al.* Dissecting the Contributions of Cooperating Gene Mutations to Cancer Phenotypes and Drug Responses with Patient-Derived iPSCs. Stem Cell Reports 2018; 10(5): 1610-24.
[http://dx.doi.org/10.1016/j.stemcr.2018.03.020] [PMID: 29681544]

[37] Sayed N, Liu C, Wu JC. Translation of Human-Induced Pluripotent Stem Cells. J Am Coll Cardiol 2016; 67(18): 2161-76.
[http://dx.doi.org/10.1016/j.jacc.2016.01.083] [PMID: 27151349]

[38] Nakatsuji N, Nakajima F, Tokunaga K. HLA-haplotype banking and iPS cells. Nat Biotechnol 2008; 26(7): 739-40.
[http://dx.doi.org/10.1038/nbt0708-739] [PMID: 18612291]

[39] Taylor CJ, Peacock S, Chaudhry AN, Bradley JA, Bolton EM. Generating an iPSC bank for HLA-matched tissue transplantation based on known donor and recipient HLA types. Cell Stem Cell 2012; 11(2): 147-52.
[http://dx.doi.org/10.1016/j.stem.2012.07.014] [PMID: 22862941]

[40] Zhao T, Zhang ZN, Rong Z, Xu Y. Immunogenicity of induced pluripotent stem cells. Nature 2011; 474(7350): 212-5.
[http://dx.doi.org/10.1038/nature10135] [PMID: 21572395]

[41] Zhao T, Zhang Z, Westenskow PD, *et al.* Humanized Mice Reveal Differential Immunogenicity of Cells Derived from Autologous Induced Pluripotent Stem Cells. Cell Stem Cell 2015; 17(3): 353-9.
[http://dx.doi.org/10.1016/j.stem.2015.07.021] [PMID: 26299572]

[42] Araki R, Uda M, Hoki Y, *et al.* Negligible immunogenicity of terminally differentiated cells derived from induced pluripotent or embryonic stem cells. Nature 2013; 494(7435): 100-4.
[http://dx.doi.org/10.1038/nature11807] [PMID: 23302801]

[43] Wu SM, Hochedlinger K. Harnessing the potential of induced pluripotent stem cells for regenerative medicine. Nat Cell Biol 2011; 13(5): 497-505.
[http://dx.doi.org/10.1038/ncb0511-497] [PMID: 21540845]

CHAPTER 14

Hemoglobinopathies

Mahnoor Asif[1], Sadia Nawaz[2,*] and Muhammad Tariq[1]

[1] *National Institute for Biotechnology and Genetic Engineering College, Pakistan Institute of Engineering and Applied Sciences (NIBGE-C, PIEAS), Faisalabad, Pakistan*

[2] *Institute of Biochemistry and Biotechnology, University of Veterinary and Animal Sciences-UVAS, Lahore-54000, Pakistan*

Abstract: Hemoglobinopathies are a group of inherited blood disorders characterized by compromised hemoglobin function. Hemoglobin is a 64kDa protein, consisting of four globin polypeptides each containing one heme molecule; blood acquires its red color from this heme molecule. Two of the four polypeptide chains are α-globin chains, whereas the other two are β and γ chains during adult and fetal life, respectively. Hemoglobin carries oxygen to respiring cells and tissues in vertebrates and defects in genes encoding this protein result in a variety of disorders, ranging from mild asymptomatic to severe fatal phenotypes. This chapter reviews various hemoglobinopathies underlying mutations in globin genes. We also provide a brief note of the traditional and contemporary diagnostic approaches and screening, both prenatal and postnatal, with a specific focus on recent advances in this regard. We have summarized various therapeutic strategies, from transfusion and iron chelation to CRISPR-driven genome editing aimed at reactivating fetal hemoglobin in adults. The chapter concludes with a brief account of the future challenges and prospects for developing a therapy for hemoglobinopathies a clinical reality.

Keywords: CVS, Hemoglobin, Hemoglobinopathies, Sickle cell anemia, Thalassemia.

1. INTRODUCTION

In 1840, Friedrich Ludwig Hünefeld accidentally discovered what he referred to as plate-like crystals in the dried blood of humans or pigs [1]. Later, Hoppe-Seyler named these crystals Hemoglobin (Hb) [2]; soon afterwards, Claude Bernard recognized them as oxygen-carrying molecules [3]. The discovery of the detailed 3-D structure of this molecule by X-ray crystallography took more than 100 years [4]. For this long-awaited discovery, Max Perutz, along with Sir John Kendrew, won the 1962 Nobel Prize in chemistry. A hemoglobin molecule consists of four

---

[*] **Corresponding author Sadia Nawaz**: Institute of Biochemistry and Biotechnology, University of Veterinary and Animal Sciences-UVAS, Lahore, Pakistan; E-mails: sadia.nawaz@uvas.edu.pk and shamiryar@hotmail.com

Syeda Marriam Bakhtiar and Erum Dilshad (Eds.)

polypeptide chains, two alpha (α) chains, each comprising 141 residues and two beta (β) chains, each containing 146 amino acids. A polypeptide chain combined with a heme constitutes a monomer or a subunit of hemoglobin. The complete molecules consists of four subunits, closely joined as in a 3D jigsaw puzzle, forming a tetramer [5]. The structure of hemoglobin is strictly conserved to maintain the affinity of Hb-O_2 [6]; aberrations during the synthesis of α or β chains result in hemoglobinopathies, a family of autosomal blood disorders, inherited in recessive fashion. Thalassemia is highly prevalent in Far East, India and in the Mediterranean areas, whereas Sickle Cell Disease (SCD) is prevalent in sub-Saharan Africa [7].

Their spread across different parts of the world, especially in the US and Europe is largely the result of migration. Globally, hemoglobinopathies have one of the highest incidences among monogenic disorders, with ~5% people carrying a disease allele. Some of the hemoglobin variants cause disease only in certain circumstances or under stress, while other variants are highly penetrant [8, 9].

1.1. Structure and Genetics of Hemoglobin Synthesis

Hemoglobin is a 64-64.5 kDa protein, carries oxygen to respirating cells and tissues, in all vertebrates except Channichthyidae [10]. Human hemoglobin consists of four globin (peptide) chains, each containing one heme molecule; blood acquires its red color from this heme molecule (Fig. **14.1**). Heme molecule is a porphyrin ring of carbon, hydrogen and nitrogen, containing an iron atom in the center like a jewel. The globin chains are produced differentially during ontogenesis; hence, these are different at various stages of life *i.e.*, embryonic, fetal and adult [11]. The adult hemoglobin molecule (HbA) has two β- and two α-globin chains whereas the predominant hemoglobin during fetal life is HbF containing two gamma (γ) globulin chains instead of β chains.

The switching of Hb F to Hb A takes place within 30 to 40 weeks of conception [12] and the transition is completed by six months postnatal life, with around 1% Hb F, $\leq$ 3% Hb A2 ($\alpha2\delta2$) and 97% Hb A ($\alpha2\beta2$) in a normal adult [13]. This switching between different hemoglobin reflects the physiological adaptation according to differing oxygen requirements during ontogenesis [12].

Globin genes are located on chromosome 11 and 16 in two remarkably conserved clusters (Fig. **14.2**). Alpha gene cluster is located on 16p13.3 whereas beta gene cluster is present on 11p15.4 [14, 15]. The mechanism underlying the expression regulation of these globin genes is not completely understood, but it is seen that at the 8th week of embryonic development, the two chains epsilon (ε) and zeta (ζ) are switched off in definitive cells and cannot be reactivated. Gamma (γ) genes undergo independent silencing, analogous to ε gene with some degree of competition, by modification in relative transcription, between β- and γ-globin genes. This relative transcription changes during development, with balance shifting from the expression of γ-globin in the fetus to β-globin gene in adults [12]. More than 1000 hemoglobinopathies have already been reported, most of which are asymptomatic. The most clinically relevant of these are SCD, Thalassemias, Erythrocytosis, Cyanosis, and Hemolytic anemias [16]. Thalassemia (208 million patients including ~4.7 million severely affected [17] and SCD (with around 3.2 million homozygous and 46 million heterozygous patients) [16] are the most common hemoglobinopathies.

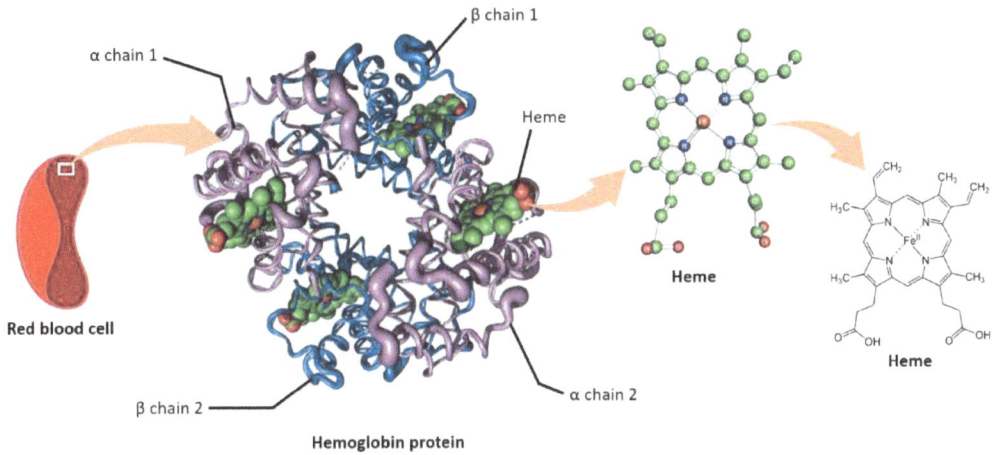

Fig. (14.1). Structure of Hemoglobin Molecule.

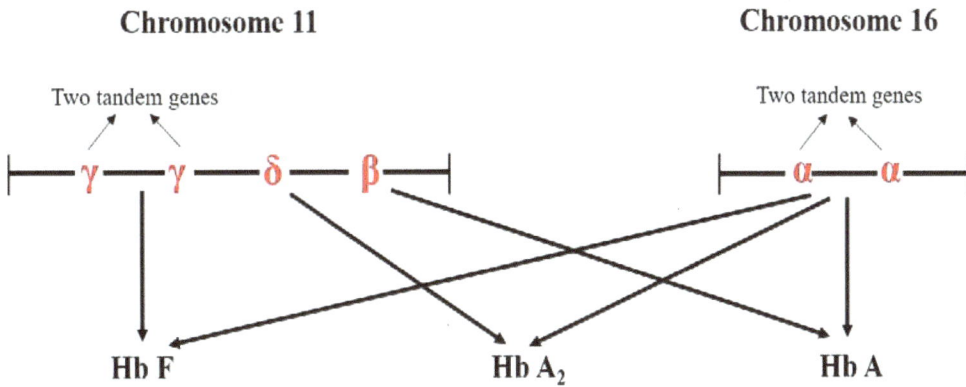

Fig. (14.2). Normal adult hemoglobin.

1.2. α-, β-, γ- and δ-Thalassemia and Related Conditions

Pathophysiology of thalassemia is rooted in the unstable synthesis of Hb that results from compromised expression of one of the main globin chains *i.e.*, α, β, γ, ε and δ [18].

α-thalassemia, underlying>100 genetic defects, results from reduced synthesis of the α chains. The severity of α-thalassemia is linked with mutations in one (α⁺) or both (α°) the α genes [19]. People with heterozygous α⁺ defects are silent carriers. Whereas, α-thalassemia minor underlies either α⁺ defects or α° defects. Abnormalities in 3 out of 4 α globin chains result in the excess of β chain tetramers (Hb H) or, at the fetal stage, γ chains (Bart's Hb), which is fatal because the absence of αglobin chains affects the oxygen transport [18, 19].

β-thalassemias is caused by defects in β-globin synthesis due to mutation(s) in the corresponding gene (>900 mutations reported to date). The disease is recessively inherited, and therefore heterozygous individuals are either asymptomatic carriers or, if they are anemic at all, the symptoms are mild or moderate (thalassemia minor); homozygous individuals develop more complex phenotypes; severely affected individuals require regular transfusion (thalassemia major) whereas those with mild disease symptoms do not require any transfusion (thalassemia intermedia). An elevated HbA2 level in heterozygous individuals present in most of the β⁺ and β° thalassemia, is the diagnostic characteristic of β-thalassemia. Heterozygous individuals with normal HbA2 levels rarely develop disease symptoms [20 - 22].

δ-thalassemia is of little therapeutic relevance except in connection with the diagnosis of the β-thalassemia, since the inheritance of δ-thalassemia, caused by impaired A2 synthesis, in *cis* or *trans* to β-thalassemia means that hemoglobin A2 may not be elevated and heterozygosity can be skipped in the diagnosis of β-thalassemia [23]. Both δ⁺ and δ° mutations exist [24].

γ-thalassemia occurs due to reduced synthesis of γchain and eventually of HbF. During late gestation, this condition is maximally manifested and, as there are usually four γ genes, clinical consequences are likely to be mild.

1.3. Sickle Cell Hemoglobin

Sickle cell anemia is marked by the presence of an abnormal hemoglobin known as hemoglobin S (HbS). HbS comprises two wild types α- and two mutant β-globin chains. An A to T substitution at the codon 6 of the β-globin changes the amino acid valine (hydrophobic) to glutamic acid (hydrophilic); this results in the formation of HbS. This substitution facilitates non-covalent polymerization (aggregation) of hemoglobin under hypoxic conditions, altering the structure and elasticity of RBCs. When oxygen pressure is restored to its normal tension, the cells are still unable to resume their native shape and, instead, undergo hemolysis; chronic damage causes hemolytic anemia. This damage is offset increased RBC production [25] and blood transfusions; this results in the induction of iron deposition and related pathological changes [26] such as sudden decrease in hematocrit (so-called aplastic crisis).

1.4. Other Hemoglobinopathies

Some variants of hemoglobin show symptoms only in certain situations or under unusual stress. Recognition of these clinically silent variants is important because their presence can blur the diagnosis.

Hemoglobin E/thalassemia has a high incidence in Bangladesh, India and Southeast Asia. The disease was previously rare in North America and Europe; however, it is now the most prevalent type of β-thalassemia in this part of the world. The disease is clinically heterogeneous with some patients presented with moderate asymptomatic anemia and others with a life-threatening severe disease requiring regular blood transfusions from early childhood [27].

Hemoglobin S/thalassemia is commonly found in Africa and Mediterranean region. Co-inheritance of these two defects is reported to lower the Mean Corpuscular Volume (MCV) and Mean Corpuscular Hemoglobin (MCH), resulting in mild type of anemia. It results in reduced hemolysis and increased total hemoglobin, rendering patients more vulnerable to vaso-occlusive and painful crises [28].

Hemoglobin C/thalassemia, too, is widespread in African and Mediterranean region. HB C, alone, usually causes moderate anemia, often asymptomatic. Hemoglobin C/β° thalassemia, however, usually causes relatively severe hemolytic anemia with enlarged spleen; hemoglobin C/β⁺ thalassemia results in milder clinical phenotype [29].

Hemoglobin D/thalassemia is commonly diagnosed in the Punjab region of India and Pakistan. It is asymptomatic in homozygous form. Hb D/β-thalassemia co-inheritance can result in mild anemia with or without mild splenomegaly, whereas patients co-segregating Hb D/ α-thalassemia usually exhibit higher Hb levels [30].

Hemoglobin O/thalassemia has been reported in Arabian Peninsula, Turkey, Bulgaria, Italy, Hungary and among Afro-Caribbean population. Homozygous individuals may be phenotypically normal with compensated hemolysis or may have recurrent jaundice anemia and splenomegaly [31].

Hb Kansas was initially reported in early 1960s as an Hb variant with a very low oxygen affinity. The disease results from an AAC to ACC change, with a resultant substitution of threonine for an asparagine at amino acid position 102 of the β-globin protein. The binding between asparagine at β102 and aspartic acid at α94, which is compromised by the mutations, is necessary for high oxygen affinity. These patients do not required any treatment because, apart from cyanosis, they remain asymptomatic [32].

2. MOLECULAR DIAGNOSIS OF HEMOGLOBINOPATHIES

Hemoglobinopathies serve as a model for molecular diagnosis of genetic disorders since these are the earliest genetic anomalies which were studied, and understood, extensively at molecular level. Therefore, there is a spectrum of PCR-based techniques used for mutation detection in globin genes; qPCR (quantitative PCR), oligonucleotide-specific amplification, oligonucleotide-specific hybridization, oligonucleotide-specific ligation, gap-PCR and restriction endonuclease analysis of amplified product [33, 34]. The choice of a mutation detection diagnostic technique depends not only on its availability in the laboratory and relevant technological knowledge, but also on the variety and nature of mutations likely to be identified. Gap-PCR, Multiplex Ligation-dependent Probe Amplification (MLPA) and Sanger Sequencing technologies are the most widely used techniques for detecting the breakpoint sequences for as yet uncharacterized deletions/duplications and deletions causing α- or β-thalassemia [33].

2.1. Hemoglobinopathy Screening in Pregnancy

PCR based prenatal diagnosis of hemoglobinopathies, analyzing DNA from chorionic villi or amniocytes, has been in use in many countries. Prenatal diagnosis of SCD using fetal DNA from extra-embryonic celomic fluid at 7th to 10th week gestation has also been practiced [35], but the high rate of miscarriage risks associated with the celocentesis procedure has limited its use. By far, PCR-based diagnosis using amniocyte and chorionic villi DNA has proved to be effective, precise and reliable [36]. Fetal samples are analyzed parallel to parental samples and controls, both positive and negative, using two different mutation detection methods whenever possible and excluding maternal DNA contamination by the analysis of informative DNA polymorphic markers. Although standard prenatal diagnosis is a complex procedure, parental mutations are commonly identified beforehand and diagnosed using inexpensive, simple and quick PCR-based methods, such as ARMS-PCR, targeting the most prevalent mutations. This approach suits for the budgets and infrastructure of underdeveloped countries [37]. PCR technologies and hybridization assays have been optimized to identify point mutations reliably using minute quantities of DNA. Less frequently, some laboratories use cell free DNA obtained from maternal peripheral blood or maternal plasma [38, 39].

2.2. Diagnosis of Hemoglobinopathies: New Scientific Advances

Despite all the scientific advances in clinical diagnostics and mutation detection methods, accurate diagnosis of hemoglobinopathies still rely on hematological findings coupled with molecular techniques. Complex phenotypes resulting from interacting co-inherited hemoglobin gene disorders command specialist knowledge of genotype/phenotype relationships. Array Comparative Genome Hybridization (aCGH) [40], Target Locus Amplification (TLA) and Next Generation Sequencing (NGS) can identify deletion/duplication breakpoints to nucleotide level [41 - 43].

NGS can detect small changes in sequence, however, because of the short sequence reads, it is unable to determine structural variants. Enrichment techniques, *e.g.*, bait capture methods, help enrich more fragments spanning the breakpoint, thereby increasing the efficiency of NGS [41, 44]. aCGH has been used to detect deletions that microscopic investigation and FISH analysis fail to detect. Differences in large deletions in paternal or maternal chromosomes can be observed by looking at SNPs (single nucleotide polymorphisms) on the array [40, 45, 46].

TLA can work without prior knowledge of the target locus because a few primers, in fact, even one, sequence tens to hundreds of kilobases of flanking DNA. This enables the identification of single nucleotide variants and breakpoint sequences of duplication/deletion/inversion [43, 47].

2.3. Recent Advances in Screening and Diagnosis of Hemoglobinopathies

Several investigative techniques have been used to define abnormal hemoglobin. These range from basic approaches, such as solubility test, alkali denaturation and acid elution test to complex tests such as hemoglobin electrophoresis, isoelectric focusing, HPLC, high voltage capillary electrophoresis and enzyme digestion coupled with mass spectroscopy [33, 34].

Routine molecular biology approaches, such as PCR screening by SSCP (Single Strand Conformation Polymorphism), CSGE (Conformation Sensitive Gel Electrophoresis), CRDB (Covalent Reverse Dot Blot hybridization), SSP (Sequence Specific Priming), ARMS (Amplification Refractory Mutation System), DGGE (Denaturant Gradient Gel Electrophoresis), Gap PCR/ Multiplex PCR, and MLPA (Multiple Ligation of Product Amplification) facilitate quick detection of variations in globin genes including small and large deletions and crossovers of these genes. Finally, SNP microarray, Sanger sequencing and NGS along with other high throughput gene-based technologies, such as dHPLC (denaturant HPLC), high resolution melting curve analysis using qPCR have reduced the turnaround time of hemoglobinopathies diagnosis in secondary and tertiary care centers [48]. Advancements in monoclonal antibodies, nanoparticle probes and lateral flow technology have made diagnosis, as point of care testing, an easy affair.

Finally, prevention of affected births by prenatal diagnosis or pre-conception screening has added yet another dimension in diagnostics. An uncontaminated fetal sample, obtained during the first trimester by aspirating amniotic fluid or by chorionic villus sampling (CVS), which is the preferred method of choice these days, is a prerequisite for successful prenatal diagnosis [38].

2.4. New Challenges in the Diagnosis of Hemoglobinopathies: Migration of Populations

Migration of people carrying hemoglobinopathy alleles, from endemic regions to countries where the disease incidence is low, dramatically modifies the distribution of mutant alleles. There are >1000 different mutant alleles described in several databases such as HbVar [49] and IthaGenes [50]. These mutations are region-specific and classified into four groups: Southeast Asian, Asian Indian, Mediterranean, and sub-Saharan African. Within a group, every country, harbors its own spectrum of hemoglobin and thalassemia variants, with a few common alleles and a greater range of low frequency alleles. The migration of carriers increases the diagnostic range of a laboratory by introducing new and novel gene variants, with a resulting pressure to upgrade and update the screening technology and diagnostic spectrum [51]. In the UK, Kurdish, Afghani and Iraqi immigrants, to name a few, posed problems for the molecular screening of β-thalassemia mutations; as a result, the diagnostic approach and mutation detection technology were changed from trivial ARMS-PCR to a more reliable and robust Sanger sequencing of the entire gene for every sample. After ten years of screening, variety and spectrum of thalassemia and hemoglobinopathy alleles in the UK have increased significantly, endorsing that the changing the screening strategy and upgrading the technology was a timely and inevitable decision [52].

3. BLOOD TRANSFUSION THERAPY IN HEMOGLOBINOPATHIES

Blood transfusion results in decreased anemia and improved survival, however, this benefit is offset by the subsequent organ damage caused by iron deposition and complications of infection with blood-borne pathogens [53]. Blood transfusions coupled with iron chelation therapy have long been used with formidable success to prolong the survival of patients with β-thalassemia. Lately, however, induction of HbF, especial in β-thalassemia intermedia, using recombinant human erythropoietin has been the focus of researchers [54]. Washed, leukocyte-free, erythrocytes are recommended for transfusions to avoid febrile and urticarial reactions and CMV infection. Alternatively, frozen-thawed RBCs are administered [55]. Current guidelines recommend a pre-transfusion hemoglobin in 9-10 g/dL range; this transfusion scheme leads to 100-200 mL/kg/year of RBC which results in a daily intake of 0.3-0.6 mg of iron per kg body weight [56, 57]. Patients have to undergo regular iron chelation therapies to have safe iron levels in the body. Cardiac status of transfusion dependent patients who receive iron chelation therapy, needs regular annual monitoring, beginning in the first decade of life [58]. Based on arterial blood pressure, diuretics, potassium-sparing agents and angiotensin-converting enzyme (ACE) inhibitors are recommended.

4. CRISPR-CAS9 GENE EDITING FOR HEMOGLOBINOPATHIES

Gene editing for the reactivation of HbF could well be a prospective therapeutic approach to β-thalassemia and SCD. In recent years, novel approaches have been devised to activate the endogenously silent γ-globin expression in order to increase HbF levels. The objective of these, and such strategies is to reactivate KLF1 and BCL11A so as to upregulate γ-globin expression [59].

There are still reservations about the efficiency of gene delivery and vector stability; there is still room for improvement in these areas. Similarly, viral titers non-oncogenic integration, variation in globin genes expression and the inconsistent contributions of the β-thalassemia phenotype and other modifiers to the effectiveness of gene transfer are the as yet addressed areas of concern [38].

Replacing DNA transfection with safer and more efficient delivery of RNA or Cas9 ribonucleoprotein complexes can further facilitate the clinical translation of these therapeutic approaches [60]. Unlike traditional approaches, which rely on viruses to deliver genetic material that randomly integrates in the genome, CRISPR-Cas9 makes precise and targeted changes to the genome. A genome editing strategy aimed to reverse switch β-to-γ-globin can potentially induce a high-level expression of the endogenous γ-globin gene at the expense of the sickle β-globin [60, 61]. Another, recent approach is CTX001 (CRISPR Therapeutics and Vertex) based cell therapy. This approach involves editing cells with CRISPR-Cas9 to disrupt BCL11A gene to increase fetal γ-globin expression. The potential of CRISPR-Cas9 system to precisely target DNA sequences, along with prospective improved efficiencies in gene-transfer and editing is expected to further boost gene therapy [60, 61]

5. CHALLENGES

Hemoglobinopathies are among the most studies and relatively well understood disorder at molecular level. Therefore, molecular therapies of these disorders designed for these disorders serve as a model of novel disease treatment. However, any gene therapy protocol for this disease is yet to be well-established. Despite extensive research, complex expression and regulation of globin genes are far from being completely understood. The expression of globin genes is tightly regulated during development; which is further complicated by tissue-specific regulation add another level regulation to it. Since the expression of globin genes also varies according to different stages during differentiation of erythroid cell line, their regulation also depends on cell type. And, finally, the coordination between α- and β-globin genes expressions adds yet another level of complexity. Nevertheless, our knowledge of the subject is accumulating exponentially and there is every reason to believe that genetic engineering will begin to heal in the near future [62].

6. FUTURE PROSPECTS

A promising strategy is based on our understanding of the pivotal role that BCL11A transcription factor plays in switching off γ-globin expression in adults; directed at triggering the synthesis of HbF by switching off the conversion of HbF to HbA [63, 64]. Downregulation of BCL11A by transiently expressing a short-hairpin RNA in the erythroid compartment offers a promising solution [65]. Alternatively, BCL11A expression can be lowered by deleting its erythrocyte specific enhancer sequence using CRISPR/Cas9-mediated genome editing [66]. Another approach to restore HbF is to re-create deletions in the β-globin locus or mutate the γ-globin promoters regulating HPFH, validated by data from clinical genetics [67]. Re-creating such HPFH mutations in adult hematopoietic stem and progenitor cells (HSPCs) by CRISPR driven genome editing increases γ-globin expression [68]; the efficiency of gene editing, however, is still subtherapeutic as compared to lentiviral vector based gene replacement. The HbF/HbA switch can also be reversed by creating a loop between the locus control region (LCR) and promoters of γ-globin, zinc-finger proteins with an effector. This will potentially upregulate the expression of γ-globin and decreasing the expression of beta S-globin alongside [69]. Contrary to gene editing, this strategy does not involve DNA cleaving and rejoining.

Genome editing holds a realistic promise for gene therapy for disease arising from globin gene variants. Once the issue of off-target effects is addressed, genome editing will become a practical option in terms of biosafety and total cost of treatment (at least for nonviral delivery of the editing machinery) [70].

CONCLUDING REMARKS

For hemoglobinopathies, gene therapy shows its safety and future efficacy in both preclinical studies and early clinical trials. However, quality, source, dosage of repopulating stem cells, suboptimal efficiency of transduction and levels of gene expression, and toxicity and effectiveness of existing conditioning regimes and an altered bone marrow microenvironment remain major limiting factors in its generalized use. Additionally, the complexity and cost associated with the development of vectors and cells, in particular in low-income countries, limit the democratization of this method. Considering the promising findings and the current excitement among both researchers and industrial supporters, these limiting factors need to be consistently tackled for gene therapy to become a therapeutic practice for hemoglobinopathies. At least some of these shortcomings can be solved by the new gene editing technologies to provide additional therapeutic options, but its efficacy and effectiveness are yet to be assessed in clinical reality [70].

CONSENT FOR PUBLICATION

Not applicable.

CONFLICT OF INTEREST

The author declares no conflict of interest, financial or otherwise.

ACKNOWLEDGEMENTS

Declared none.

REFERENCES

[1]   Hünefeld F L. Der Chemismus in der thierischen Organisation: Physiologisch-chemische Untersuchungen der materiellen Veränderungen, oder des Bildungslebens im thierischen Organismus; insbesondere des Blutbildungsprocesses, der Natur der Blut körperchen und ihrer Kernchen Ein Beitrag zur Physiologie und Heilmittellehre 1840.

[2]   Hoppe-Seyler F. Ueber die chemischen und optischen Eigenschaften des Blutfarbstoffs. Virchows Arch 1864; 29(5-6): 597-600.
[http://dx.doi.org/10.1007/BF01926067]

[3]   Bernard C. Leçons sur les effets des substances toxiques et médicamenteuses 1857.

[4]   Perutz MF, Rossmann MG, Cullis AF, Muirhead H, Will G, North ACT. Structure of haemoglobin: a three-dimensional Fourier synthesis at 5.5-A. resolution, obtained by X-ray analysis. Nature 1960; 185(4711): 416-22.
[http://dx.doi.org/10.1038/185416a0] [PMID: 18990801]

[5]   Perutz MF. Hemoglobin structure and respiratory transport. Sci Am 1978; 239(6): 92-125.
[http://dx.doi.org/10.1038/scientificamerican1278-92] [PMID: 734439]

[6]   Natarajan C, Hoffmann FG, Weber RE, Fago A, Witt CC, Storz JF. Predictable convergence in hemoglobin function has unpredictable molecular underpinnings. Science 2016; 354(6310): 336-9.
[http://dx.doi.org/10.1126/science.aaf9070] [PMID: 27846568]

[7]   Stamatoyannopoulos G. Hemoglobin switching. The Molecular Basis of Blood Diseases 2001.

[8]   Faulkner L. The Rising Global Burden of Hemoglobinopathies, A Challenge and an Opportunity for Health Care in Pakistan. Journal of Islamabad Medical Dental College 2018; 7(1): 1-4.

[9]   Modell B, Darlison M. Global epidemiology of haemoglobin disorders and derived service indicators. Bull World Health Organ 2008; 2008(6): 480-7.
[http://dx.doi.org/10.2471/BLT.06.036673] [PMID: 18568278]

[10]   Motta I, Ghiaccio V, Cosentino A, Breda L. Curing hemoglobinopathies: challenges and advances of conventional and new gene therapy approaches. Mediterr J Hematol Infect Dis 2019; 11(1): e2019067.
[http://dx.doi.org/10.4084/mjhid.2019.067] [PMID: 31700592]

[11]   Attia AM, Ibrahim FA, Abd El-Latif NA, Aziz SW, Abdelmottaleb Moussa SA, Elalfy MS. Determination of human hemoglobin derivatives. Hemoglobin 2015; 39(5): 371-4.
[PMID: 26193973]

[12]   Schechter AN. Hemoglobin research and the origins of molecular medicine. Blood 2008; 112(10): 3927-38.
[http://dx.doi.org/10.1182/blood-2008-04-078188] [PMID: 18988877]

[13]   Bain BJ. Haemoglobin and the genetics of haemoglobin synthesis 2020.
[http://dx.doi.org/10.1002/9781119579977.ch1]

[14]   Urosevic J, *et al.* Homogeneity of Hb Lepore gene in FR Yugoslavia. Balkan J Med Genet 2001; 4(1&2): 29-32.

[15]   Cao A, Galanello R. Beta-thalassemia. Genet Med 2010; 12(2): 61-76.
[http://dx.doi.org/10.1097/GIM.0b013e3181cd68ed] [PMID: 20098328]

[16]   Giordano PC. Strategies for basic laboratory diagnostics of the hemoglobinopathies in multi-ethnic societies: interpretation of results and pitfalls. Int J Lab Hematol 2013; 35(5): 465-79.
[http://dx.doi.org/10.1111/ijlh.12037] [PMID: 23217050]

[17]   He L, Rockwood AL, Agarwal AM, *et al.* Diagnosis of hemoglobinopathy and β-thalassemia by 21 tesla Fourier transform ion cyclotron resonance mass spectrometry and tandem mass spectrometry of hemoglobin from blood. Clin Chem 2019; 65(8): 986-94.
[http://dx.doi.org/10.1373/clinchem.2018.295766] [PMID: 31040099]

[18]   Steensma DP, Gibbons RJ, Higgs DR. Acquired α-thalassemia in association with myelodysplastic syndrome and other hematologic malignancies. Blood 2005; 105(2): 443-52.
[http://dx.doi.org/10.1182/blood-2004-07-2792] [PMID: 15358626]

[19]   Longo D L, Piel F B, Weatherall D J. The α-Thalassemias 2014.

[20]   Danjou F, Anni F, Galanello R. Beta-thalassemia: from genotype to phenotype. Haematologica 2011;

96(11): 1573.
[http://dx.doi.org/10.3324/haematol.2011.055962]

[21]   Daar S, Gravell D, Hussein HM, Pathare AV, Wali Y, Krishnamoorthy R. Haematological and clinical features of β-thalassaemia associated with Hb Dhofar. Eur J Haematol 2008; 80(1): 67-70.
[http://dx.doi.org/10.1111/j.1600-0609.2007.00989.x] [PMID: 18173741]

[22]   Premawardhena A, Arambepola M, Katugaha N, Weatherall DJ. Is the β thalassaemia trait of clinical importance? Br J Haematol 2008; 141(3): 407-10.
[http://dx.doi.org/10.1111/j.1365-2141.2008.07071.x] [PMID: 18341640]

[23]   Bouva MJ, Harteveld CL, van Delft P, Giordano PC. Known and new delta globin gene mutations and their diagnostic significance. Haematologica 2006; 91(1): 129-32.
[PMID: 16434382]

[24]   Huisman THJ. Gamma chain abnormal human fetal hemoglobin variants. Am J Hematol 1997; 55(3): 159-63.
[http://dx.doi.org/10.1002/(SICI)1096-8652(199707)55:3<159::AID-AJH8>3.0.CO;2-R]   [PMID: 9256297]

[25]   Mansour AK, Yahia S, El-Ashry R, Alwakeel A, Darwish A, Alrjjal K. Sickle Cell Disease (SCD) 2015.
[http://dx.doi.org/10.5772/61162]

[26]   Estcourt L J, Fortin P M, Trivella M, Hopewell S. Preoperative blood transfusions for sickle cell disease. Cochrane Database Syst Rev 2020; 7(7): CD003149.
[http://dx.doi.org/10.1002/14651858.CD003149.pub3]

[27]   Olivieri NF, Pakbaz Z, Vichinsky E. "Hb E/beta-thalassaemia: a common & clinically diverse disorder," *The Indian journal of medical research*. Hematology 2011; 134(4): 522.

[28]   Saleh-Gohari N, Mohammadi-Anaie M. Co-inheritance of sickle cell trait and thalassemia mutations in South central iran. Iran J Public Health 2012; 41(10): 81-6.
[PMID: 23304665]

[29]   Piel FB, Howes RE, Patil AP, *et al.* The distribution of haemoglobin C and its prevalence in newborns in Africa. Sci Rep 2013; 3(1): 1671.
[http://dx.doi.org/10.1038/srep01671] [PMID: 23591685]

[30]   Zakerinia M, *et al.* Hemoglobin D (Hb D Punjab/Los Angeles and Hb D Iran) and co-inheritance with alpha-and beta-thalassemia in southern Iran. Iranian Red Crescent Medical Journal 2011; 13(7): 493-8.

[31]   Hafsia R, Gouider E, Ben Moussa S, Ben Salah N, Elborji W, Hafsia A. Hemoglobin O Arab: about 20 cases. Tunis Med 2007; 85(8): 637-40.
[PMID: 18254282]

[32]   Nagayama Y, Yoshida M, Kohyama T, Matsui K. Hemoglobin Kansas as a Rare Cause of Cyanosis: A Case Report and Review of the Literature. Intern Med 2017; 56(2): 207-9.
[http://dx.doi.org/10.2169/internalmedicine.56.7349] [PMID: 28090054]

[33]   Old J, Henderson S. Molecular diagnostics for haemoglobinopathies. Expert Opin Med Diagn 2010; 4(3): 225-40.
[http://dx.doi.org/10.1517/17530051003709729] [PMID: 23488532]

[34]   Old J, Traeger-Synodinos J, Galanello R, Petrou M, Angastiniotis M. Prevention of thalassaemias and other haemoglobin disorders. Thalassaemia International Federation Publications 2005; 2: 113-6.

[35]   Makrydimas G, Georgiou I, Bouba I, Lolis D, Nicolaides K. Early prenatal diagnosis by celocentesis. 2004.
[http://dx.doi.org/10.1002/uog.1046]

[36]   Brancaleoni V, Di Pierro E, Motta I, Cappellini MD. Laboratory diagnosis of thalassemia. Int J Lab Hematol 2016; 38 (Suppl. 1): 32-40.

[http://dx.doi.org/10.1111/ijlh.12527] [PMID: 27183541]

[37]   Mahmood Baig S, Sabih D, Rahim MK, *et al.* β-Thalassemia in Pakistan. J Pediatr Hematol Oncol 2012; 34(2): 90-2.
[http://dx.doi.org/10.1097/MPH.0b013e31823752f3] [PMID: 22258353]

[38]   Traeger-Synodinos J, Harteveld CL. Preconception carrier screening and prenatal diagnosis in thalassemia and hemoglobinopathies: challenges and future perspectives. Expert Rev Mol Diagn 2017; 17(3): 281-91.
[http://dx.doi.org/10.1080/14737159.2017.1285701] [PMID: 28110577]

[39]   Weigang , *et al.* Non-invasive prenatal diagnosis for pregnancies at risk for β-thalassemia: a retrospective study. BJOG 2020.

[40]   Hupé P, Stransky N, Thiery JP, Radvanyi F, Barillot E. Analysis of array CGH data: from signal ratio to gain and loss of DNA regions. Bioinformatics 2004; 20(18): 3413-22.
[http://dx.doi.org/10.1093/bioinformatics/bth418] [PMID: 15381628]

[41]   Clark BE, Shooter C, Smith F, Brawand D, Thein SL. Next-generation sequencing as a tool for breakpoint analysis in rearrangements of the globin gene clusters. Int J Lab Hematol 2017; 39 (Suppl. 1): 111-20.
[http://dx.doi.org/10.1111/ijlh.12680] [PMID: 28447426]

[42]   Zhang H, Li C, Li J, *et al.* Next-generation sequencing improves molecular epidemiological characterization of thalassemia in Chenzhou Region, P.R. China. J Clin Lab Anal 2019; 33(4): e22845.
[http://dx.doi.org/10.1002/jcla.22845] [PMID: 30809867]

[43]   de Vree PJP, de Wit E, Yilmaz M, *et al.* Targeted sequencing by proximity ligation for comprehensive variant detection and local haplotyping. Nat Biotechnol 2014; 32(10): 1019-25.
[http://dx.doi.org/10.1038/nbt.2959] [PMID: 25129690]

[44]   Dumbrell AJ, Ferguson RM, Clark DR. Microbial community analysis by single-amplicon high-throughput next generation sequencing: data analysis–from raw output to ecology.Hydrocarbon and lipid microbiology protocols. Springer 2016; pp. 155-206.
[http://dx.doi.org/10.1007/8623_2016_228]

[45]   Shinawi M, Cheung SW. The array CGH and its clinical applications. Drug Discov Today 2008; 13(17-18): 760-70.
[http://dx.doi.org/10.1016/j.drudis.2008.06.007] [PMID: 18617013]

[46]   Phylipsen M, Chaibunruang A, Vogelaar IP, *et al.* Fine-tiling array CGH to improve diagnostics for α- and β-thalassemia rearrangements. Hum Mutat 2012; 33(1): 272-80.
[http://dx.doi.org/10.1002/humu.21612] [PMID: 21922597]

[47]   Harteveld C L. Diagnosis of haemoglobinopathies: New scientific advances. Thalassemia Reports 2018; 8(1).
[http://dx.doi.org/10.4081/thal.2018.7473]

[48]   Ghosh K, Ghosh K, Agrawal R, Nadkarni AH. Recent advances in screening and diagnosis of hemoglobinopathy. Expert Rev Hematol 2020; 13(1): 13-21.
[http://dx.doi.org/10.1080/17474086.2019.1656525] [PMID: 31432725]

[49]   Giardine B, Borg J, Viennas E, *et al.* Updates of the HbVar database of human hemoglobin variants and thalassemia mutations. Nucleic Acids Res 2014; 42(D1): D1063-9.
[http://dx.doi.org/10.1093/nar/gkt911] [PMID: 24137000]

[50]   Kountouris P, Lederer CW, Fanis P, Feleki X, Old J, Kleanthous M. IthaGenes: an interactive database for haemoglobin variations and epidemiology. PLoS One 2014; 9(7): e103020.
[http://dx.doi.org/10.1371/journal.pone.0103020] [PMID: 25058394]

[51]   Old J, *et al.* New challenges in diagnosis of haemoglobinopathies: Migration of populations. Thalassemia Reports 2018.

[52] Inusa B P, Colombatti R. European migration crises: The role of national hemoglobinopathy registries in improving patient access to care. Pediatr Blood Cancer 2017; 64(7).
[http://dx.doi.org/10.1002/pbc.26515]

[53] Prati D. Benefits and complications of regular blood transfusion in patients with beta-thalassaemia major. Vox Sang 2000; 79(3): 129-37.
[http://dx.doi.org/10.1046/j.1423-0410.2000.7930129.x] [PMID: 11111230]

[54] Chaidos A, Makis A, Hatzimichael E, *et al.* Treatment of β-thalassemia patients with recombinant human erythropoietin: effect on transfusion requirements and soluble adhesion molecules. Acta Haematol 2004; 111(4): 189-95.
[http://dx.doi.org/10.1159/000077551] [PMID: 15153710]

[55] Oliva EN, Ronco F, Marino A, Alati C, Praticò G, Nobile FJT. Iron chelation therapy associated with improvement of hematopoiesis in transfusion-dependent patients. Transfusion 2010; 50(7): 1568-70.
[http://dx.doi.org/10.1111/j.1537-2995.2010.02617.x]

[56] Cazzola M, Stefano PD, Ponchio L, *et al.* Relationship between transfusion regimen and suppression of erythropoiesis in β-thalassaemia major. Br J Haematol 1995; 89(3): 473-8.
[http://dx.doi.org/10.1111/j.1365-2141.1995.tb08351.x] [PMID: 7734344]

[57] Pasricha SR, Frazer DM, Bowden DK, Anderson GJ. Transfusion suppresses erythropoiesis and increases hepcidin in adult patients with β-thalassemia major: a longitudinal study. Blood 2013; 122(1): 124-33.
[http://dx.doi.org/10.1182/blood-2012-12-471441] [PMID: 23656728]

[58] Botzenhardt S, Li N, Chan EW, Sing CW, Wong ICK, Neubert A. Safety profiles of iron chelators in young patients with haemoglobinopathies. Eur J Haematol 2017; 98(3): 198-217.
[http://dx.doi.org/10.1111/ejh.12833] [PMID: 27893170]

[59] Chandrakasan S, Malik P. Gene therapy for hemoglobinopathies: the state of the field and the future. Hematol Oncol Clin North Am 2014; 28(2): 199-216.
[http://dx.doi.org/10.1016/j.hoc.2013.12.003] [PMID: 24589262]

[60] Antoniani C, Meneghini V, Lattanzi A, *et al.* Induction of fetal hemoglobin synthesis by CRISPR/Cas9-mediated editing of the human β-globin locus. Blood 2018; 131(17): 1960-73.
[http://dx.doi.org/10.1182/blood-2017-10-811505] [PMID: 29519807]

[61] Haematology TL. CRISPR-Cas9 gene editing for patients with haemoglobinopathies. Lancet Haematol 2019; 6(9): e438.
[http://dx.doi.org/10.1016/S2352-3026(19)30169-3] [PMID: 31471004]

[62] Pavlovic S, Ugrin M, Stojiljkovic M. Novel Therapy Approaches in β-Thalassemia Syndromes–A Role of Genetic Modifiers.Inherited hemoglobin disorders. Rijeka: InTech 2015; pp. 137-60.
[http://dx.doi.org/10.5772/61023]

[63] Smith EC, Orkin SH. Hemoglobin genetics: recent contributions of GWAS and gene editing. Hum Mol Genet 2016; 25(R2): R99-R105.
[http://dx.doi.org/10.1093/hmg/ddw170] [PMID: 27340226]

[64] Bauer DE, Orkin SH. Hemoglobin switching's surprise: the versatile transcription factor BCL11A is a master repressor of fetal hemoglobin. Curr Opin Genet Dev 2015; 33: 62-70.
[http://dx.doi.org/10.1016/j.gde.2015.08.001] [PMID: 26375765]

[65] Tsang JCH, Yu Y, Burke S, *et al.* Single-cell transcriptomic reconstruction reveals cell cycle and multi-lineage differentiation defects in Bcl11a-deficient hematopoietic stem cells. Genome Biol 2015; 16(1): 178.
[http://dx.doi.org/10.1186/s13059-015-0739-5] [PMID: 26387834]

[66] Canver MC, Smith EC, Sher F, *et al.* BCL11A enhancer dissection by Cas9-mediated *in situ* saturating mutagenesis. Nature 2015; 527(7577): 192-7.
[http://dx.doi.org/10.1038/nature15521] [PMID: 26375006]

[67]   Steinberg MH, Chui DHK, Dover GJ, Sebastiani P, Alsultan A. Fetal hemoglobin in sickle cell anemia: a glass half full? Blood 2014; 123(4): 481-5.
[http://dx.doi.org/10.1182/blood-2013-09-528067] [PMID: 24222332]

[68]   Traxler EA, Yao Y, Wang YD, *et al.* A genome-editing strategy to treat β-hemoglobinopathies that recapitulates a mutation associated with a benign genetic condition. Nat Med 2016; 22(9): 987-90.
[http://dx.doi.org/10.1038/nm.4170] [PMID: 27525524]

[69]   Breda L, Motta I, Lourenco S, *et al.* Forced chromatin looping raises fetal hemoglobin in adult sickle cells to higher levels than pharmacologic inducers. Blood 2016; 128(8): 1139-43.
[http://dx.doi.org/10.1182/blood-2016-01-691089] [PMID: 27405777]

[70]   Ferrari G, Cavazzana M, Mavilio F. Gene therapy approaches to hemoglobinopathies. Hematology/Oncology Clinics 2017; 31(5): 835-52.
[http://dx.doi.org/10.1016/j.hoc.2017.06.010]

CHAPTER 15

Metabolic Syndromes

Mahnoor Ejaz[1,*], Areena Suhail Khan[2], Faiza Naseer[3] and Alvina Gul[1]

[1] Atta-ur-Rahman School of Applied Biosciences (ASAB), National University of Sciences and Technology (NUST), Islamabad, Pakistan

[2] Department of Biosciences, COMSATS University Islamabad, Park Road, Islamabad, Pakistan

[3] Shifa College of Pharmaceutical Sciences, Shifa Tameer-e-Millat University, Islamabad, Pakistan

Abstract: Metabolic Syndromes (MetS) are recognized as a cluster of risk factors which are known to increase the likelihood of obesity, type 2 diabetes (T2D) and cardiovascular disorders (CVDs). It is significant to understand disease pathology in order to discover a pathological mechanism leading to the development of MetS. Elevated triglycerides, increased blood pressure, hyperglycemia (increased blood glucose levels), low levels of High-density lipoprotein (HDL) cholesterol and elevated waist circumference are key parameters in diagnosing MetS. Various therapeutic interventions have been developed for treating metabolic diseases like polypills which are commonly known as combination pills, along with the fixed dose combinations. In addition to pharmacological handling, surgical treatment is also showing success in treating MetS such as Bariatric treatment. With the emerging experimental techniques, gene therapy allows the replacement of a defective gene with a healthy one, which may eventually reverse the disease. Leptin Gene Therapy, ZFN Gene Editing, CRISPR/Cas9 genome editing are different platforms of gene therapy which are showing promising results in treating the metabolic disease. Novel experimental approaches and pharmacological treatments can provide a better insight into metabolic syndrome and its related complications, thereby reducing its global burden.

Keywords: CRISPR/Cas9 genome editing, CVDs, Metabolic Syndrome, Obesity, Polypills, Type 2 Diabetes.

1. INTRODUCTION

Metabolic syndrome (MetS) emerges as an epidemic and a vital public well-being concern. It is characterized not as a disorder, but as a common entity which includes a group of metabolic risk factors which are likely to increase the chances of type 2 diabetes (T2D) and cardiovascular disorders (CVD) [1]. Various other

* **Corresponding author Mahnoor Ejaz**: Atta-ur-Rahman School of Applied Biosciences (ASAB), National University of Sciences and Technology (NUST), Islamabad, Pakistan; E-mail: mahnoorejaz@hotmail.com

Syeda Marriam Bakhtiar and Erum Dilshad (Eds.)

comorbidities (like proinflammatory/prothrombic state, NAFLD, cholesterol gallstone disease, reproductive disorders) are known to be associated with MetS [2]. Several lifestyle factors including overconsumption of food, inactive lifestyle and abdominal obesity may cause MetS [1].

Although the presence of a unifying pathogenic mechanism that can help understand the disease pathophysiology is still unclear, it is extremely likely that insulin resistance and abdominal obesity play a vital role in promoting the development of MetS since studies have suggested a two-fold increased risk of CVD and a five-times increased T2D risk [3].

A number of terms are incorporated to define metabolic syndrome, and almost all of them include hypercholesterolemia, central obesity, hypertension, decreased HDL-cholesterol levels, resistance to insulin and increased plasma triglycerides [1, 4].

1.1. Background

MetS begin as a notion rather than a diagnosis. In 1920 a Swedish physician, Kylin observed a relationship among hypertension, hyperglycemia and gout, and later found visceral obesity linked to CVD and T2D [5]. In 1988, Reaven described Syndrome X as the group of risk factors for T2D and CVD- an addition of the theory of insulin resistance [6]. In 1989, Kaplan retitled the syndrome "The Deadly Quartet" adding obesity or visceral obesity as a major abnormality [7]. The syndrome was renamed once again as "The Insulin Resistance Syndrome" in 1992 [8].

1.2. Components of MetS

The idea of metabolic syndrome has numerous empirical applications, one such is the clinical assessment to categorize individuals at a greater risk of obesity, T2D or CVD as shown in Fig. (**15.1**). Therefore, it helps identify a particular subgroup of patients with a common pathophysiology. Thus, the term assists as a shorthand for clinicians for the pooled underlying biological processes [9].

1.2.1. Obesity

Various health experts assert that if obesity had not been a major public health issue that it is today, MetS would never have been put forth. By 2030, about 20% of world's population is estimated to be obese [10]. The elevated prevalence rate of obesity is linked to increase in insulin resistance and MetS [11]. The loss of insulin secretory capacity (β-cell function loss or reduced β-cell mass) along with genetic, social and environmental factors is identified to be involved in the development of the disease [12 - 15]. This universal burden insists fundamental nutrition and lifestyle modifications that are based on a sound comprehension of MetS pathology [16]. To represent abdominal obesity, measurement of body mass index (BMI) and waist circumference (WC), though widely utilized, are not the specific parameters. However, a more accurate predictor is visceral fat area (VFA) which has shown to be more strongly correlated with MetS [17].

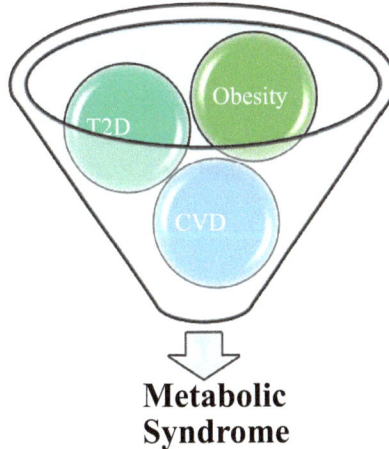

Fig. (15.1). Components of MetS. Individuals at a risk of obesity, T2D and CVD are more likely to develop MetS.

1.2.2. Type2 Diabetes

In the last 30 years, T2D prevalence has tripled, affecting millions worldwide and is predicted to rise by 54% in the next ten years [10]. T2D and MetS are known to increase the likelihood of CVD and various carcinomas [17]. Elevated blood glucose concentration marks this disorder, where defected insulin secretion is regarded as the key pathophysiological factor [11]. The degree of prevalence of T2D is one of the criteria, which is preset in all the three defined versions of MetS and hence most closely related [18]. MetS individuals have a five times greater incidence to T2D and the presence of insulin resistance has an additive effect increasing the risk 6-7 times [19]. Human body's inability to respond to elevated glucose concentration has a major role in T2D pathogenesis [20]. Loss of skeletal muscles- major insulin utilization and uptake sites increase resistance to insulin thereby elevating risk [17].

1.2.3. Atherosclerotic Cardiovascular Disease (ASCVD)

Various studies have revealed that patients with MetS are more likely to develop ASCVD [21]. It accounts for about 30% of worldwide mortality rate hence a vital health concern [22]. A higher ASCVD risk is anticipated to more features or components of MetS in an individual [23]. A combination of high plasma triacylglycerol, along with its rich remnant lipoproteins and low HDL-C, associated with small, dense LDLs is shown to increase the risk towards the disease [18]. The prevalence of ASCVD can be potentially aggravated in individuals who are likely to have inflammation in addition to MetS [22]. The risk of CVD is commonly observed in obese individuals. In fact, an interplay between enhanced levels of fasting glucose, insulin resistance, and an atherogenic lipid profile exhibits obesity as a risk factor for CVD [24].

1.3. Diagnostic Criteria For Metabolic Syndrome

Numerous groups have attempted to develop a diagnostic criterion for MetS. The first came forward in 1999 by WHO which assumed insulin resistance as the major underlying contributor. In addition, it required the presence of two other risk factors: hypertension, obesity, raised TG or low HDL [25]. The European Group for the Study of Insulin Resistance suggested an altered version which proposed the estimates of fasting insulin levels for non-diabetic subjects [26]. In 2001, a new definition was put forward by Adult Treatment Panel III stating the diagnosis when an individual has three or more of the five clinically recognizable risk factors as shown in Fig. (**15.2**) [4].

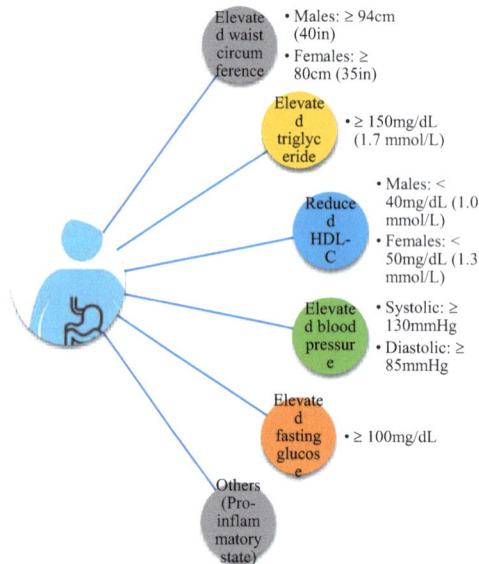

Fig. (15.2). A measure of diagnostic criteria of MetS along with their categorical cut points.

1.3.1. Clinical Measures For Diagnosis

By juggling the clinical outcomes, nearly countless number of scenarios can be derived in which individuals who do not fulfil the diagnostic criteria for MetS would be at a higher risk for obesity, T2D and CVD than would those who do. Therefore, it appears hard to maintain that a MetS diagnosis contributes unique clinical information [18].

1.3.2. Elevated Waist Circumference

Majority of people identified with MetS are categorically obese (BMI$\geq$ 30kg/m^2) [27]. Among them, individuals likely at a risk are with predominant upper body obesity [2]. The quantity of subcutaneous fat usually surpasses that of visceral fat by two to three-folds in such individuals [28]. Excess visceral and subcutaneous fat both strongly associate with MetS [29, 30]. Ectopic fat- the fat overload in tissues, appears to be highly associated with insulin resistance [31]. Excess fatty acids are either converted to ketone bodies or are re-esterified and incorporated into VLDL being released in circulation [2].

Lower body obesity also known as gluteofemoral obesity, accompanies a lesser prevalence of MetS due to a lower amount of NEFA in circulation [30]. It has been observed that adipose tissue triglycerides make up the extra body weight in obese individuals and contributes a host of bio-active peptides (adipokines) which impact MetS risk factors [2]. Another factor resulting in obese, sedentary individuals is the imbalance of energy- overnutrition, causing subsequent tissue fat accumulation. However, if curtailed, metabolic risk factors have been observed to disappear [32].

1.3.3. Elevated Triglycerides

Individuals with MetS display atherogenic dyslipidemia whose vital constituent is elevated apo B-containing lipoproteins, also including VLDL, LDL, elevated triglycerides and reduced HDL-C [2]. Several researchers consider the primary cause of ASCVD to be associated with elevated levels of apo B having lipoproteins. It has been proven through clinical trials that the risk of cardiovascular events can be reduced by lowering the levels of apo B-containing lipoproteins [33]. Hypertriglyceridemia is a condition with elevated VLDL triglycerides, commonly observed in MetS [34].

1.3.4. Low HDL-C

Reduced levels of high-density lipoprotein cholesterol (HDL-C) are another component of atherogenic dyslipidemia. A number of studies strongly associate this component with ASCVD risk [2]. It correlates to enhanced VLDL plasma triacylglycerol concentration. In insulin resistant patients, low HDL-C concentrations result from a larger VLDL pool size; the higher the transfer of cholesterol from HDL to VLDL, the reduced the concentrations of HDL-C. T2D individuals profiles reveal that the higher the measure of hyperinsulinemia, the lower the HDL-C. In nondiabetic patients, an increase in plasma insulin concentrations is correlated to greater catabolic rate of apoprotein A and reduced HDL-C concentration [18].

1.3.5. Elevated Blood Pressure

The correlation among the elevated blood pressure, insulin resistance and CVD is complex than other measures of diagnosis. A number of findings support the correlation between insulin resistance and hyperinsulinemia to hypertension [18]. Various mechanisms such as renal absorption of sodium; emerging due to insulin resistance, enlargement of intravascular volume, initiation of renin-angiotensin and sympathetic nervous system, discharge of angiotensinogen and insulin resistance, combine to explain the correlation between raised blood pressure and MetS [2].

1.3.6. Elevated Fasting Glucose

Insulin resistance is the key cause of hyperglycemia in MetS individuals. Patients with MetS have elevated plasma glucose due to a decline in the function of beta cells. However, hyperglycemia is not the primary indicator, but develops later as a result [35]. The relation between elevated fasting glucose and an increase in triacylglycerol-rich lipoproteins corresponds to insulin resistance and compensatory hyperinsulinemia [36].

1.3.7. Others (Pro-inflammatory State)

Although proinflammatory factors are not yet recognized as a diagnostic criterion, researchers reflect on their association with the group of abnormalities that make up MetS definition [18]. The presence of excessive adipose tissue stimulates macrophages, with a subsequent release of cytokines in order to trigger systemic inflammation [37]. However, overnutrition, independent of obesity may also produce inflammatory responses [38]. The obesity induced cytokines result in insulin resistance, a change in pituitary-adrenal axis, loss of beta cells of pancreas- giving rise to cardiovascular events [2].

1.3.8. Genetic Determinants of MetS

Genetic basis of MetS has a weak association, however various genome-wide scans established familial aggregation most apparent for MetS independent components [39]. Additionally, certain genes such as those who encode for leptin receptors, melanocortin receptors, neuropeptide Y, 11β-hydroxysteroid dehydrogenase, adiponectin, lipoprotein-, hormone sensitive-, hepatic- lipase, β2-β3-adrenergic receptor, TNF-α, IL1- β and the IGF1R also predispose to MetS development [40]. The composition of dietary fatty acid is suggested to modify the risk of MetS. The five phenotypes which describe MetS are recognized to have strong genetic constituents [11]. Studies which show a strong association with MetS or their linked traits are related to genes which are involved in lipid metabolism (CETP, LIPC, LPL, APOB) or are correlated with lipid levels (TRIB1, ABCB11, GCKR). And this reflection is based on the fact that lipid parameters constitute two out of five MetS criterion [40].

2. THERAPEUTICS OF METABOLIC DISORDERS

Various therapies have been developed to treat MetS, few of which are successful in treating the disease especially the pharmacological and surgical interventions, however, the gene editing based treatments have experimentally shown the potential to treat the metabolic disease.

2.1. Pharmacological Therapy

2.1.1. Polypill-Addresses More Than One Cardiometabolic Risk

Polypills or combination pills can be defined as a single formulation that contains multiple pharmacological agents in low doses for the purpose of reducing associated cardiovascular risk throughout the world. The pill consists of a statin, ACEi, diuretic and an antiplatelet agent [41 - 44]. The polypill presents potential benefits over typical pharmacotherapy. First, the minimalism and ease of utilizing an everyday pill may enhance devotion to prescription regimens and therapy [43, 44]. Second, the rejection of the demand for carrying out dosage variation may be beneficial in circumstances in which several follow-up appointments are difficult [44]. Third, for managing blood-pressure, the arrangement of several low-dose medicines instead the usage of one or more elevated-dose treatments may enhance the well-being profile, given that after effects of numerous pharmacological agents that are usually dose-dependent [41, 43].

Multiple clinical experiments are currently in progress towards the determination of the wellbeing and effectiveness of the polypill as prescriptible pharmacological agent. One such trial was carried out by Patel and associates. A randomized control trial concerning 623 accomplices from Australian customary practices was performed; the trial evaluated participants that had a launched CVD or an expected five-year CVD threat of ≥15%. These patients were given a polypill consisting of simvastatin 40mg, aspirin 75mg, lisinopril 10mg and either hydrochlorothiazide 12.5mg or atenolol 50mg [42]. The result showed a marked improvement in most parameters used to assess ASCVD upon use of the polypill therapy.

Another clinical study was conducted by Group *et al.*, (2011) to check the four components of polypill. The pill involved combination of 75mg of aspirin, 10mg of lisinopril, 20mg of simvastatin and 12.5mg of hydrochlorothiazide. 378 patients with no compelling indication but an ASCVD risk of >7.5% were selected. Side-effects were reported in 1 out of every 6 patients nonetheless the results of the trial led to the conclusion that extensive net profits would be anticipated amongst patients at an elevated risk [41]. These studies alongside many others represent how this pill may eventually replace conventional multiple drug regimens for cardiovascular disease providing ease to the patient as well as the health care system in terms of cost, compliance and disease management.

2.2. Fixed Dose Combination (FDC)

2.2.1. Diabetes

Diabetes is one of the highly popular metabolic ailments all around the world. It is categorized into two types, namely, Type1 and Type2 Diabetes (T2D) [45]. Type1 Diabetes (T1D) so-called insulin dependent diabetes is mainly triggered by shortage of Insulin produced by the β-cells in the Islets of Langerhans of pancreas. It accounts for roughly 5% of all cases in the US and is characterized by Skeletal Muscle Breakdown, Excessive breakdown of fatty acids as gluconeogenic fuels and leads to the build-up of ketoacids in blood eventually leading to a life-threatening case of Metabolic Acidosis called Diabetic Keto acidosis. The cause is still under discovery but evidence points to the disease having an auto-immune origin [46]. T2D which is caused by insulin resistance accounts for >90% of all occurrences in the US. It is a complex polygenic disease, where polymorphisms in many genes contribute to the etiology of the disease [47]. Many drugs have been developed as monotherapy for diabetes which is reviewed in Table **15.1**.

Table 15.1. Pharmacological Monotherapy against diabetes.

Drug Name	Drug Class	Mechanism of Action	Diabetes Treated
Insulin and Insulin Analogs	Exogenous Insulin	Replaces or supplements Insulin levels to induce glycemic control	Type 1, Type 2

(Table 1) cont.....

Drug Name	Drug Class	Mechanism of Action	Diabetes Treated
Pramlintide	Synthetic Amylin Analog	GLP-1 analogs. Promote Glucose-dependent insulin release, extend Gastric Emptying time	Type 2
Glyburide, Glipizide, Glimepiride	Sulfonylureas	Promote Insulin vesicle fusion and exocytosis by blocking ATP-dependent K^+ channels and increasing intracellular Ca^{2+}	Type 2
Repaglinide, nateglinide	Glinides	Stimulate Insulin Secretion in early post-prandial conditions	Type 2
Biguanides	Metformin	Reduces Hepatic Gluconeogenesis	Type 2
Pioglitazone, Rosiglitazone	Thiazolidinediones	PPAR activators, promote expression of Insulin responsive genes to induce glycemic control	Type 2
Alogliptin, Linagliptin	Dipeptidyl peptidase-4 inhibitors	Inhibit DPP-4 enzyme, prolonging incretin hormones to induce glycemic control	Type 2
Canaglifozin, Dapaglifozin	SGLT-2 inhibitors	Inhibit SGLT-2 transporter in Proximal Convulated Tubule of Nephron, preventing Glucose Reabsorption and promoting renal glucose excretion	Type 2

2.2.2. SGLT 2 Inhibitor/DPP 4 Inhibitor

FDCs have also been developed of various mono-therapeutic antidiabetic agents that have shown greater efficacy in inducing glycemic control. These FDC(s) have been developed using the agents mentioned in Table **15.1**. A recent clinical trial was conducted where Empaglifozin a SGLT-2 inhibitor was used as an additive agent in a fixed dose regimen with Linagliptin a DPP 4 inhibitor in Japanese affected people with Type2 Diabetes [48]. Their results stated that the difference from standard in HbA1c was larger with Empa/Lina than with Plc/Lina at the 24th week. Other affected people with HbA1c < 7.0% and bigger drops in fasting plasma glucose, systolic blood pressure and body weight were observed in the Empa/Lina group than in the Plc/Lina group, also the Empa/Lina was found to be well-tolerated.

2.2.3. Thiazolidinedione/DPP-4 Inhibitor

Another fixed dose arrangement of alogliptin/pioglitazone was examined in the Japanese population with Type2 diabetes. The study focused on investigating the impacts of moving from combination treatment with either alogliptin (Alo) or pioglitazone (Pio) to fixed dose combination therapy (FDCT) with alogliptin and pioglitazone (Alo-Pio FDCT). The results indicated significant improvements in

Glycosylated Hemoglobin (HbA$_{1c}$), γ-glutamyl transpeptidase (GGT) and alanine transaminase (ALT) levels after moving to Alo-Pio FDCT for 16 weeks in both the groups [14].

2.2.4. Biguanide/DPP-4 Inhibitor FDC

Alongside SGLT-2/DPP-4 inhibitor FDC other combinations of various classes of anti-diabetic drugs have been the subject of rigorous study. One such combination is Metformin XR/Gemigliptin. A randomized controlled trial conducted by Park and colleagues determined that the Pharmacodynamics, pharmacokinetic and toxicity profiles of Metformin XR/Gemigliptin FDC are quite similar to the individual PD, PK and Tox profiles of these drugs when taken alone in a tablet form [49]. Their results have proven to be a promising development in formulating a new therapeutic approach in treating Type2 Diabetes Mellitus.

2.2.5. Biguanide/α-Glucosidase Inhibitor

A conjugative therapy of Voglibose an α-glucosidase inhibitor with Metformin, a Biguanide, called Vogmet, has also been tested. The objective of the of the research was to verify the extent of post-prandial glycemic control of Vogmet as compared to Metformin monotherapy in patients that have recently developed T2DM. The study involved the comparison of Glycemic control in 187 patients aged between 20 and 70, All patients had an HbA1c levels >7.0%. The results showed that the decline in the amounts of HbA1c was -1.62%±0.07% in the vogmet group and -1.31%±0.07% in the metformin group (P=0.003), and considerably more vogmet-treated patients accomplished the mark HbA1c levels of <6.5% (P=0.002) or <7% (P=0.039). Gastrointestinal harmful happenings and hypoglycemia (%) statistically decreased in the vogmet-treated group [50]. This led to the inference that Vogmet a Bigunaide/α-Glucosidase Inhibitor is a harmless antihyperglycemic agent that regulates blood glucose level efficiently, and can be theoretically larger to metformin in terms of dropping significant glycemic limits to normal physiological values deprived of increasing the hazard of hypoglycemia.

2.2.6. Insulin Combinations

The endogenous hormone insulin is now being synthetically produced and is available in the form of sub-cutaneous and intramuscular injections. These exogenous insulin formulations are used to induce glycemic control in T1DM and T2DM. FDC(s) with insulin are now under clinical trials to determine their safety and efficacy for large scale use. Attached below is a list of synthetic Insulin preparations.

A combination therapy of Liraglutide, a GLP-1R agonist with insulin was recently investigated. This involved a multicenter, parallel-group trial, double-blind of 36 weeks where the affected patients kept on steady insulin therapy (basal/premixed/basal–bolus) were randomized 1:1 to further liraglutide 0.9 mg/day ($n = 127$) or placebo ($n = 130$). The insulin dosage was kept static for 16 weeks, and titrated on the basis of self-measured plasma glucose subsequently [51]. The HB1Ac levels were used as the standard measure of effectiveness of the Insulin/placebo and Insulin/liraglutide combination. The results suggested that the stable dose arrangement was more efficacious in reducing HbA1c than insulin alone.

Furthermore, the effectiveness of Metformin/Glimepiride combination additional to the Insulin Glargine has also been reported to be superior regimen in maintaining glycemic levels as compared to Insulin Glargine alone in affected people with T2DM. This conclusion was reached by determining the mean-reduction in HBA1c levels which were extra visible in the Metformin, Glimepiride and Insulin Glargine triple fixed dose combination regimen as compared to Insulin Glargine/Metformin and Insulin Glargine/ Glimepiride dual therapy [52].

2.2. Diabesity

Obesity has surfaced as a prominent worldwide health concern over the contemporary environmental and social alterations, preferring an encouraging energy equilibrium and weight gain. Major reasons are the inadequate physical activity, intake of high-calorie or high-fat foods, and a shift in the direction of a well-developed deskbound routine. Therefore, the total number of people who are now considered as overweight had closely doubled globally since 1980. In 2014, more than 39% of the grownups; 18 years or older, were fat with 13% of them being obese. In add-on, at least 41 million children below the age of 5 were found to be fat or obese corresponding to the World Health Organization (WHO) [53].

Diabesity is described as a mixture of T2D and obesity, with or without associated risk factors like dyslipidemia and hypertension. Hence, diabesity forms a subset of metabolic conditions. The rule for determining whether a person is obese or not uses the body mass index classification which is the ratio of the weight of an individual measured in kilograms and the height of the individual squared in m^2 as shown in Table **15.2**.

Diabesity has also been associated with exasperating other pathologies with the risk of developing ASCVD being the greatest. The risk of diabetes rises by 4.5% for each kilogram increase in body weight. Poor nutritional habits and a lack of exercise have been associated in the incidence of diabetes. These risk elements together lead to insulin endurance, hyper-insulinemia and atherogenic dyslipidemia, increased small dense LDL-C (low density lipoprotein cholesterol) and hypertriglyceridemia low HDL-C, (high density lipoprotein cholesterol).

Table 15.2. Body Mass Index Classifications for weight as per WHO guidelines

BMI/Kgm^{-2}	Classification
18.4-24.9	Average
25-29.9	Overweight
30-34.9	Class 1
25-39.9	Class 2
40+	Class 3

Various drugs are available in the market that are used to carry out glycemic control or weight loss. However, the use of one drug seems to worsen symptoms of the other pathology. For example, anti-diabetic drugs tend to cause weight gain which is an unfavorable outcome when it comes to treating a patient that suffers from Diabesity [54]. Therefore, combination therapy is the need of the hour. However, clinicians must keep in mind multiple factors such as Metabolic, psychological, and behavioral characteristics of the patient in question.

GLP 1R Agonist Combination Treatments: As GLP-1R agonists and basal insulins propose corresponding pharmacological impacts on the prandial and fasting glycemia, there is a growing clinical concern in the combinations of these two agents. The combination of exenatide (10 mg b.i.d.) with insulin glargine (a basal long-acting insulin approved in the U.S. and Europe) showed decrease in HbA1c levels, associated with insulin glargine only (−1.74% *vs.* −1.04%). Therapy including exenatide with insulin glargine led to a weight decline of −1.8 kg, although insulin glargine only headed to a weight boost of 1.0 kg [55]. Liraglutide combined with insulin degludec (IDegLira) certified in Europe is an alternative blend presently being examined for the therapy of T2D. Preliminary medical data indicate that IDegLira caused larger cuts in HbA1c (−1.9%) against insulin degludec (−1.4%) or liraglutide (−1.3%) alone. It was also found that IDegLira offered a moderate weight reduction of −0.5 kg from standard line to week 26, a −2.2-kg decrease, associated by insulin degludec [56].

2.3. Hyperthyroidism

The thyroid hormone is one of the most important chemical messengers within the body. It performs a plethora of physiological functions within the body from regulating metabolic rate to regulating temperature homeostasis and metamorphosis. Hyperthyroidism is one of the most common type of thyroid disease. Its classical presentation is called Graves' Disease and is caused by multiple factors such as complications in the Hypothalamus-pituitary, thyroid axis or adenomas [46]. Multiple treatment regimens have been developed to treat the aforementioned table that have been stated in Table **15.3**.

2.4. Methimazole/Triiodothyronine

A clinical study was conducted by Raber and colleagues in 2000 where they compared the efficacy of Methimazole/ Triiodothyronine fixed dose combination with Methimazole alone in treating the classical clinical manifestation of Hyperthyroidism-Graves' Disease. After observing a total of 112 patients out 135 for 12 months, the investigators did not observe a significant difference in remission of hyperthyroidism in patients given the fdc and patients given Methimazole alone [57].

Table 15.3. Pharmacological Monotherapy against Hyperthyroidism.

Drug Class	Mechanism of Action	Example
Iodide uptake Inhibitors	**Reduce frequency of the uptake I⁻ at the Na⁺/I⁻ symporter of the Thyroid Follicular Cells**	**Perchlorate, thiocyanate, pertechnetate**
Iodides	Reduce expression of Na^+/I^- symporter and hence reduce uptake of Iodine need to synthesize the Thyroid hormone. This phenomenon is called Wolff-Checkoff Effect	Radioactive Iodide($^{131}I^-$) and Inorganic stable Iodide ($^{127}I^-$)
Thionamides	Inhibit thyroid Peroxidase enzyme to prevent central and peripheral Thyroid Hormone synthesis	Propylthiouracil, Methimazole

Recombinant TSH/Radioiodine: Radioiodine is mainly used to treat patients with severe Goiter. Radioiodine works by releasing toxic β-particles that in turn cause destruction of Thyroid Follicular cells responsible for producing T3/T4. Recombinant TSH has been suggested as an add-on to improve the efficacy of radioiodine. An investigation was conducted to test this claim. A 2-year placebo-controlled trial was carried out using 26 Female and 2 Male patients with multinodular Goiter (MND). The patients were divided into three groups: 0.1mg rhTSH (A), 0.005mg rhTSH (B) or placebo (C). A stable activity of 1.11 GBq of (131) I was dispensed 24 h later placebo or rhTSH. The results showed that low doses of rTSH 0.005 and 0.1mg are safe, well tolerated and can be used in conjunction with radioiodine as the efficacy of radioiodine in treating MND increases [58].

Levothyroxine/Radioiodine: Another investigation was carried out where the efficacy of two fixed dose combinations levothyroxine with 150mg iodide *versus* 100mg levothyroxine joint with 100mg iodide was established. 49 individuals with euthyroid goiter; 25 men, 24 women, of age 20-43 years were cured for 12 weeks in a double-blind trial [16] revealing that together fixed dose combinations are equally effective in treating the disease.

3. SURGICAL TREATMENT

3.1. Bariatric Treatment

3.1.1. Diabesity

Gastric bypass and other weight-loss surgical treatment together is known as bariatric surgery which includes creating adjustments to the digestive system to help accelerate weight-loss. Bariatric surgery is done when nutrition and physical activity have not worked or when have severe health complications have occurred due to weight. Certain procedures restrict how much one can eat, whereas other techniques work by lowering the body's capability to absorb nutrients.

In the case of diabesity, the complexity of T2D coupled with obesity makes it difficult for conventional pharmacological therapy to be effective. Bariatric surgery, on the other hand, has shown promise. A recent clinical trial was conducted by Philip R Schauer (2012) where the usefulness of bariatric surgery in overweight individuals with diabetes was compared with Intensive Medical Therapy. They examined the efficiency of intensive medical therapy only *vs* therapeutic treatment plus Roux-en-Y gastric bypass or sleeve gastrectomy in 150 obese subjects with uncontrolled T2D [59]. Of the 150 patients, 93% finished 12 months of follow-up which revealed that the glycemic control got better in all three study groups, with an average glycated hemoglobin level (HbA1c) of 7.5±1.8% in the medical-therapy set, 6.4±0.9% in the gastric bypass set, and 6.6±1.0% in the sleeve gastrectomy set. Reduction of weight was found to be larger in the gastric bypass group and sleeve gastrectomy group (−29.4±9.0 kg and −25.1±8.5 kg, correspondingly) than in the medical-therapy group (−5.4±8.0 kg). The usage of drugs to reduce the glucose, lipid, and blood-pressure levels reduced subsequent to both surgical methods, also improved in patients obtaining medical therapy alone.

Another randomized trial was conducted out to research the special effects of surgical treatment in perversely obese adolescents with T2D by Inge and collaborators. They conducted a secondary investigation of data collected by the Teen Longitudinal Assessment of Bariatric Surgery (Teen LABS) and Treatment Options of Type 2 Diabetes in Adolescents and Youth (TODAY). Their results indicated that the average hemoglobin A1c concentration reduced from 6.8% to 5.5% in Teen LABS and risen from 6.4%-7.8% in TODAY [60]. This led to an inference that the overall glycemic control and weight loss was much more significant in individuals undergoing bariatric surgery than those who did not. However, the immediate effects of bariatric surgery are not sufficient to make a reasonable conclusion. The long-term benefits and/or harm must also be taken into consideration. A study was conducted in 2018 where the progress of obese affected people with T2D was tracked 3 years after bariatric surgery was conducted. The degree of glycemic control and weight loss was traced in 15 male and 23 female patients who had undergone Roux-en-Y gastric bypass (RYGB) surgical procedure *vs* intensive medical diabetes and management of the weight. The results showed that the RYGB group exhibited greater Glycemic control, weight deficit and lower cardiovascular risk than the IMWM group [61].

Alongside RYGB, EndoBarrier® has been developed as an alternative to pharmacotherapy for individuals suffering from obesity and T2D both. The treatment is essentially a duodenal-jejunal sleeve bypass surgery. In a study 45 patients were recruited, and 31 subjects (69%) finished the 1-year study interval. Considerable declines in weight and BMI were recorded 1-year after the device introduction had been effectively finalized. The mean HbA1c was substantially diminished followed by device insertion phase and decreases in metabolic factors such as fasting insulin and glucose points were also recorded during the research. Harmful measures were also evaluated in all subjects, the massive dissimilarity of which were described as slight [62]. Furthermore, it was also reported that use of traditional pharmacological treatment was mostly reduced and, in some cases, discontinued in patients that had opted to undergo the bariatric treatment.

3.1.2. Dyslipidemia

Coronary Heart Disease (CHD) is the prominent reason of mortality worldwide, where its incidence has been correlated with elevated levels of low-density lipoproteins (LDL) and triglycerides. There are various lipids that are metabolized, synthesized, and circulated in the body some of which are beneficial, rest maybe harmful. The order decreasing atherogenicity (ability to cause atherosclerotic heart disease) of clinically relevant lipids are LDL, chylomicrons, and High-Density Lipoprotein (HDL). Several drugs have been developed to treat dyslipidemia which are available as mono-therapeutic agents and some pharmacological classes are used in fixed dose combinations as well. Table **15.4** outlines the drugs used to treat dyslipidemia and how the drugs play role in lipid metabolism.

Table 15.4. Pharmacological Monotherapy against Dyslipidemia.

Drug Class	Example	Mechanism of Action	Therapeutic Use
HMG-coA reductase inhibitors/statins	Atorvastin, Simvastatin, Rosuvastatin	Inhibits the enzyme HMG coA reductase that catalyzes rate determining step of cholesterol synthesis	Reduces LDL Cholesterol
Niacin	Niacin	Inhibits hepatic and intracellular Lipolysis	Increases HDL Cholesterol
Fibrates	Gemfibrozil, Fenofibrate	Binds to PPARs to facilitate expression of Lipoprotein Lipase and apo AI and Apo AII	Decreases serum Triglycerides
Bile acid sequestrants	Cholestyramine, Colesevalem, Colestipol	Anion exchange resins that attach to bile-acids and bile salts enhancing their biliary excretion	Reduces LDL Cholesterol
Cholesterol absorption inhibitors	Ezetemibe	Prevents absorption of dietary cholesterol in the small intestine	Reduces LDL Cholesterol
Proprotein convertase subtilisin kexin type9 inhibitors	Alirocumab, Evolocumab	Prevents the break-down of LDL-C self-surface receptor by PCSK-9 enzyme	Reduces LDL Cholesterol
Omega 3 fatty acids	Docosahexaenoic Acid, Eicosaptenoic Acid	Nutritive	Reduces serum Triglyceride

4. GENE THERAPY

4.1. Leptin Gene Therapy

4.1.1. Diabetes

Exploration in gene transferal approaches to create interventional remedies for numerous neural illnesses has progressed at a swift rate. It is currently possible to introduce genes into cells to substitute an absent gene to modify or increase the target gene function to heal or decelerate the development of recurring ailments due to genomic abnormalities, environmental upsets and metabolic inequality.

Leptin gene therapy has entered pre-clinical trials where the central leptin therapy is being investigated for treatment in diabetic mice. Promising results have been seen in a study performed by Kojima *et al.*, (2009) which shows that after 2-3 weeks of injecting diabetic mice intracerebroventricularly a shot of recombinant adeno-associated virus vector leptin gene (rAAV-lep), it was observed that glucose levels in the blood of rAAV-lep mice began to retreat intensely by week 2-3 to coming back to normal by week 8. Moreover, the mice that were provided rAAV-lep injection did not display any observable adverse behavioral alterations or diabetic problems and the results also hinted at a restricted reappearance of pancreatic β cell function [63]. However, unanticipated side effects have been observed prompting further investigation.

4.1.2. Diabesity

For the treatment of diabesity, a pre-clinical study was carried out at the University of Chicago where the investigators used the *ob/ob* mice. These mice lack the gene for leptin and exhibited classical symptoms of diabesity. Using recombinant adenovirus vectors, the *ob/ob* gene was successfully restored in the mice. Significant improvement was observed in leptin serum levels as well as the symptoms of diabesity were also found to alleviate. The investigation proved that the *ob/ob* gene is an essential regulator of leptin levels which in-turn controls metabolism [64].

4.2. ZFN Gene Editing

Muco-polysaccharidoses (MPS) are a group of hereditary metabolic diseases where the crucial enzymes engaged in the lysosomal dependent degradation of glycosaminoglycans (GAGs) are either absent or malfunctioned. MPS I and II requires the a-L-iduronidase (IDUA) in addition to iduronate-2-sulfatase (IDS) enzymes, to function properly. Affected patients endure from multi-systemic indications and decreased life probability which can fluctuate subjecting on the type of MPS and the seriousness of the disease related variant [65].

Zinc finger nucleases (ZFNs) belong to a group of engineered DNA binding proteins that enable affected editing of the genome by producing double strand stops in DNA at user specific sites as shown in Fig. **3**. For the cure of muco-polysaccharidoses *via* gene editing ZFNs have demonstrated to be a useful approach. Sharma *et al.*, (2015) showed how site-specific incorporation of a transgene in the liver could be performed by *in-vivo* genome editing after intravenous administration using Adeno-associated virus (AAV) as the method of delivery [66]. Integration of transgenes into the albumin locus is challenging. Lately, Laoharawee *et al.*, (2018) performed an *in-vivo* experiment with the insertion of human IDS in the albumin locus of the mice liver mediated by ZFNs, which was also complemented by a dose-dependent rise in the circulating enzyme levels [67]. This IDS insertion triggered decrease of GAG level in the tissue and urine samples of MPS II mice. These findings have preceded to clinical trials exploring the safety of rising dosage concentrations of AAV vectors comprising constituents mandatory for ZFN mediated insertion of IDUA and IDS gene *in-vivo* into albumin locus of hepatocytes in liver of MPS I plus MPS II patients, individually [68]. Queries persist with regard to security owing to the off target double stranded breaks created in the genome with subsequent long-term exposure of individual to the uninhibited activity of ZNF dependent double stranded ends

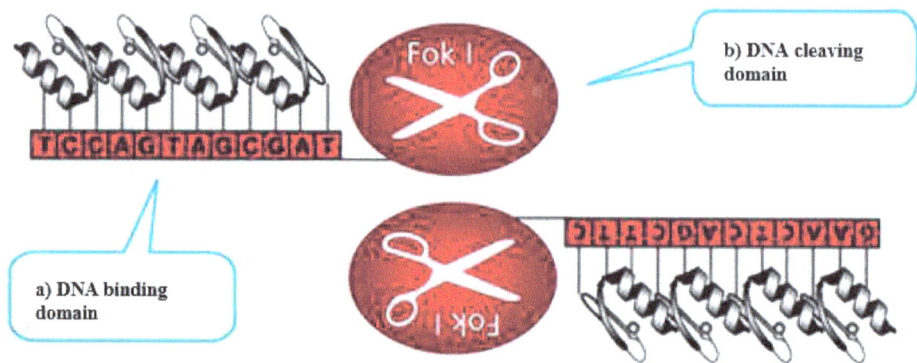

Fig. (15.3). Each ZFN comprises of two functional domains: a) DNA binding domain, b) DNA cleaving domain. First oneconsists of a sequence of two finger modules which are responsible for recognizing a unique hexamer (6 bp) sequence of DNA respectively. Both finger modules sew up reciprocally to form a ≥ 24 bpspecific zinc finger protein.The second oneincludes a nuclease domain of Fok I, which works together with the other domain to arrange like scissors.

4.3. CRISPR/ Cas9 Genome Editing

Modifying germline cells using CRISPR/ Cas9 editing has led to the creation of new animal prototypes which show promising results of how metabolic disorders can be treated. It works by deleting the disease-causing gene segment which can be identified using complementary guide RNA with the help of cas9 protein, and replacing it with the normal sequence which may eventually reverse the disease, as shown in Fig. (**4**). For treatment of MPS I, CRISPR Cas9 has been effectively utilized *in-vivo* using liposome mediated delivery and developed in enhanced IDUA expression in new-born MPS I murine [69]. Otherwise, direct addition of gene utilizing the AAV vectors (without gene editing) has been proven achievable in pre-clinical surveys for numerous MPS types [70 - 73]. This approach is being examined in various clinical trials, and latest findings using intra-cerebral delivery demonstrated promising consequences in treating the neurological deterioration of individuals with MPS IIIB [74].

A recent study shows that producing somatic mutations in murine liver cells *via* CRISPR/ Cas9 technique can create a unique model to study metabolic disease. They reveal that AAV-CRISPR can be utilized to obstruct a vital metabolic gene; low-density lipoprotein receptor (Ldlr) in mouse liver, thereby inducing atherosclerosis and hypercholesterolemia. Disrupting another metabolic gene Apolipoprotein B (ApoB) lowers the plasma cholesterol levels as a compensation thereby protecting atherosclerosis and aggravating the accumulation of hepatic fat subsequently. This model can be further used to study metabolic phenotypes using disruption of specific genes using CRISPR/ Cas9 method [75].

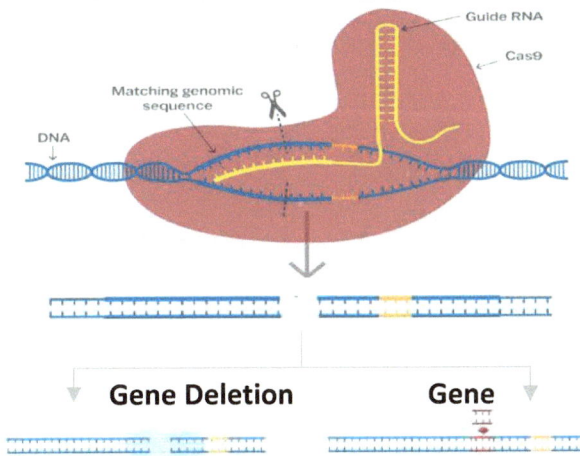

Fig. (15.4). Crispr Cas9 Gene Editing System- there are 3 components to this system namely the CRISPR RNA (crRNA), Trans-activating RNA that forms the RNA-protein complex that is needed to carry-out the immune function, CAS9 protein a multifunctional endonuclease. The endonuclease is responsible for introducing a dsbreak in the DNA of the foreign invader into various fragments.

5. GOAL OF THERAPY

Keeping in mind the discussion above, it is reasonable to suggest that the goal of the pharmacotherapy *i.e.*, polypill for ASCVD, and Fixed Dose combination is to make better the overall quality of living, decrease rate of the disease progression and prevent the onset of any future life-threatening pathology. Bariatric strategy and leptin gene therapy are treatment strategies reserved for more common metabolic disorders but only when pharmacological treatment fails, or the patient needs immediate intervention. The usage of ZFN and CRISPR Cas9 gene-therapy, albeit being mostly conducted in animal models mostly, demonstrates a "Normandy" approach where the underlying cause of the disease is the target and complete reversal in the defects at molecular and cellular level are intended to restore normal physiological function. The approach, despite being theoretically the best strategy, requires complete understanding of the condition at hand and how the condition pertains to each patient before it can be considered as an option to use. Moreover, adverse effects at the cellular and molecular such as off-target gene editing must be reduced to a minimum if not completely removed for the treatment to be considered safe enough for clinical use.

CONCLUDING REMARKS

Considering the aforementioned practices at both clinical and pre-clinical level, it is evident that significant strides have been conducted in both controlling and eradicating metabolic diseases. However, it is also evident that the complete pathophysiology of multiple diseases such as Type2 Diabetes is still unknown. FDC pharmacological therapy has been established to mainly carry out three major functions:

1. Induce prophylaxis and decrease the risk of the development of metabolic disorders as evidenced by the polypill therapy for Atherosclerotic Cardiovascular Disease [20, 43, 44, 53] and Pharmacotherapy for Hypercholesteremia [15, 76 - 79].
2. Reduce the advancement of disease and associated co-morbidities as observed in Anti-Diabetic therapy [14, 48 - 51].
3. Carry out symptomatic control and improve standard of living. It can be stated that the fixed dose combination therapy has proven to be more beneficial in terms of cost, patient compliance, therapeutic efficacy and has shown a similar of not improved safety profile as compared to traditional monotherapy in clinical practice.

Alongside pharmacological therapy, surgical intervention has been investigated as mentioned in the Bariatric Surgery section above. It has been observed that surgical intervention is preferred only when pharmacological therapy fails or when the disease has overwhelming complications or where the pharmacological agents used to treat one disease worsens the other as is in the case of Diabesity. The goal of therapy is, however, complete eradication of the metabolic disorder with little to no need for the use of drugs after the surgical procedure is complete. Still, it must be kept in mind that extensive work is required to achieve this goal. Furthermore, logistical, and patient centric factors such as cost, patient compliance and probability of failure still have to be addressed before the strategy can be considered viable for widespread use. Also, making the technology accessible not only in the first world but also in the second and third world countries where the aforementioned logistical problems are much more intricate and deeper rooted is a challenge that has to be taken up and solved.

Gene editing, mainly Leptin gene therapy and ZFN therapy, is mainly reserved for those metabolic disorders where the root cause partially or wholly is defects within the central dogma. Mutations in the genome and transcriptome of the patient eventually lead to the clinical manifestations of diseases, blood disorders and immunological deficiencies discussed above. The progression of these diseases is very rapid and there is no pharmacological cure. The main aim of this therapeutic approach is to completely rid the patient of the disease. A similar objective is that of the aforementioned CRISPR Cas9 gene surgery technique.

The problem, yet still, for the gene editing strategy is that most studies are still in the pre-clinical phase. Even though the development of humanized animal models has greatly improved our ability to understand complex disorders, it is still not enough. Furthermore, each gene editing strategy will have to be tailored according to the exact etiology of the patient's condition, bumping up costs. Challenges for example a lack of delivery system and side effects such as off-target gene editing, immunological responses to viral vectors are also issues that need to be addressed before the treatment modality can become market ready and distributed at a large scale to the mass populace.

CONSENT FOR PUBLICATION

Not applicable.

CONFLICT OF INTEREST

The author declares no conflict of interest, financial or otherwise.

ACKNOWLEDGEMENTS

Declared none.

REFERENCES

[1]   Wang HH, Lee DK, Liu M, Portincasa P, Wang DQH. Novel insights into the pathogenesis and management of the metabolic syndrome. Pediatr Gastroenterol Hepatol Nutr 2020; 23(3): 189-230.
        [http://dx.doi.org/10.5223/pghn.2020.23.3.189] [PMID: 32483543]

[2]   Grundy SM. Metabolic syndrome update. Trends Cardiovasc Med 2016; 26(4): 364-73.
        [http://dx.doi.org/10.1016/j.tcm.2015.10.004] [PMID: 26654259]

[3]   Laurent Genser M, Mariolo JRC, Rubino F. Obesity, Type 2 Diabetes, and the Metabolic Syndrome. Metabolic and Bariatric Surgery, An Issue of Surgical Clinics of North America. E-Book 2016; 96: 681.

[4]   Alberti KGMM, Zimmet P, Shaw J. IDF Epidemiology Task Force Consensus Group. The metabolic syndrome—a new worldwide definition. Lancet 2005; 366(9491): 1059-62.
        [http://dx.doi.org/10.1016/S0140-6736(05)67402-8] [PMID: 16182882]

[5]   Kylin E. Studien ueber das Hypertonie-Hyperglyka" mie-Hyperurika" miesyndrom. Zentralblatt für innere Medizin 1923; 44: 105-27.

[6]   Reaven GM. Banting lecture 1988. Role of insulin resistance in human disease. Diabetes 1988; 37(12): 1595-607.
        [http://dx.doi.org/10.2337/diab.37.12.1595] [PMID: 3056758]

[7]   Kaplan NM. The deadly quartet. Upper-body obesity, glucose intolerance, hypertriglyceridemia, and hypertension. Arch Intern Med 1989; 149(7): 1514-20.
        [http://dx.doi.org/10.1001/archinte.1989.00390070054005] [PMID: 2662932]

[8]   Ferrannini E. The ivsulin resistance syndrome. Curr Opin Nephrol Hypertens 1992; 1(2): 291-8.
        [http://dx.doi.org/10.1097/00041552-199212000-00015] [PMID: 1345629]

[9]   Huang PL. A comprehensive definition for metabolic syndrome. Dis Model Mech 2009; 2(5-6): 231-7.
        [http://dx.doi.org/10.1242/dmm.001180] [PMID: 19407331]

[10]   Julibert A, Bibiloni M, Bouzas C, *et al.* Predimed-Plus Investigators. Total and subtypes of dietary fat intake and its association with components of the metabolic syndrome in a mediterranean population at high cardiovascular risk. Nutrients 2019; 11(7): 1493.
        [http://dx.doi.org/10.3390/nu11071493] [PMID: 31261967]

[11]   Cornier MA, Dabelea D, Hernandez TL, *et al.* The metabolic syndrome. Endocr Rev 2008; 29(7): 777-822.
        [http://dx.doi.org/10.1210/er.2008-0024] [PMID: 18971485]

[12]   Green M, Arora K, Prakash S. Microbial medicine: Prebiotic and probiotic functional foods to target obesity and metabolic syndrome. Int J Mol Sci 2020; 21(8): 2890.
        [http://dx.doi.org/10.3390/ijms21082890] [PMID: 32326175]

[13]   Goodarzi MO, Taylor KD, Guo X, *et al.* Haplotypes in the lipoprotein lipase gene influence fasting insulin and discovery of a new risk haplotype. J Clin Endocrinol Metab 2007; 92(1): 293-6.
        [http://dx.doi.org/10.1210/jc.2006-1195] [PMID: 17032721]

[14]   Aoki C, Suzuki K, Kuroda H, *et al.* Fixed-dose combination of alogliptin/pioglitazone improves glycemic control in Japanese patients with type 2 diabetes mellitus independent of body mass index. Nagoya J Med Sci 2017; 79(1): 9-16.
        [PMID: 28303056]

[15]   Arai H, Yamashita S, Yokote K, Araki E, Suganami H, Ishibashi S. K-877 Study Group. Efficacy and safety of K-877, a novel selective peroxisome proliferator-activated receptor α modulator (SPPARMα), in combination with statin treatment: Two randomised, double-blind, placebo-controlled clinical trials in patients with dyslipidaemia. Atherosclerosis 2017; 261: 144-52.
        [http://dx.doi.org/10.1016/j.atherosclerosis.2017.03.032] [PMID: 28410749]

[16]   Förster G, Krummenauer F, Hansen C, Beyer J, Kahaly G. Individually dosed levothyroxine with 150 micrograms iodide versus 100 micrograms levothyroxine combined with 100 micrograms iodide. A randomized double-blind trial. Deutsche Medizinische Wochenschrift 1998; 123(22): 685-9.

[17]   Wang Q, Zheng D, Liu J, Fang L, Li Q. Skeletal muscle mass to visceral fat area ratio is an important determinant associated with type 2 diabetes and metabolic syndrome. Diabetes Metab Syndr Obes 2019; 12: 1399-407.
        [http://dx.doi.org/10.2147/DMSO.S211529] [PMID: 31616170]

[18]   Reaven GM. The metabolic syndrome: is this diagnosis necessary? Am J Clin Nutr 2006; 83(6): 1237-47.
        [http://dx.doi.org/10.1093/ajcn/83.6.1237] [PMID: 16762930]

[19]   Meigs JB, Rutter MK, Sullivan LM, Fox CS, D'Agostino RB Sr, Wilson PWF. Impact of insulin resistance on risk of type 2 diabetes and cardiovascular disease in people with metabolic syndrome. Diabetes Care 2007; 30(5): 1219-25.
        [http://dx.doi.org/10.2337/dc06-2484] [PMID: 17259468]

[20]   Nowrouzi-Sohrabi P, Hassanipour S, Sisakht M, Daryabeygi-Khotbehsara R, Savardashtaki A, Fathalipour M. The effectiveness of pistachio on glycemic control and insulin sensitivity in patients

with type 2 diabetes, prediabetes and metabolic syndrome: A systematic review and meta-analysis. Diabetes Metab Syndr 2020; 14(5): 1589-95.
[http://dx.doi.org/10.1016/j.dsx.2020.07.052] [PMID: 32947760]

[21]   Jeppesen J, Hansen TW, Rasmussen S, Ibsen H, Torp-Pedersen C, Madsbad S. Insulin resistance, the metabolic syndrome, and risk of incident cardiovascular disease: a population-based study. J Am Coll Cardiol 2007; 49(21): 2112-9.
[http://dx.doi.org/10.1016/j.jacc.2007.01.088] [PMID: 17531661]

[22]   Syauqy A, Hsu CY, Rau HH, Chao J. Association of dietary patterns with components of metabolic syndrome and inflammation among middle-aged and older adults with metabolic syndrome in Taiwan. Nutrients 2018; 10(2): 143.
[http://dx.doi.org/10.3390/nu10020143] [PMID: 29382113]

[23]   Hong Y, Jin X, Mo J, *et al.* Metabolic syndrome, its preeminent clusters, incident coronary heart disease and all-cause mortality? results of prospective analysis for the Atherosclerosis Risk in Communities study. J Intern Med 2007; 262(1): 113-22.
[http://dx.doi.org/10.1111/j.1365-2796.2007.01781.x] [PMID: 17598819]

[24]   Golabi P, Otgonsuren M, de Avila L, Sayiner M, Rafiq N, Younossi ZM. Components of metabolic syndrome increase the risk of mortality in nonalcoholic fatty liver disease (NAFLD). Medicine (Baltimore) 2018; 97(13): e0214.
[http://dx.doi.org/10.1097/MD.0000000000010214] [PMID: 29595666]

[25]   Organization WH. Definition, diagnosis and classification of diabetes mellitus and its complications: report of a WHO consultation Part 1, Diagnosis and classification of diabetes mellitus. World Health Organization 1999.

[26]   Balkau B, Charles M-A. European Group for the Study of Insulin Resistance (EGIR). Comment on the provisional report from the WHO consultation. Diabet Med 1999; 16(5): 442-3.
[http://dx.doi.org/10.1046/j.1464-5491.1999.00059.x] [PMID: 10342346]

[27]   Park YW, Zhu S, Palaniappan L, Heshka S, Carnethon MR, Heymsfield SB. The metabolic syndrome: prevalence and associated risk factor findings in the US population from the Third National Health and Nutrition Examination Survey, 1988-1994. Arch Intern Med 2003; 163(4): 427-36.
[http://dx.doi.org/10.1001/archinte.163.4.427] [PMID: 12588201]

[28]   Grundy SM, Neeland IJ, Turer AT, Vega GL. Waist circumference as measure of abdominal fat compartments. J Obes 2013; 2013: 1-9.
[http://dx.doi.org/10.1155/2013/454285] [PMID: 23762536]

[29]   Tchernof A, Després JP. Pathophysiology of human visceral obesity: an update. Physiol Rev 2013; 93(1): 359-404.
[http://dx.doi.org/10.1152/physrev.00033.2011] [PMID: 23303913]

[30]   Karpe F, Pinnick KE. Biology of upper-body and lower-body adipose tissue—link to whole-body phenotypes. Nat Rev Endocrinol 2015; 11(2): 90-100.
[http://dx.doi.org/10.1038/nrendo.2014.185] [PMID: 25365922]

[31]   Shulman GI. Ectopic fat in insulin resistance, dyslipidemia, and cardiometabolic disease. N Engl J Med 2014; 371(12): 1131-41.
[http://dx.doi.org/10.1056/NEJMra1011035] [PMID: 25229917]

[32]   Goldberg RB, Mather K. Targeting the consequences of the metabolic syndrome in the Diabetes Prevention Program. Arterioscler Thromb Vasc Biol 2012; 32(9): 2077-90.
[http://dx.doi.org/10.1161/ATVBAHA.111.241893] [PMID: 22895669]

[33]   Baigent C, Blackwell L, Emberson J, *et al.* Efficacy and safety of more intensive lowering of LDL cholesterol: a meta-analysis of data from 170,000 participants in 26 randomised trials. Elsevier 2010.

[34]   Clarenbach JJ, Grundy SM, Palacio N, Lena Vega G. Relationship of apolipoprotein B levels to the number of risk factors for metabolic syndrome. J Investig Med 2007; 55(5): 237-47.

[http://dx.doi.org/10.2310/6650.2007.00004] [PMID: 17850735]

[35]   Grundy SM. Pre-diabetes, metabolic syndrome, and cardiovascular risk. J Am Coll Cardiol 2012; 59(7): 635-43.
       [http://dx.doi.org/10.1016/j.jacc.2011.08.080] [PMID: 22322078]

[36]   Kim HS, Abbasi F, Lamendola C, McLaughlin T, Reaven GM. Effect of insulin resistance on postprandial elevations of remnant lipoprotein concentrations in postmenopausal women. Am J Clin Nutr 2001; 74(5): 592-5.
       [http://dx.doi.org/10.1093/ajcn/74.5.592] [PMID: 11684526]

[37]   Weisberg SP, Hunter D, Huber R, *et al.* CCR2 modulates inflammatory and metabolic effects of high-fat feeding. J Clin Invest 2006; 116(1): 115-24.
       [http://dx.doi.org/10.1172/JCI24335] [PMID: 16341265]

[38]   Laugerette F, Alligier M, Bastard JP, *et al.* Overfeeding increases postprandial endotoxemia in men: Inflammatory outcome may depend on LPS transporters LBP and sCD14. Mol Nutr Food Res 2014; 58(7): 1513-8.
       [http://dx.doi.org/10.1002/mnfr.201400044] [PMID: 24687809]

[39]   Terán-García M, Bouchard C. Genetics of the metabolic syndrome. Appl Physiol Nutr Metab 2007; 32(1): 89-114.
       [http://dx.doi.org/10.1139/h06-102] [PMID: 17332787]

[40]   Stančáková A, Laakso M. Genetics of metabolic syndrome. Rev Endocr Metab Disord 2014; 15(4): 243-52.
       [http://dx.doi.org/10.1007/s11154-014-9293-9] [PMID: 25124343]

[41]   Rodgers A, Patel A, Berwanger O, *et al.* PILL Collaborative Group. An international randomised placebo-controlled trial of a four-component combination pill ("polypill") in people with raised cardiovascular risk. In: Wright JM, Ed. PLoS One 2011; 6(5): e19857.
       [http://dx.doi.org/10.1371/journal.pone.0019857] [PMID: 21647425]

[42]   Patel A, Cass A, Peiris D, *et al.* Kanyini Guidelines Adherence with the Polypill (Kanyini GAP) Collaboration. A pragmatic randomized trial of a polypill-based strategy to improve use of indicated preventive treatments in people at high cardiovascular disease risk. Eur J Prev Cardiol 2015; 22(7): 920-30.
       [http://dx.doi.org/10.1177/2047487314530382] [PMID: 24676715]

[43]   Muñoz D, Uzoije P, Reynolds C, *et al.* Polypill for Cardiovascular Disease Prevention in an Underserved Population. N Engl J Med 2019; 381(12): 1114-23.
       [http://dx.doi.org/10.1056/NEJMoa1815359] [PMID: 31532959]

[44]   Soliman EZ, Mendis S, Dissanayake WP, *et al.* A Polypill for primary prevention of cardiovascular disease: A feasibility study of the World Health Organization. Trials 2011; 12(1): 3.
       [http://dx.doi.org/10.1186/1745-6215-12-3] [PMID: 21205325]

[45]   Schmidt AM. Highlighting Diabetes Mellitus. Arterioscler Thromb Vasc Biol 2018; 38(1): e1-8.
       [http://dx.doi.org/10.1161/ATVBAHA.117.310221] [PMID: 29282247]

[46]   Mencher S R, Frank G, Fishbein J. Diabetic ketoacidosis at onset of type 1 diabetes: rates and risk factors today to 15 years ago. 2019.

[47]   Pearson ER. Type 2 diabetes: a multifaceted disease. Diabetologia 2019; 62(7): 1107-12.
       [http://dx.doi.org/10.1007/s00125-019-4909-y] [PMID: 31161345]

[48]   Kawamori R, Haneda M, Suzaki K, *et al.* Empagliflozin as add-on to linagliptin in a fixed-dose combination in Japanese patients with type 2 diabetes: Glycaemic efficacy and safety profile in a 52-week, randomized, placebo-controlled trial. Diabetes Obes Metab 2018; 20(9): 2200-9.
       [http://dx.doi.org/10.1111/dom.13352] [PMID: 29766636]

[49]   Park SI, Lee H, Oh J, *et al.* A fixed-dose combination tablet of gemigliptin and metformin sustained release has comparable pharmacodynamic, pharmacokinetic, and tolerability profiles to separate

tablets in healthy subjects. Drug Des Devel Ther 2015; 9: 729-36.
[http://dx.doi.org/10.2147/DDDT.S75980] [PMID: 25678778]

[50] Oh TJ, Yu JM, Min KW, *et al.* Efficacy and Safety of Voglibose Plus Metformin in Patients with Type 2 Diabetes Mellitus: A Randomized Controlled Trial. Diabetes Metab J 2019; 43(3): 276-86.
[http://dx.doi.org/10.4093/dmj.2018.0051] [PMID: 30604594]

[51] Seino Y, Kaneko S, Fukuda S, *et al.* Combination therapy with liraglutide and insulin in Japanese patients with type 2 diabetes: A 36-week, randomized, double-blind, parallel-group trial. J Diabetes Investig 2016; 7(4): 565-73.
[http://dx.doi.org/10.1111/jdi.12457] [PMID: 27182042]

[52] Park CY, Kang JG, Chon S, *et al.* Comparison between the therapeutic effect of metformin, glimepiride and their combination as an add-on treatment to insulin glargine in uncontrolled patients with type 2 diabetes. PLoS One 2014; 9(3): e87799.
[http://dx.doi.org/10.1371/journal.pone.0087799] [PMID: 24614911]

[53] Leitner D R, Frühbeck G, Yumuk V, *et al.* Obesity and Type 2 Diabetes: Two Diseases with a Need for Combined Treatment Strategies – EASO Can Lead the Way. 2017; 10.

[54] Van Gaal L, Scheen A. Weight management in type 2 diabetes: current and emerging approaches to treatment. Diabetes Care 2015; 38(6): 1161-72.
[http://dx.doi.org/10.2337/dc14-1630] [PMID: 25998297]

[55] Buse J B, Bergenstal R M, Glass L C, *et al.* Use of Twice-Daily Exenatide in Basal Insulin–Treated Patients With Type 2 Diabetes. 2011; 12.

[56] Buse JB, Gough SC, Woo VC, Rodbard HW, Linjawi S, Poulsen P. Da mgaard, L. H., & Bode, B. W.. IDegLira, a Novel Fixed Ratio Combination of Insulin Degludec and Liraglutide, is Efficacious and Safe in Subjects with Type 2 Diabetes: A Large, Randomized Phase 3 Trial (65-OR). Nederlands Tijdschrift Voor Diabetologie 2013; 11(3): 74-5.
[http://dx.doi.org/10.1007/s12467-013-0026-6]

[57] Raber W, Kmen E, Waldhäusl W, Vierhapper H. Medical therapy of Graves' disease: effect on remission rates of methimazole alone and in combination with triiodothyronine. Eur J Endocrinol 2000; 142(2): 117-24.
[http://dx.doi.org/10.1530/eje.0.1420117] [PMID: 10664518]

[58] Cubas ER, Paz-Filho GJ, Olandoski M, *et al.* Recombinant human TSH increases the efficacy of a fixed activity of radioiodine for treatment of multinodular goitre. Int J Clin Pract 2009; 63(4): 583-90.
[http://dx.doi.org/10.1111/j.1742-1241.2008.01904.x] [PMID: 18803554]

[59] Schauer PR, Kashyap SR, Wolski K, *et al.* Bariatric surgery *versus* intensive medical therapy in obese patients with diabetes. N Engl J Med 2012; 366(17): 1567-76.
[http://dx.doi.org/10.1056/NEJMoa1200225] [PMID: 22449319]

[60] Inge T H, Laffel L M, Jenkins T M, *et al.* Comparison of Surgical and Medical Therapy for Type 2 Diabetes in Severely Obese Adolescents. JAMA Pediatr 2018; 172(5): 452-60.

[61] Simonson DC, Halperin F, Foster K, Vernon A, Goldfine AB. Clinical and Patient-Centered Outcomes in Obese Patients With Type 2 Diabetes 3 Years After Randomization to Roux-en-Y Gastric Bypass Surgery *Versus* Intensive Lifestyle Management: The SLIMM-T2D Study. Diabetes Care 2018; 41(4): 670-9.
[http://dx.doi.org/10.2337/dc17-0487] [PMID: 29432125]

[62] Patel N, Mohanaruban A, Ashrafian H, *et al.* EndoBarrier®: a safe and effective novel treatment for obesity and type 2 diabetes? Obes Surg 2018; 28(7): 1980-9.
[http://dx.doi.org/10.1007/s11695-018-3123-1] [PMID: 29450844]

[63] Kojima S, Asakawa A, Amitani H, *et al.* Central leptin gene therapy, a substitute for insulin therapy to ameliorate hyperglycemia and hyperphagia, and promote survival in insulin-deficient diabetic mice. Peptides 2009; 30(5): 962-6.

[http://dx.doi.org/10.1016/j.peptides.2009.01.007] [PMID: 19428774]

[64]   Muzzin P, Eisensmith RC, Copeland KC, Woo SLC. Correction of obesity and diabetes in genetically obese mice by leptin gene therapy. Proc Natl Acad Sci USA 1996; 93(25): 14804-8.
[http://dx.doi.org/10.1073/pnas.93.25.14804] [PMID: 8962136]

[65]   Sawamoto K, Chen HH, Alméciga-Díaz CJ, Mason RW, Tomatsu S. Gene therapy for Mucopolysaccharidoses. Mol Genet Metab 2018; 123(2): 59-68.
[http://dx.doi.org/10.1016/j.ymgme.2017.12.434] [PMID: 29295764]

[66]   Sharma R, Anguela XM, Doyon Y, *et al. In vivo* genome editing of the albumin locus as a platform for protein replacement therapy. Blood 2015; 126(15): 1777-84.
[http://dx.doi.org/10.1182/blood-2014-12-615492] [PMID: 26297739]

[67]   Laoharawee K, DeKelver RC, Podetz-Pedersen KM, *et al.* Dose-Dependent Prevention of Metabolic and Neurologic Disease in Murine MPS II by ZFN-Mediated *In Vivo* Genome Editing. Mol Ther 2018; 26(4): 1127-36.
[http://dx.doi.org/10.1016/j.ymthe.2018.03.002] [PMID: 29580682]

[68]   Therapeutics Sangamo. A Phase I / 2, Multicenter, Open-label, Single-dose, Dose-ranging Study to Assess the Safety and Tolerability of SB-318, a rAAV2/6-based Gene Transfer in Subjects With Mucopolysaccharidosis I (MPS I) (Clinical Trial Registration No. NCT02702115), 2020.

[69]   Schuh RS, Poletto É, Pasqualim G, *et al.* In vivo genome editing of mucopolysaccharidosis I mice using the CRISPR/Cas9 system. J Control Release 2018; 288: 23-33.
[http://dx.doi.org/10.1016/j.jconrel.2018.08.031] [PMID: 30170069]

[70]   Ellinwood NM, Ausseil J, Desmaris N, *et al.* Safe, efficient, and reproducible gene therapy of the brain in the dog models of Sanfilippo and Hurler syndromes. Mol Ther 2011; 19(2): 251-9.
[http://dx.doi.org/10.1038/mt.2010.265] [PMID: 21139569]

[71]   Fu H, DiRosario J, Killedar S, Zaraspe K, McCarty DM. Correction of neurological disease of mucopolysaccharidosis IIIB in adult mice by rAAV9 trans-blood-brain barrier gene delivery. Mol Ther 2011; 19(6): 1025-33.
[http://dx.doi.org/10.1038/mt.2011.34] [PMID: 21386820]

[72]   Motas S, Haurigot V, Garcia M, *et al.* CNS-directed gene therapy for the treatment of neurologic and somatic mucopolysaccharidosis type II (Hunter syndrome). JCI Insight 2016; 1(9): e86696.
[http://dx.doi.org/10.1172/jci.insight.86696] [PMID: 27699273]

[73]   Sorrentino NC, D'Orsi L, Sambri I, *et al.* A highly secreted sulphamidase engineered to cross the blood-brain barrier corrects brain lesions of mice with mucopolysaccharidoses type IIIA. EMBO Mol Med 2013; 5(5): 675-90.
[http://dx.doi.org/10.1002/emmm.201202083] [PMID: 23568409]

[74]   Tardieu M, Zérah M, Gougeon ML, *et al.* Intracerebral gene therapy in children with mucopolysaccharidosis type IIIB syndrome: an uncontrolled phase 1/2 clinical trial. Lancet Neurol 2017; 16(9): 712-20.
[http://dx.doi.org/10.1016/S1474-4422(17)30169-2] [PMID: 28713035]

[75]   Jarrett KE, Lee CM, Yeh YH, *et al.* Somatic genome editing with CRISPR/Cas9 generates and corrects a metabolic disease. Sci Rep 2017; 7(1): 44624.
[http://dx.doi.org/10.1038/srep44624]

[76]   Gumbiner B, Joh T, Liang H, *et al.* The effects of single- and multiple-dose administration of bococizumab (RN316/PF-04950615), a humanized IgG2Δa monoclonal antibody binding proprotein convertase subtilisin/kexin type 9, in hypercholesterolemic subjects treated with and without atorvastati. Cardiovasc Ther 2018; 36(1): e12309.
[http://dx.doi.org/10.1111/1755-5922.12309] [PMID: 29078037]

[77]   Hong SJ, Jeong HS, Ahn JC, *et al.* A Phase III, Multicenter, Randomized, Double-blind, Active Comparator Clinical Trial to Compare the Efficacy and Safety of Combination Therapy With

Ezetimibe and Rosuvastatin *Versus* Rosuvastatin Monotherapy in Patients With Hypercholesterolemia: I-ROSETTE (Ildong Rosuvastatin & Ezetimibe for Hypercholesterolemia) Randomized Controlled Trial. Clin Ther 2018; 40(2): 226-241.e4.
[http://dx.doi.org/10.1016/j.clinthera.2017.12.018] [PMID: 29402522]

[78]   Tarantino N, Santoro F, De Gennaro L, *et al.* Fenofibrate/simvastatin fixed-dose combination in the treatment of mixed dyslipidemia: safety, efficacy, and place in therapy. Vasc Health Risk Manag 2017; 13: 29-41.
[http://dx.doi.org/10.2147/VHRM.S95044] [PMID: 28243111]

[79]   Kim KJ, Kim SH, Yoon YW, *et al.* Effect of fixed-dose combinations of ezetimibe plus rosuvastatin in patients with primary hypercholesterolemia: MRS-ROZE (Multicenter Randomized Study of ROsuvastatin and eZEtimibe). Cardiovasc Ther 2016; 34(5): 371-82.
[http://dx.doi.org/10.1111/1755-5922.12213] [PMID: 27506635]

CHAPTER 16

Intellectual Disabilities

Zafar Ali[1,*], **Uzma Abdullah**[2] and **Ambrin Fatima**[3]

[1] *Centre for Biotechnology and Microbiology, University of Swat, Swat19130, Pakistan*

[2] *University Institute of Biochemistry and Biotechnology (UIBB), PMAS-Arid Agriculture University, Rawalpindi. Pakistan*

[3] *Department of Biological and Biomedical Sciences. The Aga Khan University, Karachi, Pakistan*

Abstract: Intellectual disability (ID) is caused by the disruption of neurodevelopmental processes. Its diagnosis and severity are defined in terms of an Intelligence Quotient score of ≤ 70. ID has diverse presentations and clinical overlaps with other cognitive disorders such as autism spectrum disorder and microcephaly. ID has a diverse etiology encompassing both environmental and genetic insults to the developing brain. The precise diagnosis is challenging but crucial for prognosis and risk assessment for future pregnancies. The suspected cases of genetic ID often follow a strategic series of tests for diagnosis. There is no effective cure for this disorder except in the cases of early diagnosed metabolic disorders. The available therapies are mostly aimed at easing the symptoms and improving the quality of life.

Keywords: Autism spectrum disorder, Genetic diagnosis, Global developmental delay, Intelligence Quotient, Microcephaly, Neurodevelopment, Supportive therapy.

1. INTRODUCTION

Human brain development is a complex process involving cellular proliferation, differentiation, migration, and integration into a cohesive circuitry. All of these processes are meticulously orchestrated and lead to a highly specialized human brain, capable of processing complex language, cognition, and emotion. On the other hand, any abnormality in these cellular processes results in neurodevelopmental disorder [1]. Intellectual Disability (ID) previously called mental retardation is a neurodevelopmental disorder and manifests as deficient cognitive functioning, adaptive behavior, and social skills compared to individual's age group. It mainly affects three different aspects of an individual's

* **Corresponding author Zafar Ali:** Centre for Biotechnology and Microbiology, University of Swat, Swat 19130, Pakistan; E-mail: zafaralibiotech@gmail.com

Syeda Marriam Bakhtiar and Erum Dilshad (Eds.)

personality; the conceptual aspects such as language, reading, writing, math, reasoning, knowledge, and memory; the social aspects that include empathy, social judgment, interpersonal communication skills, ability to make and retain friendships; the practical aspects concerning personal care, job, money handling, and organizing scholastic tasks.

The terminology used for ID is evolving; "Global Developmental Delay" is being used for children aged less than 5 years having a delay in more than one area of development namely acquisition of motor skills, speech and language, cognition, personal-social activities of daily living [2]. As these delays may be transient, around 2/3 of children diagnosed with global developmental delay may eventually be diagnosed with ID after 5 years of age [3].

The global prevalence of ID is 1-3% in the general population [4], with a higher incidence in males than females. The etiology of ID may be either genetic or non-genetic or environmental factors and both contribute comparably. The non-genetic factors include malnutrition of pregnant mothers or children, infections, toxin exposure, trauma and other obstetric complications, therefore. Genetic causes which account for almost 50% of cases include chromosome abnormalities such as aneuploidies and large deletion or duplications; point mutations and indels (small insertion and deletions) [5]. In either case, the diagnosis can be complicated because of heterogeneity of the disease both clinically and genetically.

2. DIAGNOSIS AND CLASSIFICATION OF ID

The clinical diagnosis of ID is based on an intelligence quotient (IQ) testing. It is a score derived from several different standardized tests designed to assess relative intelligence. These standardized tests include Stanford-Binet Intelligence Scale and the Wechsler Adult Intelligence Scale (WAIS) and are updated time to time. The former is used to access young children and includes both verbal and non-verbal subsets. It tests five factors namely knowledge, quantitative reasoning, visual-spatial processing, working memory, and fluid reasoning, on the other hand, is used for adults and older adolescents.

Its current version (WAIS-IV) consists of four core indexes further divided into five cores and ten supplemental subsets as shown in Fig. (**16.1**). In either case, the score of less than 70 established the diagnosis of ID [5, 7].

```
┌─────────────────────────────────────┐   ┌─────────────────────────────────────┐
│ Verbal Comprehension Index Scale    │   │ Perceptual Reasoning Index Scale    │
│   Core Subtests                     │   │   Core Subtests                     │
│     Similarities                    │   │     Block Design                    │
│     Vocabulary                      │   │     Matrix Reasoning                │
│     Information                     │   │     Visual Puzzles                  │
│   Supplemental Subtest              │   │   Supplemental Subtest              │
│     Comprehension                   │   │     Figure Weights (16-69 only)     │
│                                     │   │     Picture Completion              │
└─────────────────────────────────────┘   └─────────────────────────────────────┘
                              Full Scale
┌─────────────────────────────────────┐   ┌─────────────────────────────────────┐
│ Working Memory Index Scale          │   │ Processing Speed Index Scale        │
│   Core Subtests                     │   │   Core Subtests                     │
│     Digit Span                      │   │     Symbol Search                   │
│     Arithmetic                      │   │     Coding                          │
│   Supplemental Subtest              │   │   Supplemental Subtest              │
│     Letter-Number Sequencing (16-69 only) │     Cancellation (16-69 only)     │
└─────────────────────────────────────┘   └─────────────────────────────────────┘
```

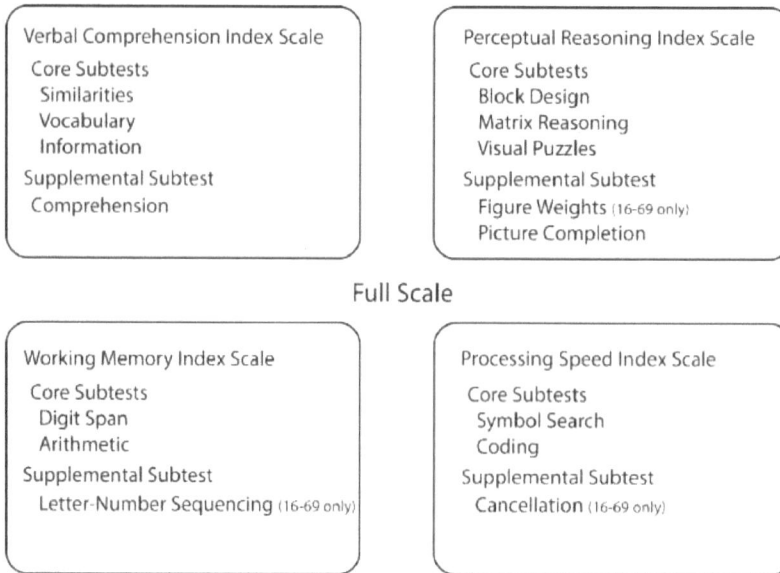

Fig. (16.1). Wechsler Adult Intelligence Scale (WAIS)- IV scale showing core and supplemental subsets of components used for assessment of Intelligence Quotient (Adopted and recreated from Wechsler 2008 [6].

Based on this IQ level, ID is classified into four subtypes. The types are mild (IQ: 55–70), moderate (IQ: 40–55), severe (IQ: 25–40) and profound (IQ< 25). Mild ID is most prevalent, accounting for almost 85% of cases, followed by the moderate ID having 10% of the patients. Severe and profound cases are the least prevalent with only 5% of the patients [8]. Based on inheritance pattern, the monogenic form of ID is divided into autosomal dominant and recessive, x-linked dominant and recessive. On the other hand, ID is grouped into non-syndromic ID and syndromic ID. In case of non-syndromic ID, ID is the sole clinical feature among the patients. While in syndromic ID, affected individuals manifest one or more clinical comorbidities along with ID. The associated comorbidities may be of dysmorphic, neurological, or systemic nature. ID may also co-occur with autism spectrum disorders (ASD), microcephaly [9 - 11].

3. AUTISM SPECTRUM DISORDERS (ASD)

ASD is a neurodevelopmental disease and is characterized by a significant impairment in social and communicative skills and abilities. It is one of the many disorders that co-occur with ID. The prevalence of comorbidity of ID with ASD ranges from 10% to 40% [12, 13]. The clinical phenotype of ASD is extremely heterogeneous in nature ranging from severe ID in patients to individuals having a normal level of IQ. Besides ID, ASD also co-occurs with epilepsy, hyperactivity, sleeping and gastrointestinal problems.

ASD is diagnosed in 1% of the pediatric population with four times higher prevalence in males [14, 15]. The inheritance pattern is complex in ASD and most of the cases follow polygenic inheritance where a combination of multiple genetic variants, each having a low risk for the disease inherits form one generation to the next. These variants are common in the general population as these variants individually do not have any effect on the fitness of the individual. However, a substantial number of cases are reported having Mendelian inheritance, where a single gene variant has a damaging effect on the individual fitness and is able to cause the disease. Cases of incomplete penetrance also exist where the disease causing rare variant is present not only in patients but it may also be present in normal individuals of the family [15].

4. MICROCEPHALY

Microcephaly is a rare disorder characterized by reduced head circumference below three standard deviations of the population mean and accompanies moderate to severe ID [16, 17]. Microcephaly can develop both prenatally and postnatally, called primary (= congenital) microcephaly and acquired or secondary microcephaly respectively. Usually, congenital microcephaly occurs as an isolated birth defect and is called primary microcephaly. It results from defective and insufficient neurogenesis [18]. It can also occur in combination with other malformations and dysmorphia and is thus called syndromic microcephaly.

In Acquired microcephaly, the head circumference of a newborn falls within the normal range but fails to grow sufficiently during postnatal development and as a result, develop microcephaly later on. It is caused by defects of the developmental process such as myelination and synapse formation owing to abnormal endosome regulation, vesicle membrane transport, or synaptic structural support. It often presents with progressive motor and cognitive impairment and seizures [19]. Currently the classification of congenital and acquired microcephaly is preferred over the previously used classification of primary and secondary microcephaly [20, 21].

Microcephaly is attributed both to environmental and genetic causes. The largest disease burden is contributed by congenital infections such as cytomegalovirus (CMV), herpes simplex virus (HSV), rubella virus, Toxoplasma gondii (*T. gondii*), and Zika Virus [22]. It can also be of genetic origin and has a very heterogenous architecture. Currently 900 OMIM phenotype entries and around

800 genes are linked to microcephaly with variable expressivity. Being very heterogeneous genetically, the etiology of microcephaly is only partially understood.

5. ETIOLOGY OF INTELLECTUAL DISABILITIES

Any interference with the normal developmental process of the human central nervous system can lead to intellectual disability. Such interference may either be genetic or environmental factors. The genetic interference may be a change in the genetic makeup of an individual in the form of monogenic mutations, chromosomal abnormalities and copy number variations (CNVs) (Fig. **16.2**). These changes cause a defect either in the nervous system or in the metabolic system. Environmental factors include but not restricted to exposure of the mother to infectious agents, excessive use of alcohol during pregnancy, and any complication both prenatally and postnatally [8, 23].

6. GENETIC FACTORS

ID is contributed by the whole spectrum of genetic abnormalities ranging from numerical or structural alterations of chromosomes and repeat expansion to single nucleotide variations. Fragile X syndrome is the most common form of X-linked ID and is caused by pathogenic variations in *FMR1* genes affecting almost 1 in every 5000 male individuals. It is caused by repeat expansion of CGG in FMR1 gene at the 5′ untranslated region. Expansion of CGG repeat may exceed 200 times causing complete silencing of the gene expression by getting methylated. FMR1 gene encodes a transcription factor required for the expression of multiple genes in the human brain, and mutations which cause ID and other behavioral abnormalities [23, 24]. Another example of monogenic genetic factor is mutations in the NF1 gene causing von Recklinghausen syndrome that is inherited in an autosomal dominant fashion. Almost 80% of children carrying NF1 gene mutation exhibit cognitive impairments [25].

Any numerical or structural alteration in chromosomes is called chromosomal abnormality. Numerical abnormality means missing or having an extra copy of a chromosome in a cell while structural abnormality refers to alteration in the structure of a chromosome through deletion, duplication translocation or inversion a part of a particular chromosome. Down syndrome is the most common example of chromosomal aberration called trisomy 21 characterized by the presence of an extra copy of chromosome 21; it affects around 0.15% of children globally. Edwards syndromes is another trisomy where chromosome 18 has an extra copy (trisomy 18) and is usually lethal early after birth [8].

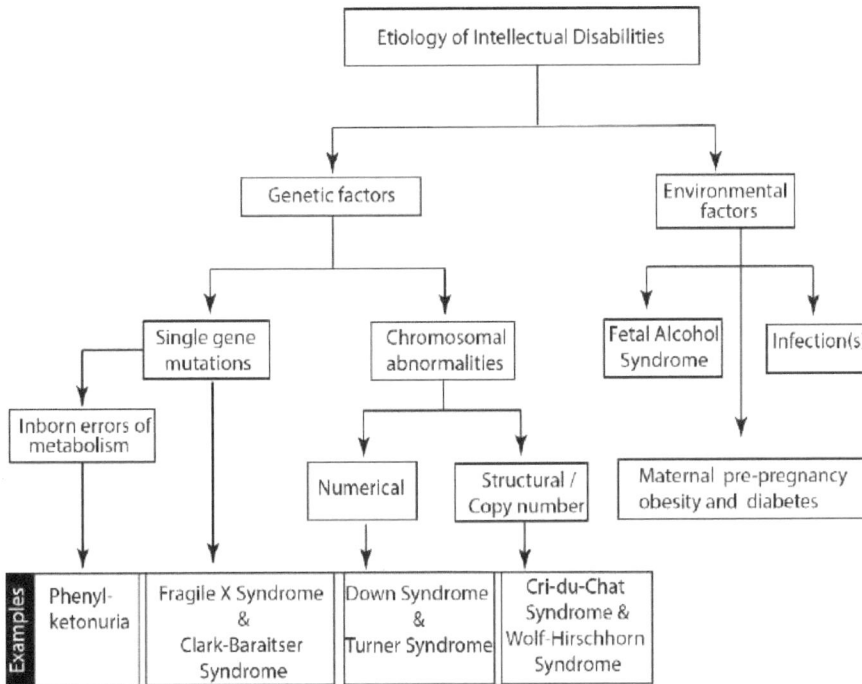

Fig. (16.2). Schematics of etiology of Intellectual Disability.

On the other hand, monosomy is a condition characterized by the presence of one copy of a chromosome pair instead of two and the most common example of this condition is Turner syndrome [26]. This is a condition where one member of the X chromosome pair is absent in females and is the only type of full monosomy that is not lethal, that is because the gene present on the other copy of X chromosome somehow compensates for the function of the missing genes. All other full forms of autosomal monosomies are lethal but the partial form may survive [27]. The patients carrying partial monosomy usually survive up to the 2nd decade of life, such as Cri-du-chat syndrome involving a microdeletion of 5p and Wolf-Hirschhorn syndrome having a 4p microdeletion [8]. Certain inborn errors of metabolism cause toxic accumulation of by-products, that damage the nervous system and cause ID. Phenylketonuria, for example, affects around 1 in every 10,000 newborn babies. This condition is characterized by the inability of the liver to convert phenylalanine into para-tyrosine. As a result, phenylalanine accumulates in the body consequently causing ID [28]. Autosomal recessive ID is genetically very diverse based on the fact that mutations in 73 candidate genes have already been identified in 136 consanguineous families having autosomal recessive mode of inheritance of non-syndromic intellectual disability. To date, the number of genes has reached to 399 which are associated with non-syndromic ID based on the data provided by OMIM and SysID (http://sysid.cmbi.umcn.nl/) [29].

7. DIAGNOSIS

ID is an integral part of both ASD and microcephaly and there may be overlapping clinical features that complicate the diagnosis. It is additionally hindered by multiple factors, particularly in developing countries, such as lack of legislation, knowledge regarding ID, appropriate training and infrastructure. Moreover, stigmatization and discrimination by the society also cause a delay in seeking diagnosis. Making a specific diagnosis imparts great benefits not only to the individual but to the family and society. It provided as relief from the uncertainty, end of the diagnostic odyssey, specific therapeutic interventions, genetic counseling, future reproductive planning and prenatal diagnosis to prevent recurrence of a disabling disorder [5].

Karyotyping has traditionally been the first genetic test, for ID cases suspected of genetic etiology. It usually involves growing lymphocytes *in vitro*, arresting the growth at metaphase and subsequently staining for visualization of bands. The numerical or structural chromosomal abnormalities are observed in 12-15% of cases with ID. Example of diseases resulting due to chromosomal abnormalities are Down syndrome, Angelman, William, 22q microdeletion, *etc* [30, 31].

Fluorescent *in situ* Hybridization (FISH) is an advancement of traditional karyotyping and proves helpful in the diagnosis of 3-5% of ID cases [31, 32]. It involves probing chromosomal spread of the patients with fluorescently labelled DNA or RNA molecules. It helps detect copy number variations and translocations. Nowadays, both karyotyping and FISH are being replaced by microarray-based technologies. Array comparative genomic hybridization (Array CGH) for example involves differential fluorescent labelling of two samples that are subsequently co-hybridized to a microarray of cloned DNA fragments, representative of the genome. It is then subjected to digital imaging and relative signal intensity is quantified that reflects the copy number gain or loss [33].

As mentioned previously, CGG repeats expansion of the FMR1 gene leading to fragile X-syndrome is very frequently observed in cases of ID and can be efficiently screened by polymerase chain reaction based tests [34]. On the other hand, in autosomal recessive cases, ID can be diagnosed by Homozygosity mapping through STR's markers and single nucleotide polymorphism (SNP) microarrays followed by sequencing of prioritized genes using Sanger sequencing approach. More than 300 genes causing ID have been identified by utilizing the above approach [33]. More importantly, genetic diagnosis can now be made in cases which previously remain undiagnosed. Thanks to Massively parallel Sequencing (MPS) technology and its application such as gene panel sequencing, whole exome sequencing and whole genome sequencing, causes of most of the ID cases can now be identified and it should be considered the first tier diagnostic assay as long as available and affordable [34]. A comprehensive strategy for genetic diagnosis of ID is outlined in Fig. (**16.3**).

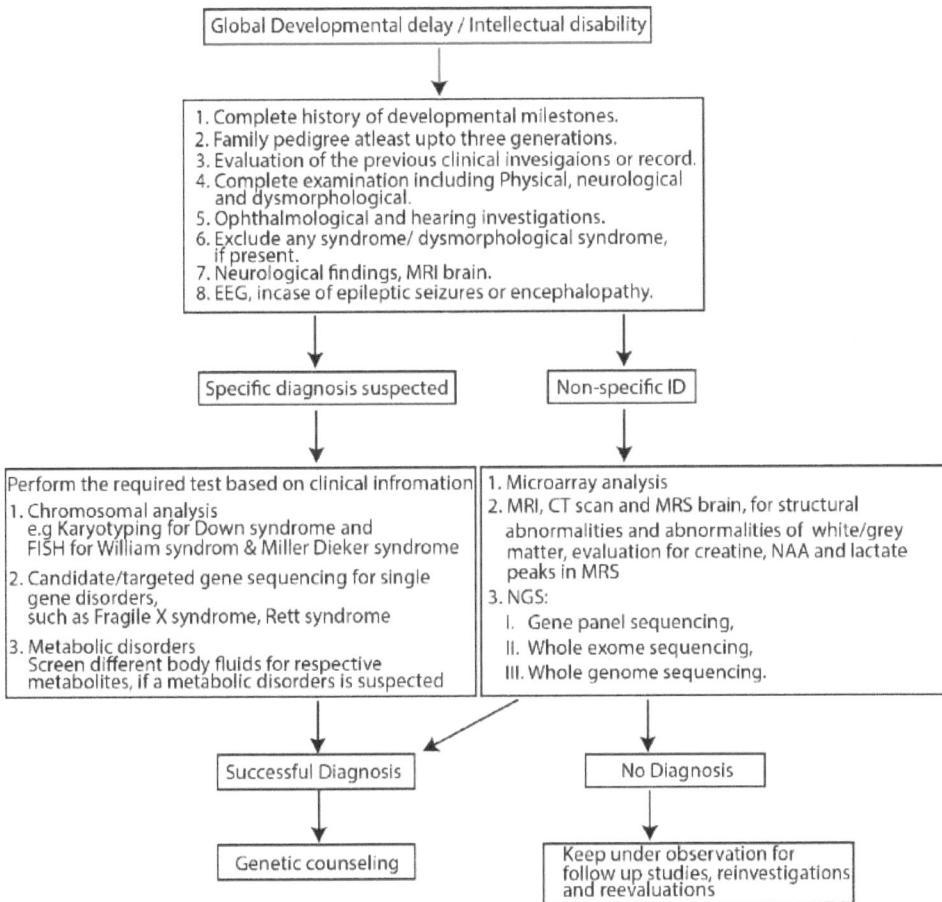

Fig. (16.3). A flow chart of general strategy for genetic diagnose a suspected case of intellectual disability (Adopted and recreated from Puri *et al.* 2016) [35] EEG: Electroencephalography, FISH: Fluorescent *In situ* hybridization, MRI Magnetic Resonance Imaging,

8. TREATMENT

There is no absolute cure for most forms of IDs except for some early diagnosed inborn errors of metabolism. In most cases, the treatment is usually symptomatic to ease the current symptoms, prevent them from further deterioration and minimize the co-morbidities. The ultimate goal is to bring some improvement in the quality of every day's life of patients. Some of the measures to improve the quality of an intellectually disabled person are discussed below in detail.

9. PSYCHOTROPIC DRUG INTERVENTIONS

The use of psychotropic drugs such as antidepressants, mood stabilizers, anxiolytics and hypnotics, antidementia drugs, and drugs for attention-deficit/hyperactivity disorder (ADHD) have a significant role in the management of comorbidities associated with IDs and psychiatric conditions [36]. Its use may not be helpful directly to treat IDs but it can have a vital role in treating behavioral and psychological abnormalities and comorbid conditions linked with IDs. For example, drugs such as Risperidone are very useful for treating aggressive, self-injurious and disruptive behaviors in kids with IDs. Similarly, the use of methylphenidate has shown a positive sign in reducing ADHD symptoms [37]. Health care personals should be careful while prescribing drugs as some patients may have comparatively high chances of side effects and they may need either an alternate or a lower dose of the same medicine. Inappropriate use of drugs has implications rather than advantages, so optimizing the use of certain drugs in certain conditions is the key to a successful therapy of patients with IDs [36]. Oxidative stress is one of the most important factors that contribute to the dysfunctional cognitive function in Down syndrome. To improve these cognitive deficits, several antioxidant molecules have been shown to be effective in preclinical studies; however, clinical trials have failed to show evidence of the efficacy of different antioxidants to improve cognitive deficits in individuals with Down syndrome. So it is highly likely that future therapeutics may combine cellular antioxidants with molecules that act on an abnormal process involved in developing symptoms of cognitive deficits in Down syndrome [38].

10. SPECIAL EDUCATION

Special education is provided to intellectually disable patients. Once diagnosed, the patients should be enrolled in special education centers. The curriculum should be designed in such a way that helps them get education and training regarding assistance, behavioral skills, vocational skills, communication skills, functional living skills, and social skills to improve their every day's life.

Activities and progress of each patient should be observed closely in the school, if a patients need extra help, his/her family can be trained to assist them at home to acquire the required skills. Family members of the patients should also be educated by the healthcare workers to understand what is intellectual disability, its management, prognosis and where to seek for help when needed [23].

11. INTERVENTION FOR INBORN ERRORS OF METABOLISM

Newborn screening for certain types of genetic diseases and inborn errors of metabolism is a routine procedure in some developed countries. Early diagnosis of an inborn error of metabolism provides the opportunity to treat such conditions through dietary restrictions. The most common example of which is those newborns identified with PKU, who are at risk of developing ID if left untreated. This condition because of the dysfunctional enzyme called Phenylalanine hydroxylase, which is unable to convert phenylalanine to tyrosine results in excessive accumulation of phenylalanine. So, if the condition is diagnosed early, the patients can be kept on a diet low in phenylalanine to prevent them from developing ID [39, 40]. Moreover a recent study shows the successful use of the drug called pegvaliase, to treat PKU in patients [40]. Another study showed a novel therapeutic intervention for PKU patients by silencing *SLC6A19*, a neutral amino acid transporter responsible for absorption of most of the free phenylalanine in the small intestine and its reuptake by renal proximal tubule cells [41]. Synthetic biotics (engineered bacterial *E.coli* strain Nissle 1917) called SYNB1618 is also designed to treat PKU in affected individuals. The bacterial strain utilizes the free phenylalanine in the upper gastrointestinal tract by converting it into either trans-cinnamic acid or phenylpyruvic acid by phenylalanine ammonia lyase and L-amino acid deaminase respectively. This study revealed a reduction of 38% of the blood phenylalanine irrespective of dietary protein intake [42, 43]. Similarly, the cognitive symptoms associated with Hurler's syndrome can also be improved by enzyme replacement therapy coupled with hematopoietic cell transplantation [44]. However, it is challenging to maintain it; irregularities may cause adverse effects on higher cognitive functions. It is worth mentioning that, enzyme replacement therapy (ERT) coupled with stem cell therapy is proven effective to improve patients' condition for Hurler syndrome (mucopolysaccharidosis type 1); in this case, very young individuals have shown improved cognition skills [45]. Additionally, phenylketonuria (PKU) is possibly treated with the dosage of BH4, a cofactor for phenylalanine hydroxylase (non-functional in PKU). Nonetheless, these treatments are temporary and prove to be effective for controlling a few symptoms of the patients [46].

11.1. GENE THERAPY

It is, to date, pre mature to uphold the fact that gene therapy is being successful for the treatment of intellectual disabilities however, the trails have started last year for genetic therapy of Angelman syndrome (AS). It is previously known that mutations in UBE3A gene can cause AS; the paternal allele of UBE3A is silenced, therefore losses of the maternal allele cause UBE3A deficient brain [47]. Later on, the silent copy of UBE3A was successfully activated using snippets of RNA in a mouse model of AS [48]. The same strategy has been used to recover the phenotype in a patient of AS. Similarly, another study carried out in a mouse model for the mutational correction of UBE3A using CRISPR Cas9 holds promising and convincing results to bring it into human trials [49]. For the genetic conditions such as Down syndrome (DS), clinicians have also followed to control gene regulation of DYRK1A (being over expressed in case of DS) by using agents such as epigallocatechin gallate - a polyphenol – for its functional modulation.

CONCLUSION

Using animal models, fragile X syndrome, Rett syndrome and tuberous sclerosis are also under investigation, however concluding remarks on the efficacy of gene therapy for these disorders might take a longer time.

CONSENT FOR PUBLICATION

Not applicable.

CONFLICT OF INTEREST

The author declares no conflict of interest, financial or otherwise.

ACKNOWLEDGEMENTS

Declared none.

REFERENCES

[1]   Hu WF, Chahrour MH, Walsh CA. The diverse genetic landscape of neurodevelopmental disorders. Annu Rev Genomics Hum Genet 2014; 15(1): 195-213.
[http://dx.doi.org/10.1146/annurev-genom-090413-025600] [PMID: 25184530]

[2]   Vasudevan P, Suri M. A clinical approach to developmental delay and intellectual disability. Clin Med (Lond) 2017; 17(6): 558-61.
[http://dx.doi.org/10.7861/clinmedicine.17-6-558] [PMID: 29196358]

[3]   Purugganan O. Intellectual Disabilities. Pediatr Rev 2018; 39(6): 299-309.
[http://dx.doi.org/10.1542/pir.2016-0116] [PMID: 29858292]

[4]   Patel D R, Apple R, Kanungo S, Akkal A. Intellectual disability: definitions, evaluation and principles

of treatment. Pediatric Medicine 2018; 1: 10.21037.

[5]   Puri R D, Tuteja M, Verma I C. Genetic Approach to Diagnosis of Intellectual Disability. Indian J Pediatr 2016; 83(10): 1141-9.
[http://dx.doi.org/10.1007/s12098-016-2205-0]

[6]   Wechsler D. Wechsler adult intelligence scale–Fourth Edition (WAIS–IV). 2008.

[7]   Patel DR, Cabral MD, Ho A, Merrick J. A clinical primer on intellectual disability. Transl Pediatr 2020; 9(S1) (Suppl. 1): S23-35.
[http://dx.doi.org/10.21037/tp.2020.02.02] [PMID: 32206581]

[8]   Parsamanesh N, Miri-Moghaddam E. Novel Insight Into Intellectual Disability; A Review Article. Gene, Cell and Tissue 2018; 5.

[9]   Wieczorek D. Autosomal dominant intellectual disability. Med Genetik 2018; 30(3): 318-22.
[http://dx.doi.org/10.1007/s11825-018-0206-2] [PMID: 30459487]

[10]   Jamra R. Genetics of autosomal recessive intellectual disability. Med Genetik 2018; 30(3): 323-7.
[http://dx.doi.org/10.1007/s11825-018-0209-z] [PMID: 30459488]

[11]   Katz G, Lazcano-Ponce E. Intellectual disability: definition, etiological factors, classification, diagnosis, treatment and prognosis. Salud Publica Mex 2008; 50 (Suppl. 2): s132-41.
[PMID: 18470340]

[12]   Wiśniowiecka-Kowalnik B, Nowakowska B A. Genetics and epigenetics of autism spectrum disorder—current evidence in the field. J Appl Genet 2019; 60: 37-47.
[http://dx.doi.org/10.1007/s13353-018-00480-w]

[13]   LoVullo S V, Matson J L. Comorbid psychopathology in adults with Autism Spectrum Disorders and intellectual disabilities. Research in Developmental Disabilities 2009; 30: 1288-96.
[http://dx.doi.org/10.1016/j.ridd.2009.05.004]

[14]   Christensen DL, Baio J, Braun KVN, *et al.* Prevalence and Characteristics of Autism Spectrum Disorder Among Children Aged 8 Years — Autism and Developmental Disabilities Monitoring Network, 11 Sites, United States, 2012. MMWR Surveill Summ 2016; 65(3): 1-23.
[http://dx.doi.org/10.15585/mmwr.ss6503a1] [PMID: 27031587]

[15]   Griesi-Oliveira K, Sertié AL. Autism spectrum disorders: an updated guide for genetic counseling. Einstein (Sao Paulo) 2017; 15(2): 233-8.
[http://dx.doi.org/10.1590/s1679-45082017rb4020] [PMID: 28767925]

[16]   Wang R, Khan A, Han S, Zhang X. Molecular analysis of 23 Pakistani families with autosomal recessive primary microcephaly using targeted next-generation sequencing. J Hum Genet 2017; 62(2): 299-304.
[http://dx.doi.org/10.1038/jhg.2016.128] [PMID: 27784895]

[17]   Makhdoom EUH, Waseem SS, Iqbal M, *et al.* Modifier Genes in Microcephaly: A Report on *WDR62*, *CEP63*, *RAD50* and *PCNT* Variants Exacerbating Disease Caused by Biallelic Mutations of *ASPM* and *CENPJ.* Genes (Basel) 2021; 12(5): 731.
[http://dx.doi.org/10.3390/genes12050731] [PMID: 34068194]

[18]   Boonsawat P, Joset P, Steindl K, *et al.* Elucidation of the phenotypic spectrum and genetic landscape in primary and secondary microcephaly. Genet Med 2019; 21(9): 2043-58.
[http://dx.doi.org/10.1038/s41436-019-0464-7] [PMID: 30842647]

[19]   Becerra-Solano LE, Mateos-Sánchez L, López-Muñoz E. Microcephaly, an etiopathogenic vision. Pediatr Neonatol 2021; 62(4): 354-60.
[http://dx.doi.org/10.1016/j.pedneo.2021.05.008] [PMID: 34112604]

[20]   DeSilva M, Munoz FM, Sell E, *et al.* Congenital microcephaly: Case definition & guidelines for data collection, analysis, and presentation of safety data after maternal immunisation. Vaccine 2017; 35(48): 6472-82.

[http://dx.doi.org/10.1016/j.vaccine.2017.01.044] [PMID: 29150052]

[21]   Marino S, Pavone P, Marino L, Rapisarda FAS, Falsaperla R. Congenital Genetic Microcephaly: Clinical Diagnostic Approach. J Pediatr Neurol 2020; 18(3): 131-4.
[http://dx.doi.org/10.1055/s-0039-1692970]

[22]   Devakumar D, Bamford A, Ferreira MU, *et al.* Infectious causes of microcephaly: epidemiology, pathogenesis, diagnosis, and management. Lancet Infect Dis 2018; 18(1): e1-e13.
[http://dx.doi.org/10.1016/S1473-3099(17)30398-5] [PMID: 28844634]

[23]   Lee K, Cascella M, Marwaha R. Intellectual Disability. StatPearls 2020. [Internet]

[24]   Jacquemont S, Berry-Kravis E, Hagerman R, *et al.* The challenges of clinical trials in fragile X syndrome. Psychopharmacology (Berl) 2014; 231(6): 1237-50.
[http://dx.doi.org/10.1007/s00213-013-3289-0] [PMID: 24173622]

[25]   Plasschaert E, Van Eylen L, Descheemaeker MJ, Noens I, Legius E, Steyaert J. Executive functioning deficits in children with neurofibromatosis type 1: The influence of intellectual and social functioning. Am J Med Genet B Neuropsychiatr Genet 2016; 171(3): 348-62.
[http://dx.doi.org/10.1002/ajmg.b.32414] [PMID: 26773288]

[26]   Morris LA, Tishelman AC, Kremen J, Ross RA. Depression in Turner Syndrome: A Systematic Review. 2020.

[27]   Fryns J P, Lukusa T P. Monosomies. 2001.

[28]   Bayat A, Møller LB, Lund AM. Diagnostics and treatment of phenylketonuria. Ugeskr Laeger 2015; 177(8)
[PMID: 25697170]

[29]   Ilyas M, Mir A, Efthymiou S, Houlden H. The genetics of intellectual disability: advancing technology and gene editing. 2020.

[30]   Devriendt K, Holvoet M, Fryns J. An etiological diagnostic survey in children attending a school for special education. Genet Couns 2003; 14: 125.

[31]   Rauch A, Hoyer J, Guth S, *et al.* Diagnostic yield of various genetic approaches in patients with unexplained developmental delay or mental retardation. Am J Med Genet A 2006; 140A(19): 2063-74.
[http://dx.doi.org/10.1002/ajmg.a.31416] [PMID: 16917849]

[32]   Baroncini A, Rivieri F, Capucci A, Croci G, Franchi F, Sensi A, *et al.* FISH screening for subtelomeric rearrangements in 219 patients with idiopathic mental retardation and normal karyotype. European Journal of Medical Genetics 2005; 48: 388-96.
[http://dx.doi.org/10.1016/j.ejmg.2005.05.002]

[33]   Vissers LELM, Gilissen C, Veltman JA. Genetic studies in intellectual disability and related disorders. 2016.
[http://dx.doi.org/10.1038/nrg3999]

[34]   Zacher P, Mayer T, Brandhoff F, *et al.* The genetic landscape of intellectual disability and epilepsy in adults and the elderly: a systematic genetic work-up of 150 individuals. Genet Med 2021; 23(8): 1492-7.
[http://dx.doi.org/10.1038/s41436-021-01153-6] [PMID: 33911214]

[35]   Puri RD, Tuteja M, Verma IC. Genetic approach to diagnosis of intellectual disability. Indian J Pediatr 2016; 83(10): 1141-9.
[http://dx.doi.org/10.1007/s12098-016-2205-0] [PMID: 27619815]

[36]   Sheehan R, Hassiotis A, Walters K, Osborn D, Strydom A, Horsfall L. Mental illness, challenging behaviour, and psychotropic drug prescribing in people with intellectual disability: UK population based cohort study. BMJ 2015; 351: h4326.

[37]   Arnold LE, Farmer C, Kraemer HC, *et al.* Moderators, mediators, and other predictors of risperidone response in children with autistic disorder and irritability. J Child Adolesc Psychopharmacol 2010;

20(2): 83-93.
[http://dx.doi.org/10.1089/cap.2009.0022] [PMID: 20415603]

[38] Rueda Revilla N, Martínez-Cué C. Antioxidants in Down Syndrome: From Preclinical Studies to Clinical Trials. Antioxidants 2020; 9(8): 692.
[http://dx.doi.org/10.3390/antiox9080692] [PMID: 32756318]

[39] Picker JD, Walsh CA. New innovations: Therapeutic opportunities for intellectual disabilities. Ann Neurol 2013; 74(3): 382-90.
[http://dx.doi.org/10.1002/ana.24002] [PMID: 24038210]

[40] Thomas J, Levy H, Amato S, Vockley J, Zori R, Dimmock D, *et al.* Pegvaliase for the treatment of phenylketonuria: Results of a long-term phase 3 clinical trial program (PRISM). Molecular Genetics and Metabolism 2018; 124: 27-38.
[http://dx.doi.org/10.1016/j.ymgme.2018.03.006]

[41] Belanger AM, Przybylska M, Gefteas E, *et al.* Inhibiting neutral amino acid transport for the treatment of phenylketonuria. JCI Insight 2018; 3(14): e121762.
[http://dx.doi.org/10.1172/jci.insight.121762] [PMID: 30046012]

[42] Isabella VM, Ha BN, Castillo MJ, *et al.* Development of a synthetic live bacterial therapeutic for the human metabolic disease phenylketonuria. Nat Biotechnol 2018; 36(9): 857-64.
[http://dx.doi.org/10.1038/nbt.4222] [PMID: 30102294]

[43] Nelson M T, Charbonneau M R, Coia H G, Castillo M J, Holt C, Greenwood E S, *et al.* Characterization of an engineered live bacterial therapeutic for the treatment of phenylketonuria in a human gut-on-a-chip. Nature Communications 2021; 12.
[http://dx.doi.org/10.1038/s41467-021-23072-5]

[44] Eisengart JB, Rudser KD, Tolar J, *et al.* Enzyme replacement is associated with better cognitive outcomes after transplant in Hurler syndrome. J Pediatr 2013; 162(2): 375-380.e1.
[http://dx.doi.org/10.1016/j.jpeds.2012.07.052] [PMID: 22974573]

[45] Eisengart JB, Rudser KD, Tolar J, Orchard PJ, Kivisto T, Ziegler RS, *et al.* Enzyme replacement is associated with better cognitive outcomes after transplant in Hurler syndrome. 2013; 162: pp. (2)375-380.e1.
[http://dx.doi.org/10.1016/j.jpeds.2012.07.052]

[46] Cerone R, Andria G, Giovannini M, Leuzzi V, Riva E, Burlina A. Testing for tetrahydrobiopterin responsiveness in patients with hyperphenylalaninemia due to phenylalanine hydroxylase deficiency. Adv Ther 2013; 30(3): 212-28.
[http://dx.doi.org/10.1007/s12325-013-0011-x] [PMID: 23436109]

[47] Albrecht U, Sutcliffe JS, Cattanach BM, *et al.* Imprinted expression of the murine Angelman syndrome gene, Ube3a, in hippocampal and Purkinje neurons. Nat Genet 1997; 17(1): 75-8.
[http://dx.doi.org/10.1038/ng0997-75] [PMID: 9288101]

[48] Bailus BJ, Pyles B, McAlister MM, *et al.* Protein delivery of an artificial transcription factor restores widespread Ube3a expression in an Angelman syndrome mouse brain. Mol Ther 2016; 24(3): 548-55.
[http://dx.doi.org/10.1038/mt.2015.236] [PMID: 26727042]

[49] Wolter JM, Mao H, Fragola G, *et al.* Cas9 gene therapy for Angelman syndrome traps Ube3a-ATS long non-coding RNA. Nature 2020; 587(7833): 281-4.
[http://dx.doi.org/10.1038/s41586-020-2835-2] [PMID: 33087932]

CHAPTER 17

Primary Microcephaly and Schizophrenia: Genetics, Diagnostics and Current Therapeutics

Iram Anjum[1,*], Aysha Saeed[1], Komal Aslam[1,2], Bibi Nazia Murtaza[3] and Shahid Mahmood Baig[4]

[1] *Department of Biotechnology, Kinnaird College for Women, Lahore, Pakistan*

[2] *Department of Biotechnology, Lahore College for Women University, Lahore, Pakistan*

[3] *Department of Zoology, Abbottabad University of Science and Technology, Abbottabad, Pakistan*

[4] *Pakistan Science Foundation, Islamabad, Pakistan*

Abstract: Intellectual disabilities (ID) are among the most common genetic disabilities worldwide. Over the last two decades, ID has especially drawn special scientific interest being the key to understanding normal brain development, growth, and functioning. Here, we discuss two intellectual disabilities to better understand the emerging trends in disease diagnosis as well as the therapies available for their management. Primary microcephaly (MCPH) is a monogenic genetic disorder with twenty-eight loci (MCPH1-MCPH28) mapped so far with all the causative genes being elucidated as well. The role of these genes in disease prognosis along with their association with various MCPH-linked phenotypes plays an important role in the molecular diagnosis of the disease. As there is no cure/treatment yet available to enlarge a congenitally small brain, management modalities in use include physical, speech and occupational therapies as well as psychological and genetic counselling to not only reduce the incidence of the disorder but also to help families cope better. The second intellectual disability being discussed here is schizophrenia which is a multifactorial disorder owing to its complex and extremely heterogeneous etiology. Although various environmental factors play an important role, the genetic factors have been identified to play the most pivotal role in disease presentation as to date, 19 loci (SCZD1-SCZD19) have been linked to schizophrenia. However, underlying genes for only six of these loci have been mapped along with 10 other genes that are either linked to schizophrenia or show susceptibility to it. Diagnosis of schizophrenia needs careful consideration and various tests and tools currently employed for complete diagnosis have been discussed here. The management options for schizophrenia include pharmacological, non-pharmacological and intracranial therapies. These disorders shed light on the important role omics technologies have played not only in better understanding of the disease prognosis but also assisting in disease diagnosis and treatment modalities too.

* **Corresponding author Iram Anjum**: Department of Biotechnology, Kinnaird College for Women, Lahore, Pakistan; E-mail: iram.anjum@kinnaird.edu.pk

Keywords: Cortical development, Dopamine pathways, Genetic heterogeneity, Genotype-phenotype associations, Occipitofrontal head circumference (OFC), Primary microcephaly (MCPH), Schizophrenia.

1. INTRODUCTION

Intellectual disabilities have also attracted a lot of scientific inquisitiveness since ancient times, as Hippocrates in the fifth century BC, proposed a physiological insight and identified intellectual disability as a neurodevelopmental defect and explained it as a defect caused by irregularities in the four humors of the cerebrum.

People with intellectual disabilities (ID) have since long been a target of public isolation and humiliation. Not only the early influential Greek and Roman scholars used to belittle such people, but till very recently, individuals with such disabilities have been tagged as mentally retarded. However, the term mental retardation has now been replaced by intellectual disability, owing to the offensive nature of the term as well as the negativity surrounding it.

However, the degree of intellectual disability is variable ranging from mild to severe and people with intellectual disabilities can learn new skills, although slower than their normal counterparts, depending on the severity of the condition. The underlying mechanisms causing intellectual diseases are complex and though many factors may contribute, their etiology can be mainly divided into two categories, *genetic abnormalities* (*e.g.* gene mutations, copy number variations and chromosomal aberrations) and *environmental* factors, which include maternal exposure to toxins, delivery and postnatal complications as well as traumas after birth [1].

To better understand the intellectual diseases, their etiology, diagnoses as well as the current therapeutics, here we discuss two intellectual diseases, primary microcephaly having a predominantly genetic etiology and schizophrenia being a multifactorial complex disorder.

2. PRIMARY MICROCEPHALY

Primary microcephaly or *microcephaly vera* or *microcephaly primary hereditary* (MCPH; OMIM 251200) is a congenital neurodevelopmental condition, characterized by a smaller head (at least -2 standard deviations at birth below the mean accounting for the age, sex and ethnicity) accompanied with non-progressive mild to severe intellectual disability. The smaller head characteristic of this disorder explains the Greek origins of the term, *i.e.*, μικρό and κεφάλι meaning small and head respectively. It is essentially a disorder of the neocortex involving not only abnormal neuronal migration but also a reduction in the number of neurons in the developing neocortex [2, 3].

2.1. Clinical Attributes

Although the head circumference (HC) of MCPH individuals is at least -2 standard deviations (SD) at birth, it has been observed that most MCPH affected have HC > -4 SD, six months postnatally below the individuals of the same age and sex, meanwhile their femur length remains within 2 SD of the normal range. The HC measurement, which is also termed occipitofrontal circumference (OFC), is considered a direct indication of brain growth, and a key step in the assessment of childhood development and growth. If the head circumference is less than 4 SD, severe mental retardation is observed. Apart from a smaller head size, the symptoms of microcephaly may include seizures, developmental delays like a delayed speech, sitting, walking, and standing as well as cognitive impairments and intellectual delay. Other symptoms include high-pitched cry, hearing defects and vision problems. The severity of these symptoms varies and could be life-long and sometimes even be life threatening. However, it has also been observed that some affected persons may even show no symptoms at all except a smaller than average head circumference [2 - 4].

2.2. Types of Microcephaly

Primary microcephaly is one of the two types of microcephaly categorized based on the time and factors contributing to the smaller head [5]. Primary microcephaly is present at birth which can either be an inherited condition or the result of a malfunction during pregnancy. Generally, genetic abnormalities interfering with the expansion of the cerebral cortex during the development of the fetus cause primary microcephaly. Reasons for PM other than genetic may include any infection which may be passed from the mother to the fetus during pregnancy such as toxoplasmosis, German measles (rubella), cytomegalovirus, chickenpox (varicella), and zika virus. Exposure of a baby in the womb to alcohol, drugs or any toxic chemical can also lead to brain abnormalities.

Secondary microcephaly as opposed to its counterpart develops postnatally from an insult to an otherwise well-formed central nervous system. It is characterized by a remarkably low number of neuronal dendrites as well as synaptic connections. Environmental factors which most likely contribute are disruptive brain injuries, teratogen exposure, ischemic stroke, *etc.* affecting the postnatal development of the brain and thus secondary microcephaly.

2.3. Incidence

Although primary microcephaly is a very rare genetic disorder, its birth incidence varies from 1.3 to as high as 150/100,000 worldwide. This disparity in incidence across the globe is based on the populations dynamics as well as the HC criteria used to describe primary microcephaly, for example, the incidence of primary microcephaly in Holland (a non-consanguineous population) has been calculated to be 1/250,000, in contrast to 1/10,000 in Asian and Arab populations who practice a higher than the global rate of consanguinity [4].

2.4. Genetics of Primary Microcephaly

There is a huge significance of understanding the underlying genetics causing abnormal development of the brain, thus, explaining the immense attention primary microcephaly has drawn from the scientific community worldwide in the last two decades. MCPH displays great genetic heterogeneity and as of August 2021, twenty-eight genetic loci have been mapped to primary microcephaly, with all underlying genes (*Microcephalin, WDR62, CDK5RAP2, CASC5, ASPM, CENPJ, STIL, CEP135, CEP152, ZNF335, PHC, CENPE, CDK6, SASS6, ANKLE2, MFSD2A, CIT, WDFY3, COPB2, KIF14, NCAPD2, NCAPD3, NCAPH, NUP37, MAP11, LMNB1, LMNB2 and RRP7A*) also been elucidated [2, 3, 6 - 10]. Primary microcephaly is mostly inherited in autosomal recessive patterns and all genes follow the pattern of inheritance except for *WDFY3, LMNB1* and *LMNB2* that follow the autosomal dominant mode of inheritance [2, 3, 7]. The first microcephalic gene was mapped in 2002 and expeditious research in unraveling the genetics of this disorder has led to the identification of twenty-seven more genes in the last two decades (Table **17.1**).

Table 17.1. Timeline of MCPH genes, Mendelian inheritance in man (MIM) number, chromosomal location, mode of inheritance (MOI) and functions.

TIMELINE	GENE	MIM #	LOCATION	MOI*	FUNCTION
2002	*Microcephalin*	607117	8p23.1	AR	Chromosome condensation, Cell cycle checkpoint regulator, DNA damage response
2002	*ASPM*	605481	1q31	AR	Centriole biogenesis, Spindle orientation, Cytokinesis, Wnt signaling
2005	*CDK5RAP2*	608201	9q33	AR	Pericentriolar material scaffold, Microtubule nucleation, Centriolar engagement, Cytokinesis, Spindle orientation
2005	*CENPJ*	609279	13q12	AR	Centriole biogenesis, Pericentriolar material tethering

(Table 1) cont.....

TIMELINE	GENE	MIM #	LOCATION	MOI*	FUNCTION
2009	STIL	181590	1p33	AR	Centriole biogenesis, Pericentriolar material scaffold, Microtubule nucleation, Spindle orientation
2010	WDR62	613583	19q13	AR	Centriole biogenesis, Spindle orientation
2010	CEP152	613529	15q21	AR	Centriole biogenesis
2012	CASC5	609173	15q14	AR	Kinetochore attachment, Mitotic checkpoint complex regulation
2012	CEP135	611423	4q12	AR	Centriole biogenesis
2012	ZNF335	610827	20q13	AR	Transcriptional regulation
2013	PHC1	602978	12p13	AR	Chromatin remodeling
2013	CDK6	603368	7q21	AR	Cell cycle checkpoint regulation
2014	CENPE	117143	4q24	AR	Kinetochore attachment, Mitotic checkpoint complex regulator
2014	SASS-6	609321	1p21	AR	Centriole biogenesis
2014	ANKLE2	616062	12q24	AR	Nuclear envelop disassembly
2015	MFSD2A	614397	1p34	AR	BBB lipid transporter, Cell cycle checkpoint regulator
2016	CIT	605629	12q24	AR	Microtubule nucleation, Cytokinesis, Spindle orientation
2016	WDFY3	617485	4q21	AD	Wnt signaling
2016	NCAPD2	615638	12p13	AR	Chromosome condensation, Sister chromatid disentanglement
2016	NCAPD3	609276	11q25	AR	Kinetochore attachment, Mitotic checkpoint complex regulation
2016	NCAPH	602332	2q11	AR	Kinetochore attachment, Mitotic checkpoint complex regulation
2017	COPB2	606990	3q23	AR	Cell cycle checkpoint regulator, Cellular trafficking
2017	KIF14	611279	1q31	AR	Cytokinesis, Microtubule network stabilizer
2018	NUP37	609264	7q22	AR	Nuclear pore complex, kinetochore attachment
2019	MAP11	618350	7q22	AR	Cytokinesis, Microtubule network stabilizer
2020	LMNB1	150340	5q23	AD	Nuclear envelope stability
2021	LMNB2	150341	19p13	AD	Nuclear and chromatin structure stability
2021	RRP7A	-	22q13.1-13.2	AR	rRNA regulation, Primary cilia resorption, Cell cycle progression

2.5. Diagnosis

Primary microcephaly can be diagnosed before or after birth. During pregnancy, microcephaly can be diagnosed through prenatal ultrasound as early as 30 weeks, but sometimes goes unnoticed till the third trimester [11]. The neonatal diagnosis of primary microcephaly is usually done by physical examination of the head size, being the most common diagnostic tool, measured in the first 24 hours of birth as per WHO criteria. However, the complete diagnosis of PM can only be established by not just physical examination but brain and cellular imaging as well as molecular analysis to know the precise underlying cause (Fig. **17.1**).

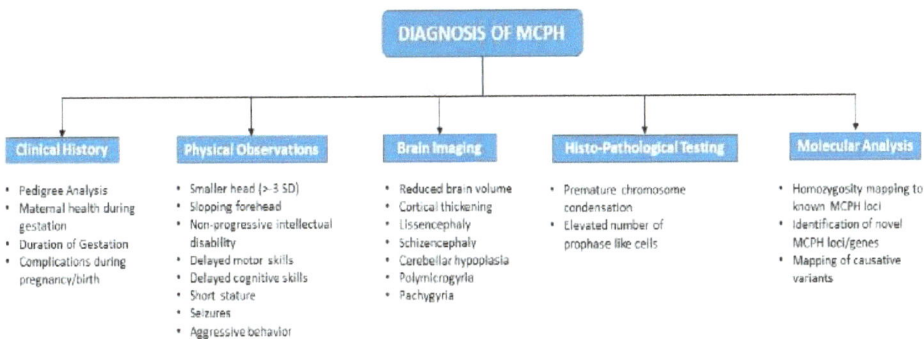

Fig (17.1). The criteria used for clinical, histopathological and molecular diagnosis of MCPH. The pedigree information is collected and information regarding gestational/birth complications is gathered to establish the mode of inheritance as well as to rule out the environmental factors leading to disease presentation.

Amongst other clinical diagnostic criteria, the intellectual disability resulting due to primary microcephaly is non-progressive and the IQ of the affected individuals ranges between 30 and 70-80. The delay in motor skills is usually observed with delayed developmental milestones like sitting, standing and walking. The other characteristics (seizures, short stature *etc.*) are not commonly observed in all MCPH patients and are sometimes more associated with some MCPH causative genes than others.

To further confirm the clinical diagnosis and evaluate the simplification of the gyral pattern, typical of primary microcephaly, magnetic resonance imaging (MRI) and computed tomography scan (CT) can also be employed [5]. The molecular diagnosis of primary microcephaly is quite challenging though, owing to the extremely heterogeneous nature of the disorder [3, 12]. Linkage studies have been implied since the first decade of microcephaly research to identify the genome location linked to microcephaly. Once linkage is established, conventional sequencing can be used to identify the causative variant, which is also confirmed by restriction enzymes.

Currently gene panels are an effective tool for identification of underlying culprit gene. However, these panels require regular upgradation too, due to the rapidly growing number of MCPH causative genes.

As a second tier of gene identification, the deletion/duplication panels are also being used by various research groups. If the underlying cause still remains undiscovered, whole exome sequencing (WES) is performed, sequencing the coding genome to identify the homozygous variant. Some studies have included high-resolution chromosomal microarray analysis (CMA) combined with exon sequencing to identify the novel copy number variants (CNV). If WES too does not reveal any molecular explanation, whole genome sequencing (WGS) is considered [3, 5]. All these diagnostic approaches are being used to get a precise molecular picture of the disorder but they still need improvement as many of the MCPH families are still without an underlying causative gene identified. There is also a need to improve the already available genotype-phenotype correlations and thus lead to better disease-gene associations to aid diagnose of the disease (Table **17.2**).

Table 17.2. List of loci/genes linked to schizophrenia, Mendelian inheritance in man (MIM) #, chromosomal location, mode of inheritance (MOI) and functions of the mapped genes.

LOCUS	PHENOTYPE	GENE	LOCUS/GENE MIM #	CHROMOSOMAL LOCATION	MOI*	GENE FUNCTION
SCZD1	SCHIZOPHRENIA 1	-	181510	5q23-q35	AD	
SCZD2	SCHIZOPHRENIA 2	-	603342	11q14-q21	AD	
SCZD3	SCHIZOPHRENIA 3	-	600511	6p23	AD	
SCZD4	SUSCEPTIBILITY TO SCHIZOPHRENIA 4	PRODH	606810	22q11.21	AD	Involved in proline degradation
SCZD5	SCHIZOPHRENIA 5	-	603175	6q13-q26	AD	
SCZD6	SCHIZOPHRENIA 6	-	603013	8p21	AD	
SCZD7	SCHIZOPHRENIA 7	-	603176	13q32	AD	
SCZD8	SCHIZOPHRENIA 8	-	603206	18p	AD	
SCZD9	SUSCEPTIBILITY TO SCHIZOPHRENIA 9	DISC1	605210	1q42.2	AD	Involved in neurite outgrowth and cortical development
SCZD10	SUSCEPTIBILITY TO SCHIZOPHRENIA 10	-	-	15q15	AD	
SCZD11	SCHIZOPHRENIA 11	-	608078	10q22.3	AD	
SCZD12	SCHIZOPHRENIA 12	-	608543	1p36.2	AD	
SCZD13	SUSCEPTIBILITY TO SCHIZOPHRENIA 13	-	-	15q13	-	
SCZD14	SUSCEPTIBILITY TO SCHIZOPHRENIA 14	-	-	2q32.1	-	
SCZD15	SUSCEPTIBILITY TO SCHIZOPHRENIA 15	SHANK3	606230	22q13.33	AD	Involved in synapse formation and dendritic spine maturation
SCZD16	SUSCEPTIBILITY TO SCHIZOPHRENIA 16	-	-	7q36.3	-	
SCZD17	SUSCEPTIBILITY TO SCHIZOPHRENIA 17	NRXN1	600565	2p16.3	-	Involved in synapse formation and subsequent neurotransmission
SCZD18	SUSCEPTIBILITY TO SCHIZOPHRENIA 18	SLC1A1	133550	9p24.2	-	Involved in glutamate and aspartate transportation, termination of glutamate post-synaptic action and maintains extracellular glutamate levels within normal range
SCZD19	SUSCEPTIBILITY TO SCHIZOPHRENIA 19	RBM12	607179	20q11.22	AD	Encodes RNA-binding motifs, transmembrane domains and proline-rich regions
	SCHIZOPHRENIA	DAOA	607408	13q33.2	AD	Involved in degradation of g liotransmitter D-serine as well as in mitochondrial function and dendritic arborization
	SCHIZOPHRENIA	APOL2	607252	22q12.3	AD	Involved in cytoplasmic movement of lipids and facilitates lipid binding to organelles
	SCHIZOPHRENIA	APOL4	607254	22q12.3	AD	Involved in reverse cholesterol transportation from peripheral cells to liver as well as lipid transportation all over the body
	SUSCEPTIBILITY TO SCHIZOPHRENIA	MTHFR	607093	1p36.22	AD	Involved in remethylation of homocysteine to methionine
	SUSCEPTIBILITY TO SCHIZOPHRENIA	CHI3L1	601525	1q32.1	AD	Involved in inflammation and tissue remodeling
	SUSCEPTIBILITY TO SCHIZOPHRENIA	SYN2	600755	3p25.2	AD	Involved in synaptic transmission by selectively binding to synaptic vesicles in the presynaptic terminal
	SUSCEPTIBILITY TO SCHIZOPHRENIA	DRD3	126451	3q13.31	AD	Encodes dopamine receptors
	SUSCEPTIBILITY TO SCHIZOPHRENIA	HTR2A	182135	13q14.2	AD	Encodes serotonin receptors
	SUSCEPTIBILITY TO SCHIZOPHRENIA	COMT	116790	22q11.21	AD	Involved in O-methylation of dopamine, epinephrine and nor-epinephrine and metabolism of catechol drugs
	SUSCEPTIBILITY TO SCHIZOPHRENIA	RTN4R	605566	22q11.21	AD	Involved in inhibition of axonal growth and regulation of axonal regeneration and CNS plasticity

SCHIZOPHRENIA LINKED GENES

It is now evident that intellectual disability is the most common MPCH associated phenotype (observed in 24 MCPH genes) followed by cortical malformations observed in 20 of the 28 MCPH genes. Short stature seems to have lost its exclusivity to MCPH1 locus and is now observed associated with 12 loci. The widest phenotype spectrum has been observed by *ASPM* (MCPH5) and *LMNB1* (MCPH26). However, low body weight (*COPB2*), clinodactyly (*NUP37*) and limb hypertonia (*NCAPD3*), have yet been associated with a single MCPH gene only. Blood disorders like leukemia (*ASPM* and *CDK5RAP2*) and anemia (*ANKLE2* and *LMNB2*) are now also linked with MCPH phenotype. This genotype phenotype correlation is essential to help point towards a precise a correct molecular diagnosis and also facilitate future gene identification for causing primary microcephaly.

2.6. Management

No cure for primary microcephaly is yet available as it is not possible to return the microcephalic brain to a normal size, and thus no treatment modalities can be offered to the affected families. However, the following lifelong management skills can help in reducing the severity of associated conditions and the following therapies can be offered to better manage this condition:

Physical therapy: to improve their motor coordination, movement and strength.

Speech therapy: to enable the microcephalics to communicate better. Speech is another hurdle in their social integration as their speech is either restricted to single words or short sentences or is very poorly conveyed. Speech therapy can thus ensure the social integration microcephaly in society.

Occupational therapy: to help increase the functional independence of these patients. Despite having mild to severe intellectual disability, people affected by microcephaly mostly retain a good memory and can be given vocational trainings (such as of crafts) to lead them to a less-dependent life.

3. SCHIZOPHRENIA

The term schizophrenia was coined by Eugen Bleuler in 1908 and finds its origin in Greek with σχίζειν means *splitting* and φρήν, φρεν- stands for *mind*, roughly meaning splitting of mind [13]. Schizophrenia (SCZD; OMIM 181500) is a multifactorial mental illness encompassing a wide range of symptoms such as delusions, hallucinations, unorganized behavior, disordered speech, severe emotional inadequacy along with many other psychiatric symptoms. Some patients also experience cognitive symptoms as inability to concentrate and or manage daily life tasks. Due to its multifactorial nature, several factors contribute to the progression of the disease [13, 14].

3.1. Clinical Attributes

Schizophrenia is a psychotic disorder with a variety of manifestations in affected individuals. It often develops in young adults with no history of split personality disorder but the affected individuals have disrupted thoughts and imaginations. The patients of schizophrenia are not able to build normal social relationships and neither can they participate in social events. Widely the symptoms of schizophrenia have been categorized as *positive, negative* and *cognitive* [14, 15].

Positive Symptoms: These symptoms are classified as positive as they are not usually seen in healthy individuals. Schizophrenic patients with these symptoms are very easily distinguishable from normal individuals owing to these additional behaviors. Positive symptoms include hallucinations, delusions, thinking disorders and sometimes movement disorders too. Although positive symptoms have a more serious presentation at times, but may remain unnoticed otherwise. Moreover, some patients may experience recurring spikes of these symptoms while others may have a more stable and prolonged presentation [15].

Negative Symptoms: Negative symptoms include speech problems, heavy voice, flat face (absence of facial expressions) as well as difficulty in planning or sticking to a task. Some patients may even experience alogia (lack of verbal communication due to disruption in normal thinking patterns) and anhedonia (*i.e.* inability to feel pleasant/happy emotions). These symptoms may also lead to emotional difficulty as well as social withdrawal. However, these symptoms are sometimes not easy to identify as part of schizophrenia, as these symptoms may be confused with depression or other psychological conditions [15].

Cognitive Symptoms: Cognitive symptoms include difficulty in decision-making along with impulsive behavior. The degree of cognitive symptoms can be assessed by how well the affected individuals can perform their duties. Such symptoms are mostly detected with certain medical tests as it is otherwise difficult to identify them [15].

Schizophrenia is a multifactorial disorder as many different factors may contribute to the development of this disorder. According to a recent study, it has been found that schizophrenia begins *in utero* and the critical time for development of schizophrenia is the second trimester of pregnancy as this is the crucial time of neurodevelopment. Any excessive stress, maternal infections or other complications such as gestational diabetes, emergency caesarian section, excessive bleeding, low birth weight or asphyxia could also cause schizophrenia [16].

There are many hypotheses related to the pathogenesis of schizophrenia. Several studies predict that schizophrenia develops as the delicate balance in various neurotransmitter pathways is disturbed *e.g.* hyperactivity of dopaminergic, serotonergic and alpha-adrenergic pathways as opposed to hypoactivity of glutaminergic and GABA pathways leads to schizophrenia [17].

The hypothesis of neurochemical abnormalities suggests that the psychiatric manifestations of the disease are due to the imbalance of important neurotransmitters such as dopamine, serotonin, glutamate, and gamma aminobutyric acid (GABA). Abnormal activity of dopamine has been linked with various schizophrenia symptoms at the sites of dopamine receptors (specifically D2). Endrogenous dopamine has been involved in four dopaminergic pathways which are associated with symptoms of schizophrenia namely nigrostriate pathway, mesolimbic pathway, mesocortical pathway and the tuberoinfundibular pathway [17] (Fig. **17.2**).

The *Nigrostriatal pathway* comes from the substantial nigra and ends in the nucleus of caudates. The low dopamine levels in the extrapyramidal system are thought to affect the motor symptom. The *Mesolimbic pathway* plays an important role in the presentation of positive symptoms when dopamine is present in excessive amount. It extends from the ventral tegmental area (VTA) to limbic area. The negative symptoms arise due to low mesocortical dopamine levels derived from the *Mesocortical pathway*. The blockage of the *Tuberoinfundibular pathway* causes an increase in prolactin levels due to reduced *Tuberoinfundibular* dopamine access and results in symptoms such as aménorrhea and deteriorated libido. Evidence that N-methyl-d-aspartate (NMDA) receptor antagonists intensify positive and negative symptoms in schizophrenia suggests the potential role of glutaminergic hypoactivity. The serotonergic hyperactivity has also been observed to perform an important role in the development of schizophrenia. Hence, it can be concluded that an increase or a decrease in the neurotransmitter levels of serotonin, dopamine, and glutamate gives rise to this disorder. Other studies also suggest the development of schizophrenia due to an imbalanced neurotransmission of GABA, aspartate, and glycine neurotransmitter [17].

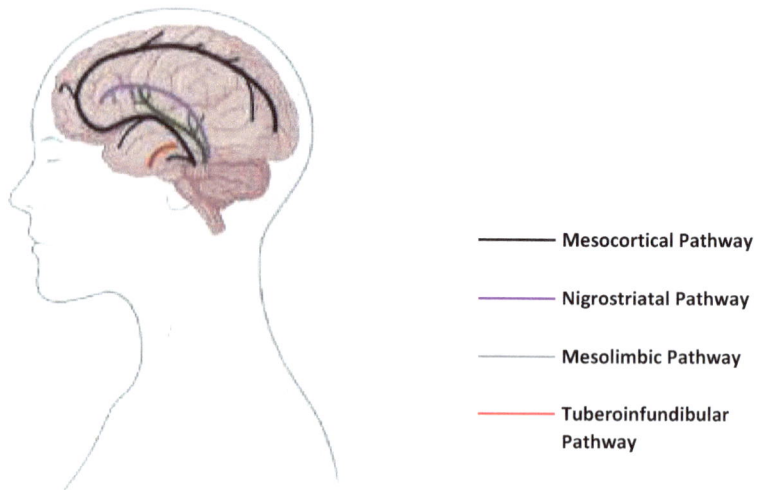

Fig. (17.2). Dopamine pathways relevant to schizophrenic symptoms.

As multiple environmental factors play an important role in the development of schizophrenia, it has been observed that social factors as migrant vs. local, urban vs. rural increase the risk of developing schizophrenia. Others factors that have been observed to lead to schizophrenia include the malnutrition of mother during pregnancy as well as maternal infections like toxoplasmosis, rubella *etc.* Another interesting association is the annual season a baby is born, as birth during late winter and early spring is prone to schizophrenia, owing probably to elevated risk of intrauterine viral exposure. All these early environmental risks seem to influence the development of brain and thus cause this disorder.

All these risk factors collectively point to an association of biological, psychological and social risk factors that drive even more divergent development of the disorder [16, 17].

3.2. Types of Schizophrenia

Schizophrenia can be categorized in the following types based on the of pattern of appearance of symptoms [18].

3.2.1. Paranoid Schizophrenia

It is characterized mainly by positive symptoms like anger, anxiety, and hostile behavior. The patients may also experience delusions and often hear audio hallucinations. However, there could be none or very few other prominent symptoms like disordered speech, flat/ catatonic or disorganized behavior.

3.2.2. Disorganized Schizophrenia

This type of schizophrenia is also known as *Hebephrenic schizophrenia* and is characterized mainly by disorganized symptoms like disorganized language and behaviors and inappropriate emotions.

3.2.3. Catatonic Schizophrenia

Catatonic schizophrenia is now regarded as a rare form as it results from untreated schizophrenia. Thus, an earlier intervention and treatment may result in less frequent occurrence of this type. It is marked by increased severity of two or more symptoms with significant disturbance in movements, as affected with this form may move continuously whereas some may remain immobile. Similarly, they may speak all the day while others may remain silent for hours up to several days.

3.2.4. Undifferentiated Schizophrenia

Undifferentiated schizophrenia does not fit in any of the preceding three categories as the affected individuals display symptoms of more than one type of schizophrenia. These people experience significant illusions, hallucinations, disorderly speech and even catatonic conduct. Their symptoms cannot be categorized as belonging to positive, negative, disorganized or catatonic, rather are they are a combination of all these.

3.2.5. Residual Schizophrenia

This is a very tricky type and is used to describe a patient who was previously diagnosed with schizophrenia but does not have any prominent symptoms currently like illusions, hallucinations, unorganized speech or distorted behavior. The intensity of the disorder is lessened in the later stages for this type.

3.3. Incidence

Schizophrenia is commonly observed in adults aged between 20-54 years of age. Its incidence has been found to be very variable and ranges between 8/1000 to as high as 43/1000. A recent study has revealed a gender disparity too in the prevalence of schizophrenia as it was observed that it is 76% more common in males than females with the per 1000 individuals respectively [19].

3.4. Genetics of Schizophrenia

Although diverse factors lead up to disease prognosis, making schizophrenia a polygenic disorder, however, the heritability of schizophrenia has been calculated to be as high as 80%, implying genetic factors as the most important factor causing this disorder [20]. Genetically, schizophrenia is not only extremely heterogeneous but also very complex disorder, owing to the many genes susceptible for schizophrenia which interact with environmental factors and cause disease prognosis. Genome wide association studies have identified more than 100 genetic loci that could cause schizophrenia. It is not believed that genetic factors causing schizophrenia are comprised of single nucleotide polymorphisms (SNPs) as well as highly penetrating copy number variants [20].

Among other factors, changes in immune system have also been found to increase risk, being further endorsed by schizophrenia susceptible locus at the major histocompatibility complex (MHC) on chromosome 6 [20].

However, till April 2021, there are 19 loci (SCZD1-SCZD19) linked to or susceptible to schizophrenia in the OMIM (online Mendelian inheritance in man) database. Six of these loci have their genes identified (*PRODH, DISC1, SHANK3, NRXN1, SLC1A1* and *RBM12*) while others are still not elucidated. Apart from these loci, several studies have identified almost 10 genes (*DAOA, APOL2, APOL4, MTHFR, CHI3L1, SYN2, DRD3, HTR2A, COMT* and *RTN4R*) that either cause schizophrenia or are still susceptible to cause this disorder (Table **17.2**).

All the genes mapped so far as being either linked to or susceptible to cause schizophrenia follow an autosomal dominant manner, thus explaining the higher heritability of this disorder. It has thus been observed that the degree of relatedness increases the risk of developing schizophrenia, as the prevalence is almost 1% in unrelated spouses and increases up to 44% in case of monozygotic twins.

3.5. Diagnosis

In order to diagnose schizophrenia both historical and collateral data are essential. It is important to confirm that the symptoms represent schizophrenia, since not all psychosis is schizophrenia. There are different diagnostic tools and tests available for schizophrenia.

Medical history and physical examination should be performed by an expert clinician in case schizophrenia is suspected as it primarily has a clinical diagnosis. Specific laboratory tests include urea and electrolytes levels, HIV/syphilis serology tests, serum calcium levels, thyroid function tests, blood glucose levels, 24-hour cortisol levels and urine toxicology screening tests.

Since schizophrenia is linked to brain changes that mostly involve reflection, emotions, actions, speech, and behavioral adaptations, radiographic investigations like computed tomography (CT scan) and magnetic resonance imaging (MRI) may help confirm the diagnosis while excluding other possible causes.

Using these tools, structural brain differences have been identified in chronic schizophrenia patients which are absent in the brains of controls. These structural variations include changes in gray and white matter, non-localized changes in temporal lobe volumes and more specifically abnormality in the superior temporal gyrus and the temporal and frontal lobe white-matter connections [15].

If no clear-cut physical evidence is observed, the patient should be referred to a psychologist or psychiatrist specialized in diagnosing and treating mental illnesses. In order to evaluate the patient for schizophrenia, these experts use a designed interview and other assessment tools. A thorough system review and mental condition examination should be performed by experts in which behavior, mood, speech, cognition, insight and evidence of delusions or formal disorders of the mind are assessed. A comprehensive mental history is also taken by using organized questionnaire for evaluation [15]. According to the fifth edition of the American Psychiatric Association's Diagnostic and Statistical Manual (DSM-5), schizophrenia can be formally diagnosed for a patient if there are at least two of the following five symptoms (at least one of the symptoms to be among the first three listed below) lasting for at least six months:

- delusions
- hallucinations
- disorganized speech
- catatonic behavior
- negative symptoms

Some candidate diagnostic biomarkers for schizophrenia have been discovered using metabolomic methods as it was found that biofluid metabolites are associated with this disorder and can be used as a diagnostic tool [18]. These biomarkers include neurophysiological markers (*e.g.*, smooth pursuit eye movement dysfunction) neuroimaging markers (*e.g.*, fronto-cerebellar/striat--thalamic gray matter deficit) and cognitive markers (*e.g.*, verbal memory deficit, cortical or subcortical cognitive type).

3.6. Management

The lifelong symptoms of schizophrenia require both management and treatment. In order to effectively treat schizophrenia, collaboration with a psychiatrist is important as it is not very different from other chronic psychological conditions and a psychiatrist can easily differentiate between the conditions. The following therapies are currently in use for treating schizophrenia:

Pharmacological Therapies: Pharmacologic intervention is only one facet of the treatment. Some common pharmacological therapies are:

D2-receptor Blockers: All current schizophrenia pharmacology treatments are based on D2-receptor blockers. Positron emission tomography (PET) studies in affected patients have shown that more than 60% of the dopamine D2 receptors are required for this treatment approach. Generally a higher level of D2 (above 80%) explains the common adverse impacts and proposes a therapeutic treatment window [21].

Anti-inflammatory Therapies: As many studies have revealed that the neuroimmune dysfunction (rather than simple immune dysfunction) causes schizophrenia, anti-inflammatory therapies are being repurposed for the therapeutics applications of schizophrenia [22].

Antipsychotic Medication: Chlorpromazine an antipsychotic medication, was developed in 1950s and continues till date as a medication for treatment of schizophrenia. Unfortunately, some studies revealed that some patients (about 20% to as much as 50%) do not respond to this treatment and even develop treatment resistant schizophrenia (TRS) [17]. Currently, Clozapine being FDA approved medication is used for treatment-resistant schizophrenia but is of limited benefits [17]. Novel long-acting injectable antipsychotics have also been formulated now for the treatment of schizophrenia due to their distinctive pharmacokinetic and pharmacodynamic profiles. This allows better control of titration to recommended dosage, stability in drug plasma level, avoidance of first-pass metabolism as well as ensures effective medication delivery. These drugs when administered in combination with second-generation antipsychotic (SGA) drugs, are known as second-generation antipsychotic long acting injectable (SGA-LAIs). Hopefully, these drugs using novel mechanism of action will be approved soon, not only to treat schizophrenia linked symptoms but also to reduce the risk of adverse side-effects associated with such drugs, subsequently enhancing the functional outcomes for the patients in long term [15].

Intracranial Therapies: Deep brain stimulation (DBS) is a novel surgical procedure of intracranial therapy which targets the specific regions of the brain directly. However, it is not a direct choice of treatment as it is invasive and has additional risks of hardware malfunctions.

Non-pharmacological Therapies: Non-pharmacological therapies are also known as psychotherapeutic approaches and may be classified as individual, group and cognitive behavioral. Psychotherapies are introduced to lessen the symptom burdens of schizophrenia, are non-invasive but time consuming and at times very expensive [15].

CONCLUSION

These therapies can be used in addition to medication but not a replacement. For the treatment of schizophrenia, various psychiatric therapies such as counselling, personal therapies, social skill therapies, involvement of family, and cognitive behavioral therapies are being used [17].

CONSENT FOR PUBLICATION

Not applicable.

CONFLICT OF INTEREST

The author declares no conflict of interest, financial or otherwise.

ACKNOWLEDGEMENTS

Declared none.

REFERENCES

[1]   Linn J G, Chuaqui J, Wilson D R, Arredondo E. The Global Impact of Intellectual Disabilityand. Int J Childbirth Edu 2019; 34.

[2]   Xu S, Wu X, Peng B, Cao S-L, Xu X. Primary microcephaly with an unstable genome. Genome Instability & Disease 2020; pp. 1-30.

[3]   Jean F, Stuart A, Tarailo-Graovac M. Dissecting the genetic and etiological causes of primary microcephaly. Front Neurol 2020; 11: 570830.

[4]   Faheem M, Naseer MI, Rasool M, *et al.* Molecular genetics of human primary microcephaly: an overview. BMC Med Genomics 2015; 8(S1) (Suppl. 1): S4.
        [http://dx.doi.org/10.1186/1755-8794-8-S1-S4] [PMID: 25951892]

[5]   Boonsawat P, Joset P, Steindl K, *et al.* Elucidation of the phenotypic spectrum and genetic landscape in primary and secondary microcephaly. Genet Med 2019; 21(9): 2043-58.
        [http://dx.doi.org/10.1038/s41436-019-0464-7] [PMID: 30842647]

[6]   Cristofoli F, Moss T, Moore HW, *et al. De novo* variants in LMNB1 cause pronounced syndromic microcephaly and disruption of nuclear envelope integrity. Am J Hum Genet 2020; 107(4): 753-62.
        [http://dx.doi.org/10.1016/j.ajhg.2020.08.015] [PMID: 32910914]

[7]   Parry DA, Martin CA, Greene P, *et al.* Heterozygous lamin B1 and lamin B2 variants cause primary

microcephaly and define a novel laminopathy. Genet Med 2021; 23(2): 408-14.
[http://dx.doi.org/10.1038/s41436-020-00980-3] [PMID: 33033404]

[8]   Barbelanne M, Tsang WY. Molecular and cellular basis of autosomal recessive primary microcephaly. 2014.
[http://dx.doi.org/10.1155/2014/547986]

[9]   Makhdoom EUH, Waseem SS, Iqbal M, *et al.* Modifier Genes in Microcephaly: A Report on *WDR62, CEP63, RAD50* and *PCNT* Variants Exacerbating Disease Caused by Biallelic Mutations of *ASPM* and *CENPJ.* Genes (Basel) 2021; 12(5): 731.
[http://dx.doi.org/10.3390/genes12050731] [PMID: 34068194]

[10]   Farooq M, Lindbæk L, Krogh N, *et al.* RRP7A links primary microcephaly to dysfunction of ribosome biogenesis, resorption of primary cilia, and neurogenesis. Nat Commun 2020; 11(1): 5816.
[http://dx.doi.org/10.1038/s41467-020-19658-0] [PMID: 33199730]

[11]   Shaheen R, Maddirevula S, Ewida N, *et al.* Genomic and phenotypic delineation of congenital microcephaly. Genet Med 2019; 21(3): 545-52.
[http://dx.doi.org/10.1038/s41436-018-0140-3] [PMID: 30214071]

[12]   Sajid Hussain M, Marriam Bakhtiar S, Farooq M, *et al.* Genetic heterogeneity in Pakistani microcephaly families. Clin Genet 2013; 83(5): 446-51.
[http://dx.doi.org/10.1111/j.1399-0004.2012.01932.x] [PMID: 22775483]

[13]   Yeragani VK, Ashok AH, Baugh J. Paul Eugen Bleuler and the origin of the term schizophrenia (SCHIZOPRENIEGRUPPE). Indian J Psychiatry 2012; 54(1): 95-6.
[http://dx.doi.org/10.4103/0019-5545.94660] [PMID: 22556451]

[14]   Dipiro JT, Talbert RL, Yee GC, Matzke GR, Wells BG, Posey LM. 2014.

[15]   Correll CU, Schooler NR. Negative symptoms in schizophrenia: a review and clinical guide for recognition, assessment, and treatment. Neuropsychiatr Dis Treat 2020; 16: 519-34.
[http://dx.doi.org/10.2147/NDT.S225643] [PMID: 32110026]

[16]   Girdler SJ, Confino JE, Woesner ME. Exercise as a treatment for schizophrenia: a review. Psychopharmacol Bull 2019; 49(1): 56-69.
[PMID: 30858639]

[17]   Patel KR, Cherian J, Gohil K, Atkinson D. Schizophrenia: overview and treatment options. P&T 2014; 39(9): 638-45.
[PMID: 25210417]

[18]   Jablensky A. The diagnostic concept of schizophrenia: its history, evolution, and future prospects. Dialogues Clin Neurosci 2010; 12(3): 271-87.
[http://dx.doi.org/10.31887/DCNS.2010.12.3/ajablensky] [PMID: 20954425]

[19]   Orrico-Sánchez A, López-Lacort M, Muñoz-Quiles C, Sanfélix-Gimeno G, Díez-Domingo J. Epidemiology of schizophrenia and its management over 8-years period using real-world data in Spain. BMC Psychiatry 2020; 20(1): 149.
[http://dx.doi.org/10.1186/s12888-020-02538-8] [PMID: 32248839]

[20]   Gejman PV, Sanders AR, Duan J. The role of genetics in the etiology of schizophrenia. Psychiatr Clin North Am 2010; 33(1): 35-66.
[http://dx.doi.org/10.1016/j.psc.2009.12.003] [PMID: 20159339]

[21]   Kapur S, Zipursky R, Jones C, Remington G, Houle S. Relationship between dopamine D(2) occupancy, clinical response, and side effects: a double-blind PET study of first-episode schizophrenia. Am J Psychiatry 2000; 157(4): 514-20.
[http://dx.doi.org/10.1176/appi.ajp.157.4.514] [PMID: 10739409]

[22]   Khandaker GM, Cousins L, Deakin J, Lennox BR, Yolken R, Jones PB. Inflammation and immunity in schizophrenia: implications for pathophysiology and treatment. Lancet Psychiatry 2015; 2(3): 258-70.
[http://dx.doi.org/10.1016/S2215-0366(14)00122-9] [PMID: 26359903]

SUBJECT INDEX

A

Abnormalities 32, 33, 34, 38, 40, 41, 229, 247, 269, 273, 284, 285, 292, 296
  behavioral 273
  congenital 33
  genetic 38, 41, 284, 285
  neurochemical 292
  renal 33
Acid(s) 82, 83, 96, 122, 160, 194, 197, 200, 203, 204, 229, 231, 246, 249, 257, 278
  aspartic 231
  eicosaptenoic 257
  fatty 160, 246, 249, 257
  folic 197
  glutamic 229
  glycolic 83
  hyaluronic 204
  lactobionic 197
  nucleic 122, 194, 200, 203
  organic 160
  phenylpyruvic 278
  polyglycolic 82
  ribonucleic 96
  trans-cinnamic 278
  urocanic 197
Adeno-associated virus 258
Adiponectin 248
Adipose tissues 104, 204
Age, advanced maternal 30, 33
Agents 248, 250, 251
  antiplatelet 248
  harmless antihyperglycemic 251
  mono-therapeutic antidiabetic 250
Alanine transaminase 251
Alzheimer's disease 35, 70, 116, 144, 218
Amino acids 61, 97, 98, 99, 117, 160, 167, 227
  genetically-encoded 97
Amniocentesis 32, 37, 41, 48, 81
Amniocytes 231
Amniotic fluid stem cells (AFSCs) 81

Amplification refractory mutation system 233
Amyotrophic lateral sclerosis 70
Analysis 22, 36, 47, 129
  cytogenetic 36
  dermatoglyphic 47
  genomic 129
  silico 22
  spectrometry 169
Anastomosis 203
  nerve 203
Anemia 230, 290
  moderate asymptomatic 230
Angelman syndrome 279
Angiogenesis 86
Angiotensin-converting enzyme (ACE) 234
Angiotensinogen 247
Ankylosing spondylitis 66, 67
Anomalies 22, 87, 88
  diaphyseal segmental 87
  neurogenetic 22
Antibodies 98, 126, 162, 197
  enzyme-conjugated 98
Anti-citrullinated protein/peptide antibodies (ACPAs) 115
Anti-diabetic therapy 261
Apert's syndrome 19
Apoprotein 247
Applications 4, 5, 9, 21, 23, 63, 64, 65, 83, 120, 121, 124, 139, 146, 148, 157, 177, 185, 205, 216
  of induced pluripotent stem cells 216
  of metaomics techniques 139
  of pharmacogenomics 177
  orthotopic 205
  systematic 185
AR cytokinesis 287
ARMS-PCR assay 17
Arthroplasty 190
Atherosclerotic cardiovascular disease (ASCVD) 244, 245, 246, 249, 260, 261
Autism spectrum disorders (ASD) 103, 218, 269, 271, 272, 275